PHARMACOLOGY - RESEARCH, SAFETY TESTING AND REGULATION

CHONDROITIN SULFATE

STRUCTURE, USES AND HEALTH IMPLICATIONS

PHARMACOLOGY - RESEARCH, SAFETY TESTING AND REGULATION

Additional books in this series can be found on Nova's website under the Series tab.

Additional e-books in this series can be found on Nova's website under the e-book tab.

BIOCHEMISTRY RESEARCH TRENDS

Additional books in this series can be found on Nova's website under the Series tab.

Additional e-books in this series can be found on Nova's website under the e-book tab.

PHARMACOLOGY - RESEARCH, SAFETY TESTING AND REGULATION

CHONDROITIN SULFATE

STRUCTURE, USES AND HEALTH IMPLICATIONS

VITOR H. POMIN

EDITOR

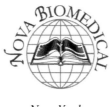

New York

For permission to use material from this book please contact us:
Telephone 631-231-7269; Fax 631-231-8175
Web Site: http://www.novapublishers.com

NOTICE TO THE READER

The Publisher has taken reasonable care in the preparation of this book, but makes no expressed or implied warranty of any kind and assumes no responsibility for any errors or omissions. No liability is assumed for incidental or consequential damages in connection with or arising out of information contained in this book. The Publisher shall not be liable for any special, consequential, or exemplary damages resulting, in whole or in part, from the readers' use of, or reliance upon, this material. Any parts of this book based on government reports are so indicated and copyright is claimed for those parts to the extent applicable to compilations of such works.

Independent verification should be sought for any data, advice or recommendations contained in this book. In addition, no responsibility is assumed by the publisher for any injury and/or damage to persons or property arising from any methods, products, instructions, ideas or otherwise contained in this publication.

This publication is designed to provide accurate and authoritative information with regard to the subject matter covered herein. It is sold with the clear understanding that the Publisher is not engaged in rendering legal or any other professional services. If legal or any other expert assistance is required, the services of a competent person should be sought. FROM A DECLARATION OF PARTICIPANTS JOINTLY ADOPTED BY A COMMITTEE OF THE AMERICAN BAR ASSOCIATION AND A COMMITTEE OF PUBLISHERS.

Additional color graphics may be available in the e-book version of this book.

Library of Congress Cataloging-in-Publication Data

ISBN: 978-1-62808-490-0

Library of Congress Control Number: 2013943516

Published by Nova Science Publishers, Inc. † New York

Contents

Preface

Chondroitin sulfate (CS) is the most abundant glycosaminoglycan (GAG) of the human body. Besides its natural occurrence as side chains in physiologically active proteoglycans localized at the extracellular matrices and/or at cell surfaces, this GAG can also be found in marine organisms with differential structures and functions, such as the anticoagulant fucosylated chondroitin sulfate isolated from sea-cucumbers. In addition, CSs isolated from vertebrate sources, such as shark and whale cartilages, are used as a biomedical ingredient for alternative medicinal therapies of osteoarthritis, osteoarthrosis, and possibly osteoporosis. CS formulations for oral administration are also employed as a nutraceutical to prevent lesions or degenerations of joint cartilages, especially in those people susceptible to physical impacts of their knees, like athletes, soccer players and dancers. In terms of structure, this GAG can show different sulfation patterns that vary accordingly with the types of cell, tissue, organism, and pathological conditions. However, the saccharide backbone of CS is always made up of alternating galactosamine and an uronic acid unit, regardless the source or condition. This book presents a compilation of some of the recent achievements obtained by scientific research on CS. Overall the most relevant areas and sub-areas regarding the science of this GAG type are somewhat discussed herein. The major areas include biology, biotechnology, physiology, chemistry and pharmacology. Specific sub-areas are biosynthesis, chemical and enzymatic modifications, extraction methods, occurrence and abundance, *in vitro* enzymatic degradations, structural diversity versus functions, disease-related mechanisms, physiological roles, medical applications and novel methods of structural characterization. The contributing authors of this publication are internationally recognized leaders in the field. All these features contribute significantly to the quality of this publication.

Chapter 1 - Chondroitin sulfate (CS) is a polysaccharide ubiquitously distributed in connective tissues and on cell surfaces of both vertebrates and invertebrates. It consists of a disaccharide repeating unit, composed of glucuronic acid and *N*-acetyl-galactosamine, whose hydroxyl groups, during polymerization, undergo sulfation to a various extent. Sulfation pattern is tissue/age specific, and is able to encode functional information. For this reason, it is tightly regulated *in vivo*. Since CS polysaccharides are involved in a myriad of biological processes, their chemical and chemo-enzymatic manipulation is an emerging topic, that has already allowed the obtainment of CS polysaccharide products with potential tailored biomedical applications. In this chapter the authors present a review of chemical and chemo-enzymatic methods for the controlled modification of CS structure. In dependence of the kind of structural modification, the reviewed works are divided into two areas, covering, respectively, the following topics: 1) CS sulfation pattern modifications by regioselective sulfation or de-sulfation reactions; 2) CS functionalizations other than sulfation pattern modifications, with a specific attention to cross-linking reactions.

Chapter 2 - The constructions of chondroitin sulfate oligosaccharides using the chemoenzymatic procedures were investigated. Enzymatically prepared alkyne-containing chondroitin sulfate repeating disaccharide and ligated to the azide polyethylene glycol by click chemistry. Then, utilizing the pegylated disaccharide as an acceptor for the transglycosylation reaction of bovine testicular hyaluronidase, chondroitin sulfate oligosaccharides were successfully constructed on the polyethylene glycol. These synthesized chondroitin sulfate oligosaccharides will be clarify novel biological activities, and various medicinal treatment applications can be expected. The authors believe the present method will contribute to the development glycosaminoglycan glycobiology and technology.

Chapter 3 - The world industrial production of chondroitin sulfate uses animal tissue sources as raw materials: CS is extracted with long and complex procedures that start with the recovery of CS from the cartilaginous tissues, by the break of the linkage with the proteoglycan protein core, and continue with numerous steps of purifications for the complete removal of all the contaminants. Shark fins, bovine, porcine or chicken trachea are actually the most commonly used sources but, according to the different origins, CS structure could vary in terms of molecular weight, type and grade of sulfation. A biotechnological-chemical strategy has recently gained attention as a new, alternative, promising way to produce CS. The process consists of three main steps: fermentative production of a chondroitin-like polysaccharide by capsulated bacteria, its purification from the fermentation broth and then site specific chain sulfation. The extractive and the biotechnological process approaches resulted completely different from a productive point of view: in the "top-down-like" extractive process CS chains of the desired specific sulfation patterns and chain lengths are obtained after diverse steps of purification; in the "bottom-up-like" biotechnological approach the process could be designed to obtain structural tailored cut molecules. In this chapter both productive schemes are described, underlining the different nature of the starting materials and comparing the diverse structural transformations occurring during the two processes up to obtain CS as final product.

Chapter 4 - Enzymes like lyases and hydrolyses that degrade chondroitin sulfates are well-known to reproducibly release just certain oligosaccharide types in terms of their sulfation patterns. Here, the authors have characterized the disaccharides and hexasaccharides produced from enzymatic digestions of chondoritin sulfates A and C when treated with bacterial chondroitinases ABC and C and ovine testicular hyaluronidase. The structural characterization was based on nuclear magnetic resonance spectroscopy combined with mass spectrometry. These chemically well-defined oligosaccharides were obtained by a combination of size-exclusion chromatography and strong-anion exchange chromatography of the products generated from limited digestions of chondoritin sulfates A and C. The amounts of released products were measured and the endolytic versus exolytic activities were confirmed for each enzyme type. The catalytic directionality was also determined through MS experiments by using chemically modified products at their reducing terminus. Analysis based on the structures of the released products indicates the preferential enzymatic sites of cleavage in terms of sulfation patterns. In all, 15 chondroitin sulfate hexasaccharide structures have been produced and structurally characterized. These may serve as a useful library of chondroitin sulfates to be assayed in future biological or physicochemical assays.

Chapter 5 - Mucopolysaccharides such as keratan sulfate, dermatan sulfate, heparan sulfate, heparin, and chondroitin sulfate are heterogeneous sulfated polysaccharides. Chondroitin sulfate contains primarily alternating N-acetylgalactosamine (both sulfated and unsulfated) and glucuronic acid residues, and is most commonly found as chondroitin-6-sulfate and chondroitin-4-sulfate, which differ in the position of the sulfate group on the N-acetylgalactosamine residues. Mucopolysaccharides are degraded in the lysosome by the sequential action of multiple enzymes. For example, chondroitin-6-sulfate degradation occurs primarily due to the enzymes N-acetylgalactosamine-6-sulfatase (GALNS), β-hexosaminidase, and β-glucuronidase. This chapter focuses on the degradation of chondroitin sulfate by the human lysosomal enzyme GALNS, and on the relationship of GALNS to the lysosomal storage disease mucopolysaccharidosis IV A (also known as MPS IV A and Morquio A). Loss of activity of the GALNS enzyme leads to accumulation of chondroitin-6-sulfate and keratan sulfate, which leads to development of disease. Substrate accumulation leads to a range of disease symptoms, including dysostosis multiplex, joint mobility, hearing, vision and cardiovascular impairment. There are no approved therapies for MPS IV A; however enzyme replacement therapy using recombinant GALNS glycoprotein is currently in Phase III clinical trials in the United States. To better understand the molecular basis for the disease, the authors recently determined the three-dimensional structure of GALNS by X-ray crystallography. The three-dimensional structure of GALNS shows a catalytic gem diol nucleophile derived from enzymatic modification of a cysteine side chain in the active site. GALNS contains a large indentation around the active site, with many basic amino acid residues allowing charged interactions with the negatively charged substrates chondroitin-6-sulfate and keratan sulfate. In order to understand the effect on the protein due to disease-causing mutations, 120 missense mutations were mapped onto the GALNS structure. Most of these mutations are buried in the core of the protein, suggesting that in the majority of MPS IV A patients, GALNS activity loss in is due to misfolding of the protein. The active site of GALNS falls at the base of a deep trench; thus GALNS may be a suitable target for rational design of small molecule therapeutics.

Chapter 6 - Chondroitin sulfate (CS) is a symptomatic slow-acting drug for osteoarthritis (OA) widely used for the treatment of this highly prevalent disease, which is mainly characterized by articular cartilage degradation. However, little is known about its mechanism of action and recent large-scale clinical trials have reported variable results on OA symptoms. Proteomic applications to pharmacological issues are termed pharmacoproteomics. In the field of OA research, quantitative proteomics technologies are demonstrating a very interesting power for studying the molecular effect of some drugs employed to treat OA patients, such as CS and glucosamine sulfate (GS). Herein, the authors present results on the modulations in the intracellular proteome and secretome of human articular cartilage cells treated with these drugs. An analysis of the effect of CS from different origin and purity using two complementary proteomic approaches (DIGE and SILAC) shows that the three different CS compounds have diverse effects on the intracellular and extracellular human chondrocytes proteomes. Each of the studied compounds induced a characteristic protein profile in OA chondrocytes. CS from porcine origin displayed the widest effect, but increased the cartilage oligomeric matrix protein and some catabolic or inflammatory factors like interstitial collagenase, stromelysin-1 and pentraxin-related protein. CS from bovine origin, on the other hand, increased a number of structural proteins, growth factors and ECM proteins. Pharmacoproteomic approaches can also be useful to analyze the differences between simple and combined administration by proteomic analysis of normal human articular chondrocytes (HACs). A gel-based proteomic study using HACs stimulated with IL-1β and treated with CS, alone or in combination with GS, shows a number of target proteins and points out the different mechanisms of action of these drugs. Regarding their predicted biological function, 35% of the proteins modulated by GS are involved in signal transduction pathways, 15% in redox and stress response, and 25% in protein synthesis and folding processes. Interestingly, CS affects mainly energy production (31%) and metabolic pathways (13%), decreasing the expression levels of ten proteins. Finally, an analysis of secretomes from normal chondrocytes stimulated with IL1β, demonstrated how CS reduces inflammation directly, by decreasing the presence of several complement components (CFAB, C1S, CO3, and C1R) and also indirectly, by increasing proteins such as tumour necrosis factor-inducible gene 6 protein (TSG6). Moreover, a strong CS-dependent increase of an angiogenesis inhibitor, thrombospondin 1 (TSP-1), was found in this analysis. In summary, pharmacoproteomic studies of CS demonstrate that CS from porcine origin induces the activation of inflammatory and catabolic pathways, while bovine CS induces an anti-inflammatory and anabolic response. In addition, they unravel novel molecular evidences of the anti-angiogenic, anti-inflammatory, and anti-catabolic properties of CS in the presence of pro-inflammatory stimuli. The overall goal of this review is to gather most of the available information about pharmacoproteomic studies of CS and also to discuss the clinical usefulness of proteomics and the perspectives for CS use in OA management.

Chapter 7 - Growth factors (GFs) are a group of biologically active polypeptides produced by the body that can stimulate cellular division, growth, and differentiation. Through the regulation of these key biological functions GFs participate in the development and homeostasis of tissues throughout life and are implicated in numerous pathological processes. Chondroitin sulfate (CS) is a glycosaminoglycan composed of repeating disaccharides of N-acetylgalactosamine and d-glucuronic acid or l-iduronic acid in the case of dermatan sulfate (DS/CS-B), with various sulfation patterns. CS chains, covalently bound into proteoglycan (PGs) core proteins, are located to the extracellular space, at the cell membrane and also intracellularly. Through elegant feedback mechanisms CS can influence cellular processes by regulating the presentation and availability of growth factors to cells, matricine signaling. This chapter focuses on the role of CS/DS in the regulation of growth factor signaling pathways crucial to development and tissue homeostasis as well as to disease conditions.

Chapter 8 - Marine organisms are a rich source of sulfated polysaccharides with unique structures. Fucosylated chondroitin sulfate (FucCS) from the sea cucumber *Ludwigothuria grisea* is one of these unusual molecules since it shows a saccharide backbone similar to the regular chondroitin sulfate from mammals, however, with uneven branches of sulfated fucosyl units. Besides the uncommon structures of marine polysaccharides, they also may exhibit important therapeutic properties when assayed in clinical systems that resemble parts of the human physiology. The mostly studied and highly desirable therapeutic action of FucCS is its anticoagulant and antithrombotic activity. The capacity for these activities is mainly attributed to the presence of the branching fucosyl unit since the regular chondroitin sulfate composed only of the alternating galactosamine and glucuronic acid backbone is devoid of these biological actions. Earlier, it was considered that the anticoagulant activities of FucCS was driven mainly by a catalytic serpin-dependent mechanism likewise the mammalian heparins. Its serpin-dependent anticoagulant action relies on promoting thrombin and/or factor Xa inhibition by their specific natural inhibitors (the serpins antithrombin and heparin cofactor II). However, unlikely heparins, the FucCS proved still capable in promoting coagulation inhibition when using serpin-free plasmas. This puzzle observation was further investigated and clearly demonstrated that the echinoderm FucCS has an unusual serpin-independent anticoagulant effect by inhibiting the formation of factor Xa and/or thrombin through the pro-coagulant tenase and prothrombinase complexes, respectively. The marine FucCS with unusual anticoagulant mechanism opens clearly new perspectives for the development of new antithrombotic drugs, especially in clinical cases of related serpins-compromised patients.

Chapter 9 - Chondroitin sulfate (CS) is a negatively charged linear glycosaminoglycan (GAG) composed of individual sulfated monosaccharides. CS is an essential component of the extracellular matrix of soft and connective tissues and is a structural unit of large macromolecules, proteoglycans, such as aggrecan and versican, organized in a 3D bottle-brush architecture. Sulfation of CS allows water uptake providing tissue hydration and contributing to the osmotic pressure and compressive resistance. Elegant 3D organization of CS in proteoglycans provides an additional contribution to compressive stiffness of the tissue due to electro repulsive forces between CS molecules. With age and degeneration, GAG content in tissue is reduced due to low cell activity and increased enzymatic attacks, which results in a host of mechanical, hydration and nutritional deficits to tissue function. This, in turn, can manifest in pain, joint stiffness and loss of mobility. Most common examples of tissue degeneration associated with loss of GAG content are osteoarthritis and intervertebral disc degeneration. Conservative treatments of these diseases include physical exercise to reduce mechanical stress on joints and analgesics to reduce pain, or even surgical joint replacements or disc fusions in severe cases. However, these methods do not address underlying cause of the problem. Therefore, there have been increased efforts in developing alternative strategies which aim to restore structural integrity of the degenerated tissue. Application of CS to restore reduced GAG content is one of the potential ways to treat degenerated tissue. Most well-known approach, which has undergone clinical trials, involves an oral administration of CS, however it does not provide a local effect, and long-time hydration/restoration effects are limited due to diffusion of low-molecular weight CS out of the tissue. Other ongoing research efforts include studies on effect of chondroitin sulfate and its sulfation chemistry on cell synthetic activity in tissue; various chondroitin-hyaluronic acid-collagen scaffolds to mimic extracellular matrix; organization of CS in larger aggregates to mimic natural proteoglycans and their effect on biological and mechanical tissue function. An overview of these research initiatives will be provided in the current article.

Chapter 10 - Schizophrenia is a chronic psychiatric illness known to affect approximately 1% of the population. Genetic and early life environmental factors conjure to disrupt distinct neuronal and glial populations in several cortical and subcortical brain regions. The resulting clinical symptoms emerge in late adolescence to early adulthood, preceded by a prodromal syndrome. Recent evidence points to a role for chondroitin sulfate proteoglycans (CSPGs) in the pathophysiology of schizophrenia. The authors' group has shown large increases of CSPG expression in glial cells accompanied by reductions of perineuronal nets (PNNs) in the medial temporal lobe of subjects with schizophrenia. Similar findings in the prefrontal cortex and olfactory epithelium suggest that CSPG abnormalities may be widespread in this disease. Genetic studies reporting associations of polymorphisms for specific CSPG genes, including PTPRZ1, neuroglycan-C and neurocan with schizophrenia, and recent animal studies examining the effects of abnormal CSPG expression or sulfation on brain development and function, lend further support for CSPG abnormalities in this disorder. In this chapter the authors discuss these findings and their potential relevance to core aspects of the pathophysiology of schizophrenia, such as brain development, myelination and regulation of key neurotransmitter systems including the glutamatergic, GABAergic and dopaminergic systems. The authors put forth the hypothesis that altered CSPG expression may contribute to a number of critical components of the pathophysiology of schizophrenia, including altered neuronal migration and connectivity, neural circuit plasticity, synaptic regulation, and electrical oscillatory rhythms observed in this disorder.

Chapter 11 - The structural studies of chondroitin sulfates (CSs) have mostly been based on the use of NMR spectroscopy, particularly from the information of the ^{1}H- and ^{13}C-atoms. Nevertheless, a new scope has recently emerged. This concerns the extraction of data from the much less used isotope nitrogen-15. Despite its low abundance and very weak magnetic sensitivity, NMR technology has progressed, and nowadays research more based on the ^{15}N-nuclear properties has demonstrated to be relatively easy accomplishable for the retrieval of structural, conformational and dynamic information of CSs. The use of ^{15}N-related chemical shifts has proved to be quite diagnostic to the proper recognition of the CS types. Development of isotopic labeling methods for CS molecules has been implemented. Structural sequencing of sulfation patterns (4- and/or 6-substitutions), and anomeric ratio determination in CS-derived oligosaccharides were proved to be possible when analyses are focused on specific ^{15}N-chemical shifts. Moreover, this type of information can be achieved in a much simpler and straightforward way as compared to the more common NMR methods involving the ^{1}H- and/or ^{13}C-nuclei. The 3D-structural prediction of unsulfated CS determined by high-field ^{15}N-NMR points towards the conception of little effect of 4-sulfation on the backbone conformation. This chapter aims at describing the recent achievements made in structural analysis of CSs by the novel ^{15}N-NMR approach.

In: Chondroitin Sulfate
Editor: Vitor H. Pomin

ISBN: 978-1-62808-490-0
© 2013 Nova Science Publishers, Inc.

Chapter 1

Chemical and Chemoenzymatic Manipulation of Chondroitin Sulfate Polysaccharides

Emiliano Bedini[*] *and Michelangelo Parrilli*
Department of Chemical Sciences, University of Naples "Federico II", Naples, Italy

Abstract

Chondroitin sulfate (CS) is a polysaccharide ubiquitously distributed in connective tissues and on cell surfaces of both vertebrates and invertebrates. It consists of a disaccharide repeating unit, composed of glucuronic acid and *N*-acetyl-galactosamine, whose hydroxyl groups, during polymerization, undergo sulfation to a various extent. Sulfation pattern is tissue/age specific, and is able to encode functional information. For this reason, it is tightly regulated *in vivo*. Since CS polysaccharides are involved in a myriad of biological processes, their chemical and chemo-enzymatic manipulation is an emerging topic, that has already allowed the obtainment of CS polysaccharide products with potential tailored biomedical applications. In this chapter we present a review of chemical and chemo-enzymatic methods for the controlled modification of CS structure. In dependence of the kind of structural modification, the reviewed works are divided into two areas, covering, respectively, the following topics: 1) CS sulfation pattern modifications by regioselective sulfation or de-sulfation reactions; 2) CS functionalizations other than sulfation pattern modifications, with a specific attention to cross-linking reactions.

Introduction

Glycosaminoglycans (GAGs) are a class of complex macromolecules ubiquitously distributed in extracellular matrices and at cell surfaces, with a high biological significance,

[*] E-mail address: ebedini@unina.it.

as they interact with a huge number of proteins involved in physiological and pathological processes. From a structural point of view, GAGs are highly negatively charged polysaccharides, with a molecular weight usually ranging between 10 and 100 kDa. GAGs could be divided into two subclasses: sulfated GAGs – including chondroitin sulfate (CS), dermatan sulfate (DS), keratan sulfate (KS), heparin and heparin sulfate (HS) – and unsulfated GAGs, namely hyaluronic acid (HA). GAGs consist of disaccharide building blocks, usually containing an uronic (glucuronic or L-iduronic acid) acid and an aminosugar (glucosamine or galactosamine). The recurrence of a single or more distinct disaccharide units dozens to hundreds times generates the macromolecular structure of the GAGs. Their structure is often even more complicated by the presence of some substituents on the carbohydrate backbone: acetyl groups on the nitrogen atoms of the aminosugars and, in the case of sulfated GAGs, sulfate groups again on aminosugar nitrogen atoms and/or on the hydroxyl oxygen atoms of the sugars. Interestingly, at physiological pH both uronic acids and sulfate groups are not protonated, thus conferring a very high negative charge density to sulfated GAGs (heparin possesses the highest negative charge density of any known biomolecule).

Chondroitin sulfate (CS) is a sulfated GAG constituted of glucuronic acid (GlcA) and *N*-acetyl-galactosamine (GalNAc), linked together through alternating β-1→3 and β-1→4 glycosidic bonds, to give a polysaccharide with a 4)-β-GlcA-(1→3)-β-GalNAc-(1→ disaccharide repeating unit. During the *in vivo* biopolymerization process, the polysaccharide is sulfated to some extent. Depending on the position of sulfate group substitutions, several disaccharide subunits could be identified in the backbone of natural CSs. The most common sulfation patterns are listed in Figure 1. The positions 4 and/or 6 of the GalNAc units are most commonly sulfated while positions 2 and 3 of the GlcA units are more rarely substituted with sulfate groups. [1]

CS polysaccharides isolated from sea cucumbers (*Echinodermata*) present an additional, unique characteristic, that is the presence of a sulfated fucose (Fuc) branch at position 3 of GlcA units. [2] Different kinds of sea cucumbers from the seawaters of different geographical zones present fucosylated CS polysaccharides with different Fuc branches. Indeed, a variation in both the number (1 or 2) of Fuc units composing the branch and its sulfation pattern could be observed. [3] A general structure of fucosylated CSs isolated up to now from sea cucumbers is depicted in Figure 2. However, more details about the range of known natural CS structures could be found in chapter 11.

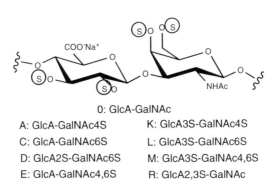

0: GlcA-GalNAc

A: GlcA-GalNAc4S	K: GlcA3S-GalNAc4S
C: GlcA-GalNAc6S	L: GlcA3S-GalNAc6S
D: GlcA2S-GalNAc6S	M: GlcA3S-GalNAc4,6S
E: GlcA-GalNAc4,6S	R: GlcA2,3S-GalNAc

Figure 1. Disaccharide subunits found in natural CSs.

CSs extracted from animal sources often possess a combination of different sulfation patterns. Recent studies suggested that CS may be capable of encoding functional information in a sequence-specific manner, mainly through the sequence of sulfate sites pattern on the saccharide backbone. [4] This sequence seems to be strictly regulated *in vivo* and is tissue/age specific. It also depends on the physiological or pathological state of the organism. However, the details of this "sulfation code" have yet to be fully elucidated

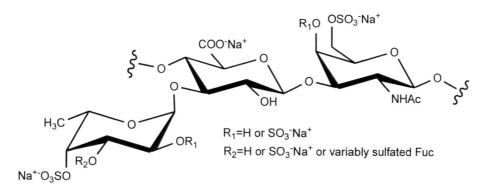

Figure 2. General structure of natural fucosylated CSs.

CSs isolated from natural sources have some applications as therapeutics. In particular, the CS polysaccharide predominantly composed of A and C disaccharide subunits (CS-A,C) isolated from bovine and porcine nasal septa and tracheas, poultry bones, and shark cartilages are employed for the medium-long term treatment of osteoarthritic patients. It is marketed primarily as a dietary supplement for pain and inflammation relief in tibiofibular osteoarthritis [5] as well as for related diseases affecting the joints. It is also used as component of viscoelastic solutions used as surgical aids in cataract extraction and intraocular lens implantation procedures, as well as ingredient for skin moisturizers and creams for the treatment of burns. Other pharmaceutical applications – as an antiviral against herpes simplex virus type I, an antimalarial, a tissue regeneration factor for central nervous system and liver, an anticancer, have been recently proposed for CSs, in relation to different size and/or sulfation pattern. [6] Furthermore, in recent years, fucosylated CSs have been shown to possess very interesting and unique anticoagulant and antithrombotic activities. [7] This has strongly suggested some fucosylated CSs as potential candidates for the replacement of heparin as anticoagulant and antithrombotic drug. [8]

The high biomedical interest in CSs prompted many efforts of several carbohydrate chemists aimed at opening a synthetic access to oligosaccharide fragments representative of CS biological features. Several CS di- to octasaccharide fragments have been prepared in the last two decades. Some comprehensive reviews appeared in literature, describing the synthetic approaches employed to this aim. [9-12]

In this chapter we review the achievements on a somehow different topic, that is the modification of the structure of natural CS and chondroitin polysaccharides. In general, the fine chemical derivatization of the polysaccharides through chemo-, regio- and stereoselective reactions is an emerging area, that has recently allowed the obtainment – from vegetal, algal or microbial sources – of a relevant number of products with a defined chemical structure and interesting physical and biological properties. [13, 14] Here we present the results in this field regarding CS polysaccharides. The reviewed works are divided into two areas, covering, respectively, the following topics: 1) CS sulfation pattern modifications by regioselective sulfation or de-sulfation reactions; 2) CS polysaccharides functionalization other than sulfation pattern modifications, with a specific attention to cross-linking reactions.

Sulfation and Desulfation Reactions

Some chemical and chemoenzymatic methods for the modification of the sulfation pattern in CS polysaccharides were reported. Early attempts used sulfuric or chlorosulfuric acid, [15, 16] affording polysaccharide structures with an increased sulfation index ($SO_3H/COOH$ molar ratio) with respect to the natural polysaccharides used as starting materials. A non-negligible depolymerization was contemporarily observed, due to the strong acid character of the reagents, provoking the cleavage of the glycosidic bonds connecting GlcA and GalNAc units in the polysaccharide backbone. Nonetheless, by treating the triethylamine salt of CS extracted from bovine intestinal mucosa or from shark cartilage with chlorosulfonic acid in N,N-dimethylformamide (DMF) for 1h at 50°C, it was possible to obtain CS polysaccharides with a significant increase in sulfation index and without a too extensive depolymerization (Figure 3). [17]

Starting material	Starting ➤ obtained molecular weight (kDa)	Starting ➤ obtained sulfation index ($SO_3H/COOH$ molar ratio)
CS-A,C from bovine intestinal mucosa	26.6 ➤ 11.7	1.08 ➤ 3.20
CS-A,C,D from shark cartilage	45.0 ➤ 10.1-17.9	1.21 ➤ 1.62-2.85

Figure 3. Analytical data for natural CSs and their sulfation products ($ClSO_3H$, DMF, 50°C, 1h).

A milder and generally used approach to the chemical sulfation of glycosaminoglycans relies upon the use of sulfuric trioxide adducts with tertiary amines or amides in aprotic solvents, such as pyridine, DMF or dimethyl sulfoxide (DMSO). [18] By employing sulfur trioxide-pyridine complex (15 molar equivalents per mole of available hydroxyl group) in DMF, it was possible to introduce additional sulfate groups on CS-A,C from bovine tracheal cartilage (sulfation index increased from 1.0 to 2.5-4.0 depending on reaction temperature ranging from 0 to 40°C). Under these conditions, no glycosidic linkage breakdown occurred, as observed by a slight increase of the molecular weight in the resulting CSs, consistent with the mass of the added sulfate groups. [19] Interestingly, the per-O-sulfated chondroitin polysaccharide (sulfation index = 4.0) obtained conducting this reaction at 40°C for 1 hour, presented a conformational change on its GlcA residues. These units, usually residing in the $^4C_1$ form in natural CSs, had a $^1C_4$ conformation at 30°C and a $^2S_0$ one at 60°C, similarly to the preferred conformation of 2-O-sulfo-iduronate residue most commonly found in heparin (Figure 4). Per-O-sulfated chondroitin was studied for its potential high antithrombotic activity as well as for the treatment of degenerative joint disease. Unfortunately, this product can induce a strong allergic-type response due to immunological cross-reactivity with heparin. [20] Indeed, per-*O*-sulfated chondroitin was recently identified as a contaminant in heparin lots, [21] where it was added to increase fraudulently the anticoagulant titer of the preparation. The administration of such contaminated lots caused a cluster of serious adverse events, including 200 deaths in United States alone. [22]

In order to increase the sulfation index of natural CSs and contemporarily to avoid per-*O*-sulfation, regioselective sulfation reactions were firstly studied. Nagasawa and co-workers studied the reaction of the tributylammonium salt of natural CSs with variable amounts of sulfur trioxide-pyridine complex in DMF at 0°C for 1 hour. [23] Under such mild reaction conditions, a regioselective sulfation on the primary hydroxyl at *O*-6 position of GalNAc residues was possible (Figure 5). By conducting the reaction with 2-8 molar equivalents of sulfur trioxide-pyridine complex per available hydroxyl group, the conversion of CS-A,C from whale cartilage into a CS-A,C,E polymer containing up to 66% CS-E disaccharide subunits was accomplished, as demonstrated by a liquid chromatography analysis after a chondroitinase ABC digestion of the obtained polymer. Analogously, a CS-A,C,D polymer from shark cartilage could be converted into CS-C,D,E. Furthermore, the data reported in Figure 5 suggest that, among secondary hydroxyls, sulfation occurred only on GlcA units and to a very limited extent, whereas sulfation at *O*-4 position could be not detected at all. It could be concluded that sulfation regioselectivity is in the order GalNAc-*O*-6 >> GlcA-*O*-2 > GlcA-*O*-3 ≈ GalNAc-*O*-4. Nonetheless, this order was obtained by an analysis relying upon a chondroitinase ABC digestion, that is known to underestimate the sulfate group content at position *O*-3 of GlcA residues. [24]

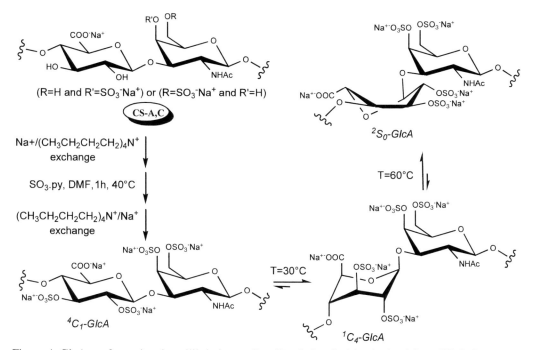

Figure 4. GlcA conformational equilibria in per-O-sulfated chondroitin obtained from CS-A,C.

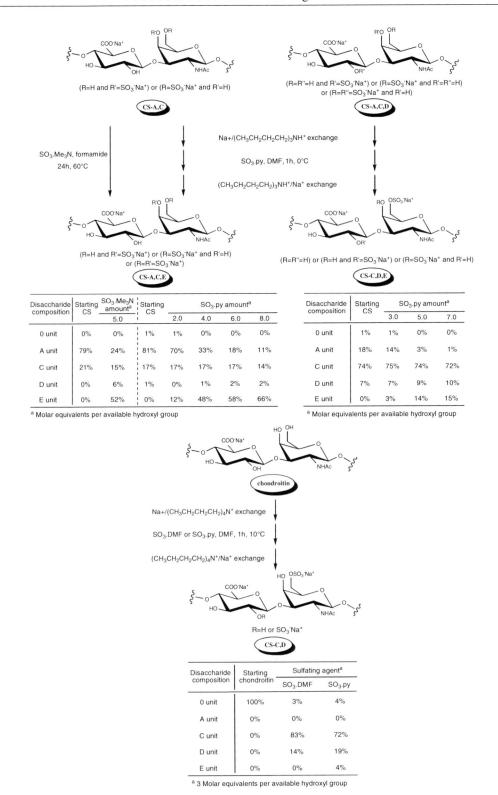

Figure 5. Regioselective sulfation with sulfur trioxide complexes.

The regioselective sulfation of the primary hydroxyl at *O*-6 position of GalNAc units was accomplished also with other sulfur trioxide complexes, such as sulfur trioxide-trimethylamine and sulfur trioxide-DMF. Since triethylamine possesses a higher Lewis base strength with respect to both DMF and pyridine, the reactivity of sulfur trioxide-trimethylamine is lower than the other complexes and therefore harsher reaction conditions are usually needed even for regioselective sulfations. Indeed, CS-A,C from bovine tracheal cartilage was treated with sulfur trioxide-trimethylamine complex (5 molar equivalents per available hydroxyl group) in formamide at 60°C for 24 hours to afford a CS-A,C,E polymer containing up to 52% E disaccharide subunits. [25] Analogously, the tetrabutylammonium salt of unsulfated chondroitin from microbial sources [26, 27] was treated with 3 molar equivalents of sulfur trioxide-DMF (or, again, of sulfur trioxide-pyridine) complex per available hydroxyl group in DMF at 10°C for 1 hour, affording a CS-C,D polymer containing sulfate groups not only at *O*-6 position of GalNAc units but also at *O*-2 position of GlcA residues, although the latter resulted in minor amounts (Figure 5). [28]

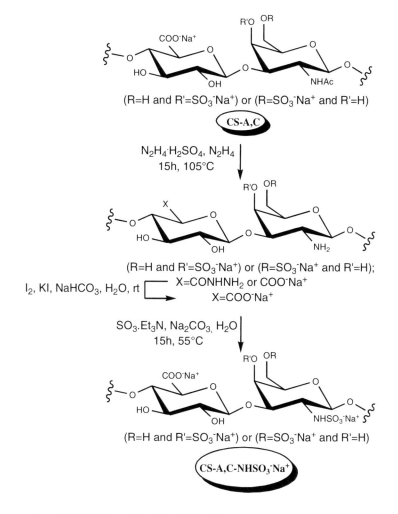

Figure 6. Conversion of CS-A,C into *N*-sulfated-CS-A,C.

When sulfation was conducted with sulfur trioxide complexes in water, a chemoselectivity on nitrogen *versus* oxygen atoms was achieved. In particular, Linhardt and co-workers treated a CS-A,C polymer firstly with anhydrous hydrazine in the presence of hydrazine sulfate in order to cleave the acetamido group of GalNAc residues (Figure 6). The resulting polysaccharide presented an hydrazine amide moiety on some GlcA residues, that could be cleaved by oxidation with iodine. After these two steps, the *N*-deacetylated polymer showed an intact sulfation pattern on *O*-4 and *O*-6-position of GalNAc residues, that demonstrated the stability of sulfate groups to hydrazinolysis. The free amine was then *N*-sulfated chemoselectively by treatment with sulfur trioxide-triethylamine complex in aqueous sodium carbonate solution at 55°C for 15 hours, affording a CS-A,C-NHSO$_3^-$Na$^+$ polymer. [29]

Regioselective sulfations of CSs were achieved not only by chemical methods but also through enzymatic processes employing specific sulfotransferases. Habuchi and co-workers reported the regioselective sulfation of a CS-A polysaccharide from whale cartilage at *O*-6-position of GalNAc units by incubating the polymer with a GalNAc4S-6-*O*-sulfotransferase (GalNAc4S-6ST) purified by squid cartilage, [30] in the presence of the cofactor 3'-phosphoadenosine 5'-phosphosulphate (PAPS). A CS-A,E polysaccharide with up to 43% E disaccharide subunits was obtained (Figure 7). [31] Similarly, a recombinant squid GalNAc4S-6ST could catalyze the conversion of the CS-A,D tetrasaccharide sequences contained in CS from shark cartilage [32] into CS-E,D ones. [33] Furthermore, a recombinant human GlcA-2-*O*-sulfotransferase (GlcA-2ST) showed some activity in the selective sulfation at *O*-2 position of GlcA residues exclusively contained in C subunits of CS-A,C, whereas no 2-*O*-sulfation of unsulfated disaccharide subunits and little or no sulfation of A disaccharide residues was observed. [34]

The selective sulfation at the non-reducing end of CS polymers was also accomplished through an enzymatic reaction. A recombinant human GalNAc4S-6ST was able to convert the non-reducing A disaccharide terminus of CS-polysaccharides rich in A subunits into a CS-E terminal sequence. [35] The employment of enzymatic sulfation reactions is limited by the very low scale of the reported syntheses and by the availability of sulfotransferases and cofactor PAPS. Nonetheless, a method to reduce the cost of PAPS synthesis has been very recently proposed, [36] thus opening an avenue to progressively scale-up enzyme-based syntheses of complex GAG molecules. [37]

Regioselective desulfation reactions on natural CSs were also studied as an alternative approach to gain regioselectively sulfated CS polysaccharides. A chemical method to obtain a regioselective desulfation at the primary hydroxyls was developed using *N*,*O*-bis(trimethylsilyl)acetamide (BTSA). By treating the pyridinium salt of CS-A,C with this reagent in pyridine at 60°C for 2 hours, the loss of sulfate groups concerned exclusively the position *O*-6 of GalNAc units, thus affording a CS-A polysaccharide. [38] Analogously, the treatment of a semi-synthetic per-*O*-sulfated chondroitin with BTSA at 70°C for 5 hours allowed again a selective 6-*O*-desulfation, furnishing an unprecedented CS polymer with a GlcA2,3S-GalNAc4S disaccharide repeating unit. [39] Interestingly, no cleavage of glycosidic bonds was observed in both cases, whereas typical reactions for global desulfation − solvolysis in aprotic solvents such as DMSO, DMF, pyridine [40] or DMSO containing small amounts of water or methanol − [41, 42] were always accompanied by a considerable depolymerization. An enzymatic method for selective desulfation at position 4 of GalNAc units has been very recently developed, employing a sulfatase from the human commensal bacterium *Bacteroides thetaiotaomicron*. [43]

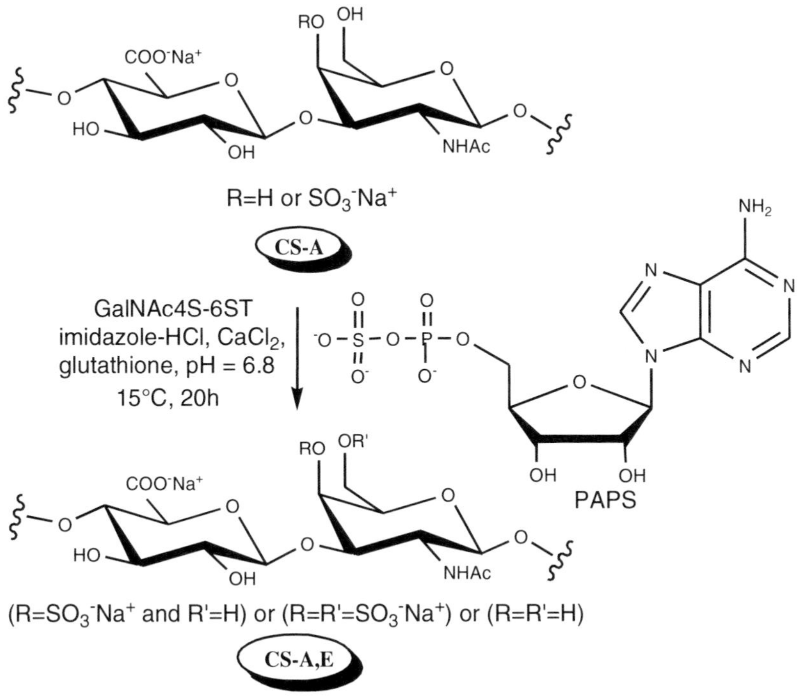

Figure 7. Enzymatic conversion of CS-A into CS-A,E.

Disaccharide composition	Starting CS	GalNAc4S-6ST amount[a]	
		90 ng	180 ng
0 unit	18%	19%	19%
A unit	78%	51%	34%
C unit	3%	4%	3%
E unit	0%	25%	43%

[a] Referred to a 3×10^{-5} cpm CS reaction

In the last years, the obtainment of regioselectively sulfated CS polysaccharides from natural unsulfated chondroitin has been also achieved, through multi-step strategies relying upon the regioselective protection of a chondroitin exopolysaccharide followed by sulfation of the unprotected hydroxyls and final global deprotection. As starting compound, unsulfated chondroitin could be easily obtained by microbial sources. Indeed, some bacteria that produce chondroitin and chondroitin-like capsular polysaccharides have been reviewed. [44, 45] Among them, *Pasteurella multocida* type F produces an unsulfated chondroitin polymer, [46] whereas *Escherichia coli* O5:K4:H4 synthesizes a capsular polysaccharide possessing an unsulfated chondroitin backbone with the additional presence of a β-fructose branch linked at

O-3 position of GlcA units. [26] After early results in producing the latter polysaccharide in fermentation experiments, [27] the optimization of both medium design and cultivation conditions together with the development of fed-batch fermentation strategies, have very recently allowed a significant upscale in unsulfated chondroitin production from microbial sources. [47, 48] Indeed, a fermentation broth of *Escherichia coli* O5:K4:H4 obtained by a fed–batch process was subjected to microfiltration, protease treatment, diafiltration of the harvested broth, and mild hydrolysis of the β-fructose branch with aqueous acetic acid, [49] thus affording, on a multigram-scale, the pure unsulfated chondroitin polysaccharide free of any toxic lipopolysaccharide contaminant. [50] More details about biotechnological production and purification of unsulfated chondroitin from microbial sources could be found in chapter 3.

A plethora of protecting groups were employed in the total syntheses of CS oligosaccharides from GlcNAc and GlcA monosaccharide starting materials, [9-12] nonetheless their application on polysaccharide species imposes some strict constrains, because their regioselective installation had to involve well defined hydroxyl position(s) in each repeating unit and, at the same time, the glycosidic linkages had to survive unaltered during the protection–deprotection reactions. A benzylidene protection was firstly reported on unsulfated chondroitin as well as on its methyl ester derivative **1**, obtained in turn by mild esterification with acetyl chloride in methanol at room temperature. Two derivatives (polysaccharides **2** and **3** in Figure 8) carrying a benzylidene ring at *O*-4 and *O*-6 positions of GalNAc units were obtained by subsequent treatment with α,α-dimethoxytoluene in DMF under acid catalysis with *p*-toluenesulfonic acid at 70°C. An acetylation of the hydroxyl functions at *O*-2 and *O*-3 positions of GlcA units with acetic anhydride, triethylamine and 4-dimethylamino-pyridine (DMAP) in CH_3CN, followed by acid cleavage of the benzylidene ring with aqueous acetic acid, afforded the polysaccharide intermediates **6** and **7** possessing free alcohol functions on GalNAc residues exclusively. Thus, a sulfation of **6** or **7** with sulfur trioxide-pyridine complex in DMF at 50°C, followed by ester protecting group hydrolysis with aqueous sodium hydroxide, afforded two CS-E polysaccharides in a global 44-49% mass yield, whereas a milder sulfation at 0°C furnished, after ester cleavage, CSs prevalently constituted of C disaccharide subunits in a global 44-50% mass yield. Furthermore, polysaccharide **6** or **7** were protected on the less sterically demanding *O*-6 position with a bulky trityl group, thus giving intermediates **8** and **9**, respectively, with an alcoholic group exclusively at *O*-4 position of GalNAc residues. After sulfation and full deprotection under aqueous acid and then alkaline conditions, CS polymers with up to 71% A subunits were obtained in a global 19-22% mass yield. [51] In all cases, a non-negligible decrease of the weight-averaged molecular weight (M_w) was observed: starting unsulfated chondroitin possessed a M_w=45 kDa, that decreased to a M_w=6.4-13.3 kDa in the obtained CSs, due to the acid character of some of the employed reagents, that cleaved the glycosidic linkages of the polysaccharides to some extent.

Recently, the cleavage of the 4,6-benzylidene rings on GalNAc residues was alternatively conducted under oxidative conditions, instead of hydrolytic ones. Indeed, by treating polysaccharide **4** with sodium bromate and sodium hydrosulfite in an hetereogeneous ethyl acetate/water mixture, [52] a non-regioselective oxidative opening of the benzylidene rings was observed, furnishing intermediate **10**, possessing a single free alcoholic function per disaccharide subunit, randomly distributed between position *O*-4 and *O*-6 of GalNAc residues. (Figure 8) Polysaccharide **10** was then per-*O*-sulfated with sulfur trioxide-pyridine complex in DMF and then fully deprotected to give a CS polysaccharide possessing both A and C disaccharide subunits, randomly distributed in the same polymer chain, in a rather high yield (80% mass yield from unsulfated chondroitin). [53, 54] Interestingly, a close resemblance between this product and two lots of pharmacological CS-A,C was demonstrated by 1D- and 2D-NMR spectroscopy techniques as well as HPLC analysis of chondroitinase ABC digest. Furthermore, the M_w of this semi-synthetic CS (17.3 kDa) was demonstrated, through high-performance size-exclusion chromatography combined with a triple detector array (HP-SEC-TDA), [55, 56] to be higher than the previously obtained semi-synthetic CSs (Figure 8) and very close to that of pharmacological CSs (16.8 kDa), which has been shown to be more bioavailable and thus more efficient in osteoarthritis treatment than naturally occurring high-molecular-weight CSs. [57] These features proposed this semi-synthetic CS-A,C as a valuable candidate for the replacement of CS-A,C animal-sourced drugs, that actually present several problems. Apart from obvious ethical problems in producing it from animal sources (bovine and porcine nasal septa and tracheas, poultry bones, and shark cartilages), the fact that one of the most common source is the bovine trachea involves a risk of safety problems associated with transmissible infectious agents, such as bovine spongiform encephalopathy. Furthermore, the purity, and, above all, the sulfation pattern of CS-A,C products are not always strictly monitored, [58] although a too high sulfate content, such as in per-*O*-sulfated chondroitin, can induce a strong allergic-type response, [20] and recently caused 200 deaths in United States [22] as a contaminant in heparin lots. [21]

Very recently, an orthoester ring was investigated as protecting group for GalNAc *O*-4,6 diol alternative to benzylidene. The tetrabutylammonium salt of unsulfated chondroitin as well as methyl ester **1** were treated with trimethyl orthoacetate in DMF at 50-70°C in the presence of β-camphor-10-sulfonic acid as acid catalyst. The two obtained derivatives (polysaccharides **12** and **13** in Figure 9) were then acetylated to furnish derivatives **14** and **15**, that were in turn subjected to orthoester hydrolysis under acid conditions with aqueous 57-90% acetic acid at rt-60°C. After sulfation with sulfur trioxide-pyridine complex in DMF and then full deprotection under aqueous alkaline conditions, CS-A,C polymers with a variable A,C disaccharide subunits ratio were obtained. [59] The authors suggested that the prevalence of sulfate groups at positions 4 or 6 of GalNAc residues was due to temperature and acid concentration of the orthoester hydrolysis reaction, that could steer the regioselectivity of ring opening, thus affording a free hydroxyl mainly at position 4 or 6 of GalNAc units in derivatives **16** and **17**. However, structural characterization of these and any other intermediate was not reported.

A slight modification of the semi-synthetic strategy relying upon the orthoester protection opened an access to CS polysaccharides containing sulfate groups not only on GalNAc residues but also on GlcA units. [60, 61] In particular, by conducting the orthoester ring installation and its cleavage in a one-pot fashion and omitting the acetylation in between, chondroitin derivative **18** with only one acetyl protecting group randomly distributed between position *O*-4 and *O*-6 of GalNAc units was obtained (Figure 10). Sulfation of **18** with sulfur trioxide-pyridine complex at 50°C in DMF furnished CS polysaccharide **19** possessing per-*O*-sulfated GlcA units and an additional sulfate group per disaccharide subunit randomly distributed between position *O*-4 and *O*-6 of GalNAc residues (4-sulfate/6-sulfate ratio = 1.4:1).

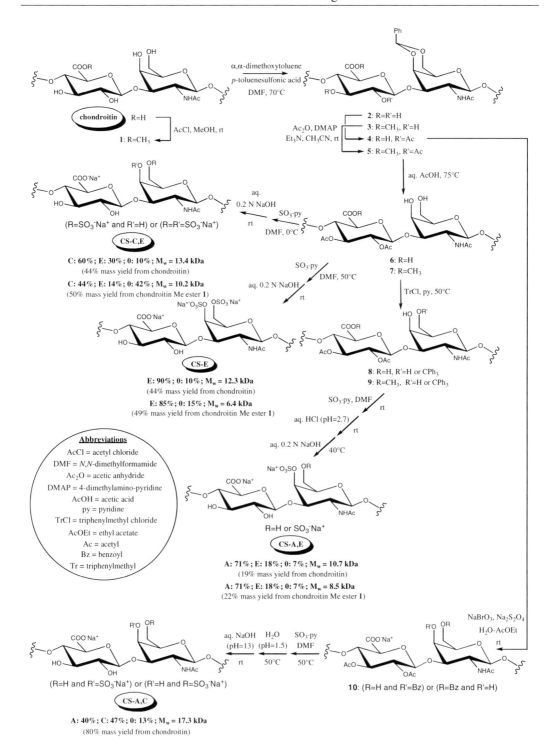

Figure 8. Semi-synthesis of CSs from unsulfated chondroitin through benzylidene protection.

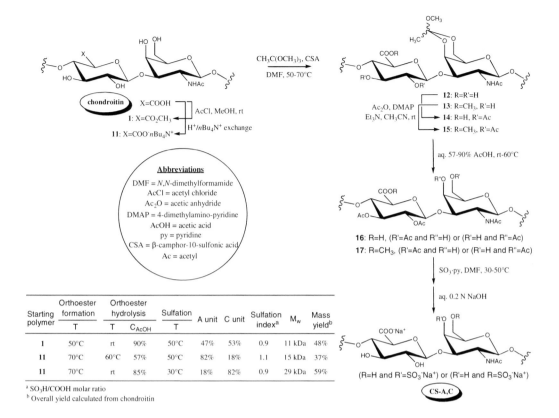

Figure 9. Semi-synthesis of CSs from unsulfated chondroitin through orthoester protection.

By subjecting unsulfated chondroitin to an orthoester ring installation-acetylation-orthoester ring cleavage sequence in a one-pot fashion, derivative **20** was obtained. Its per-*O*-sulfation, followed by deprotection under alkaline conditions, giving a CS polysaccharide with four different disaccharide subunits, possessing A, C, K, and L sulfation profiles in a 2.1:2.3:1:1.2 ratio (Figure 10). This is the only strategy reported up to now, affording a CS polymer with GlcA units sulfated exclusively at their *O*-3 position. Such subunits have been detected in CSs isolated from squid and king crab cartilages as well as from squid liver integuments. [24, 62, 63] These CSs have been shown to promote neurite outgrowth in the central nervous system [64] and to bind heparin-binding growth/differentiation factors. [65]

The obtainment of a CS polysaccharide possessing K and L disaccharide subunits was firstly ascribed to a non-quantitative acetylation at position 3 of the GlcA units in the orthoesterification-acetylation-orthoester cleavage one-pot sequence. Nonetheless, several powerful acylation conditions were tested (Figure 10) and in every case the obtained CS polysaccharide contained sulfate groups at *O*-3 position of GlcA units to a certain extent. Alternatively, a transient protection at *O*-3 position of some GlcA units through an acyclic orthoester group during orthoester ring installation was hypothesized (intermediate **21**), similarly to the acyclic acetal moieties formed on Glc units during acetalation of dextrans. [66] Acyclic acetals showed a shorter half-life in acid and even neutral aqueous solution with respect to their cyclic analogues. Similarly, the acyclic orthoester moiety in **21** should be too labile to survive upon isolation on derivative **12-13**, whereas it could be stable in base solution during the acetylation reaction and then cleaved in the final acid hydrolysis step of the one-pot sequence, thus giving derivative **20** carrying a free hydroxyl group at position *O*-3 of some GlcA units. However, work is in progress to elucidate this point in full details. [67] In Figure 11 the conversions between CS polysaccharides through sulfation/desulfation reactions presented in this chapter are summarized.

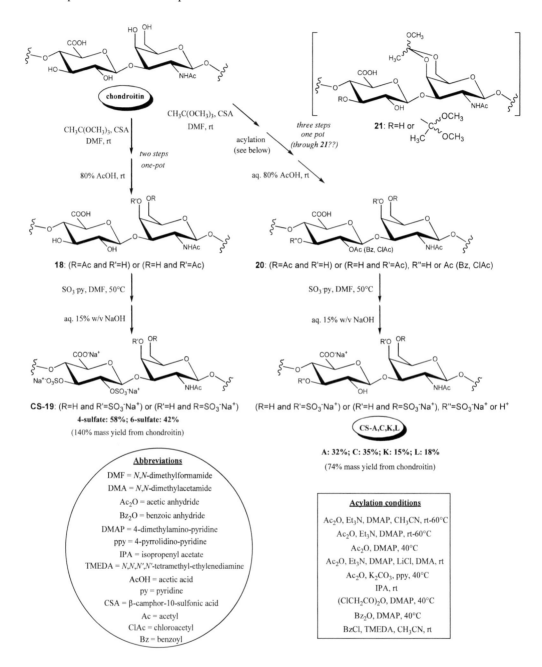

Figure 10. Semi-synthesis of CSs containing sulfated GlcA units from unsulfated chondroitin through orthoester protection.

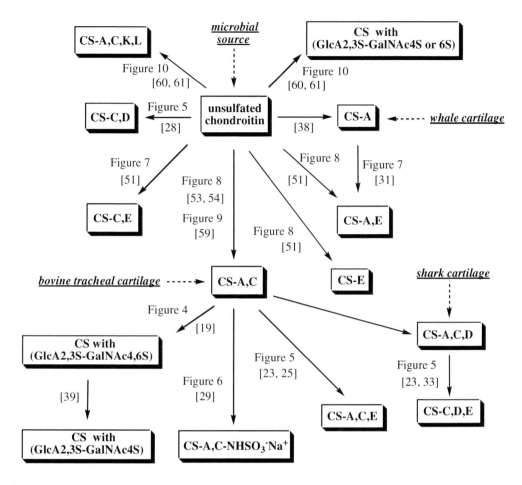

Figure 11. Summary of conversions between chondroitin and CS polysaccharides through sulfation/desulfation reactions.

Other Reactions

The multi-functionality of GAGs, CS included, offered several opportunities to carbohydrate chemists to install non-native moieties on their structures. [68, 69] N-acetyl groups of CS-A,C from bovine tracheal cartilage were cleaved by hydrazinolysis without concomitant depolymerization, as already cited above. [29] The resulting free amino groups were acylated with several acyl anhydrides giving N-propionyl-, N-butyryl-, N-hexanoyl and N-benzoyl-CS-A,C. [70] N-formyl-CS-A,C was also obtained, but, since the respective anhydride is not available, a different acylating system was chosen. Formic acid was converted into an activated ester by reaction with N-(3-dimethylaminopropyl)-N'-ethylcarbodiimide hydrochloride (EDCI) and then coupled one-pot with CS-A,C. The resulting N-formyl derivative was then treated with aqueous NaOH in order to restore any carboxyl group that reacted with EDC. Unnatural N-acyl-CS-A,C derivatives were subjected to chondroitinase ABC digestion, showing that N-formyl, N-hexanoyl and N-benzoyl derivatives were completely resistant, whereas N-propionyl and N-butyryl ones underwent digestion, albeit at much slower rates than native CS-A,C.

Most chemical manipulations on CSs, other than sulfation/desulfation reactions, concerned the carboxyl group of GlcA units. Its conversion into an amide group was described by Danishefsky and Siskovic already more than forty years ago. [71] They treated a mixture of CS-A or CS-C and glycine methyl ester with EDCI in slightly acid aqueous solution (pH=4.75). After saponification of the methyl ester groups, CS derivatives **21** and **22** with 33-36% glycine groups were obtained. (Figure12) When the reaction of CS-C carboxyl groups with EDCI was performed in the absence of any nucleophile, the intermediate *O*-acylisourea **23** was isolated. [72] Interestingly, CS derivative **23**, as well as a heparin acylisourea analogue, showed inhibition of myeloma and breast cancer cell proliferation by induction of apoptosis both *in vitro* and in mice, without causing apparent toxicity to adjacent normal tissues. [73] *O*-Acylisourea moieties of derivative **23** could be reduced to hydroxymethyl groups by treatment with aqueous sodium borohydride at 50°C for 2 hours, thus giving polysaccharide **24** possessing Glc units in place of GlcA ones. Derivative **23** was also treated with aqueous sodium carbonate, that hydrolyzed the most part of *O*-acylisourea moieties back to carboxyl functions, whereas a residual 10% rearranged to give *N*-acylurea groups. [72]

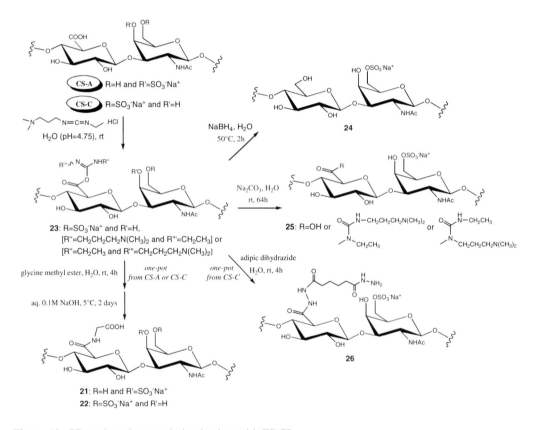

Figure 12. CSs carboxyl group derivatization with EDCI.

Carboxyl group modification was also extensively used to cross-link CS polymer chains into networks, that are able to absorb large amount of water and find several biomedical applications in the field of tissue engineering. [74, 75] One of the first results on this topic was reported by Prestwich and co-workers, that treated CS-C with adipic dihydrazide in the presence again of EDCI at pH=4.75 to obtain derivative **26** (Figure 12), carrying a pendant hydrazide functionality, that could react with poly(ethylene glycol) (PEG)-propiondialdehyde at neutral pH in few minutes giving CS-C network **27** (Figure 13). This cross-linked polymer formed flexible, hydratable hydrogel films, that were evaluated for wound healing ability in mice. [76] Analogously, CS-A was cross-linked by reaction with 1,12-diaminododecane in DMSO in the presence of dicyclohexylcarbodiimide (DCC) as GlcA carboxyl groups activator. [77]

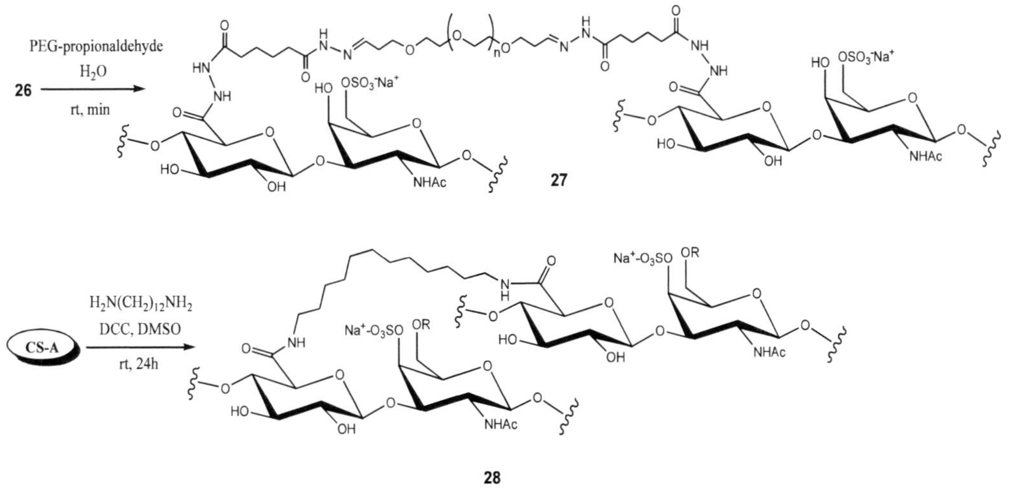

Figure 13. CSs chemical cross-linking.

CS-A,C networks were obtained also by employing PEG-diglycidyl ether as cross-linking agent in a reaction conducted in aqueous 1M NaOH at rt overnight. The reaction was not studied in details, however it was proposed a non-regioselective involvement of both GalNAc and GlcA hydroxyl groups to act as nucleophiles and attack the epoxide rings on PEG-diglycidyl ether. The obtained hydrogels were studied as drug delivery vehicles. [78,79]

Very recently, a chemoenzymatic strategy to cross-link a CS-C polysaccharide was proposed. The reaction of carboxyl groups of CS-C with tyramine in the presence of EDCI and *N*-hydroxysuccinimide (NHS) in 2-morpholinoethane sulphonic acid (MES) aqueous buffer (pH=6.0) and DMF afforded derivative **29**, possessing up to 40% of GlcA units carrying a tyramide function (Figure 14). The tyrosine moieties of **29** were then oxidized enzymatically by tyrosinase in the presence of oxygen in phosphate buffered saline (PBS) to give the cross-linked product **30** through an *o*-quinone intermediate. Network **30** was demonstrated to possess some favourable characteristics, such as high elasticity, biodegradability, interconnected porous structure, good biocompatibility, for drug delivery and tissue engineering applications. [80]

CS networks were obtained by photoinitiated cross-linking too. CS-A was functionalized with methacrylate groups by reacting it with methacrylic anhydride in aqueous NaOH solution (pH=10) at 60°C for 24 hours, affording CS derivative **31** with up to 25% methacryl substituents per disaccharide subunit randomly distributed between *O*-6 position of GalNAc units and *O*-2,3 positions of GlcA residues (Figure 15). [81] Derivatization of CS-A was performed under alternative reaction conditions with glycidyl methacrylate (GMA) in PBS at

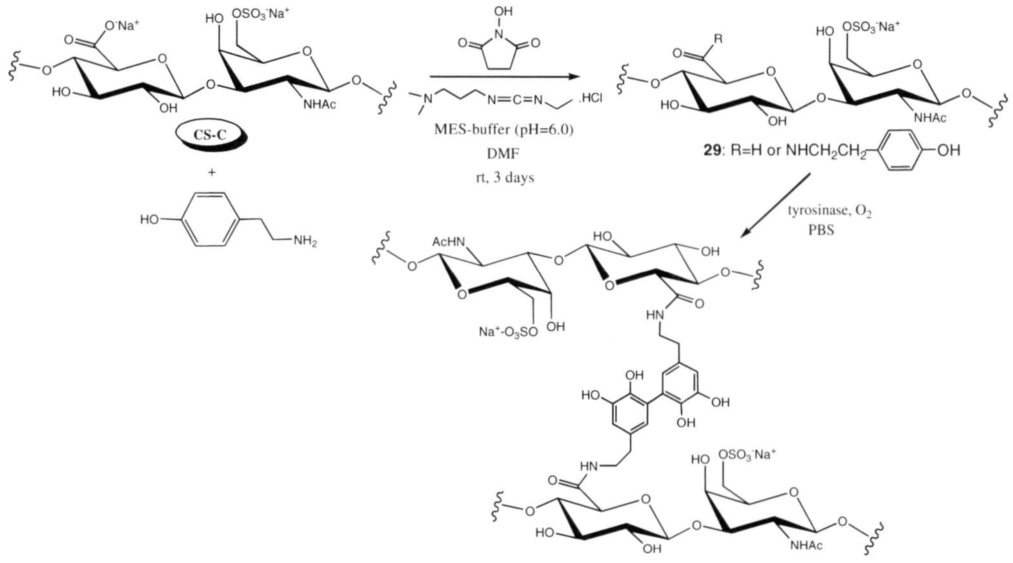

Figure 14. CS-C chemoenzymatic cross-linking.

pH=7.4 at rt. [82] This reaction was studied in details, revealing that transesterification between CS-A and GMA − producing **31** − proceeded rapidly and reached the balance in one day. The system pH value then began to decrease due to the slower methacrylate hydrolysis producing methacrylic acid. At lowered pH (6.4) transesterification terminated and the slowest epoxide ring opening reaction started. In the long term (15 days), the accumulation of product **32**, carrying methacrylate functions only on carboxyl and sulfate groups, was enabled. A 12% incorporation of methacrylate groups into CS-A was observed. Both derivatives **31** and **32** were cross-linked by UV-irradiation with 365-nm light in the presence of a biocompatible photoinitiator, giving hydrogels useful for cartilage tissue engineering [83]. Furthermore, derivative **32** was subjected to oxidative cleavage of the vicinal diol moiety in GlcA units with sodium periodate to form aldehyde groups along the polysaccharide backbone. The obtained multifunctional CS-A derivative **33** was used as a "tissue primer" for repair of cartilage defects. Elisseeff and coworkers demonstrated that **33** was able to anchor the amine groups present on tissue proteins through a Schiff-base linkage with its aldehyde groups, and contemporarily to form a hydrogel network by *in vivo* photoinitiated cross-linking of methacryl groups. [84]

Methacrylated derivative **32** was photochemically cross-linked in the presence of double-bond functionalized polymers, acting as linkers between CS chains. Hydrogel network thus obtained by a mixture of **32** and PEG-diacrylate was used as an encapsulation medium for mesenchymal stem cells for chondrogenic differentiation. [85] Hydrogels obtained by mixing methacrylated CS **31** and polyvinyl-alcohol [81] or PEG-dimethacrylate, [86] polyacrylamide or poly(*N,N*-dimethyl acrylamide) [87] under photopolymerization conditions were reported too. Other photo-crosslinked CS materials were obtained by UV-irradiation of CS tetraalkylammonium salts, that were previously non-regioselectively functionalized at their free hydroxyls with activated 7-coumaryloxyacetic acid. [88]

The cross-linking of CS polysaccharides in the presence of polymer spacers was accomplished through Schiff-base linkages too. Oxidative cleavage on GlcA diols was performed on native CS-A with sodium periodate as already described for derivative **31**. The obtained aldehyde-functionalized CS-A derivative was cross-linked with polyvinyl alcohol covinylamine, and simultaneously anchored to amine groups present on tissue proteins, as already described for CS derivative **33**. This material was shown *ex vivo* to be an effective adhesive for sealing corneal incisions. [89]

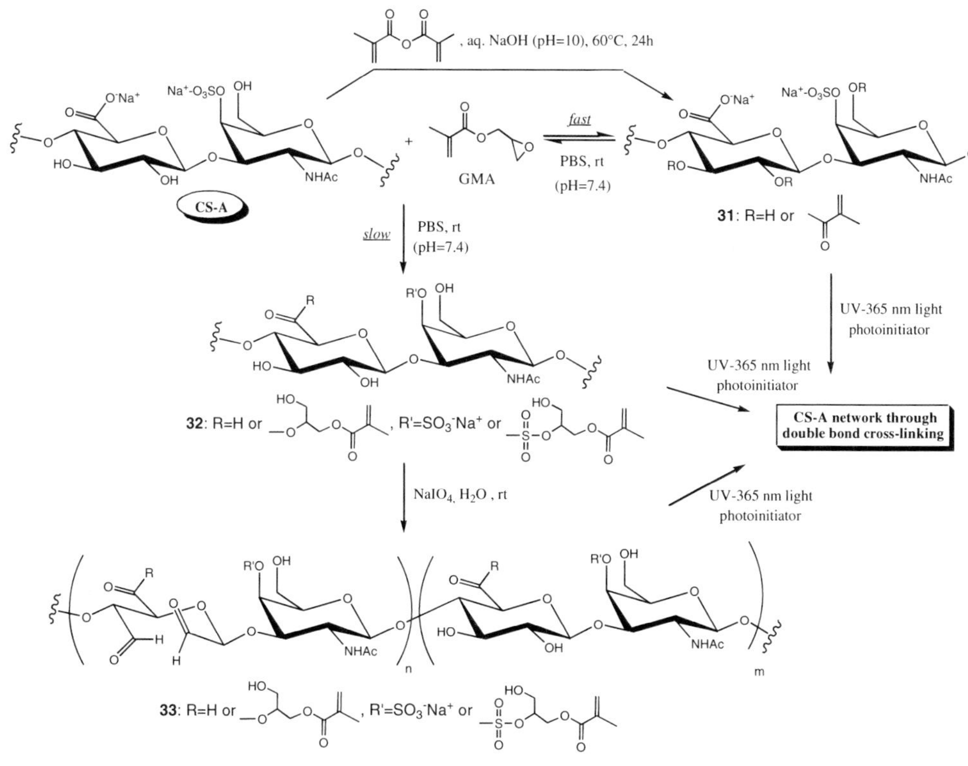

Figure 15. CS-A photoinitiated cross-linking.

The cross-linking of CS-C with another GAG, such as heparin, was accomplished through a thiol-ene coupling. CS-C was reacted with 3,3'-dithiobis(propanoic hydrazide) in the presence of EDCI at pH=4.75, followed by cleavage of the disulfide bond with dithiothreitol (DTT) at pH=8.5 in order to have a free thiol group (Figure 16). The obtained derivative **34** contained 63% GlcA units linked to a thiol-functionalized appendage. Analogously, heparin was subjected to the same protocol to give thiol-appended heparin derivative **35**. By mixing **34** and **35** in different ratios in the presence of PEG-diacrylate in different concentrations in Dulbecco's phosphate buffered saline (DBS) at rt for few minutes, an array of cross-linked hydrogels were obtained. They showed interesting properties as injectable materials for controlled release of heparin-binding growth factors *in vivo*. [90]

CS polysaccharides were cross-linked with proteins, such as collagen, [91] gelatin, [92] and collagen-elastin, [93] through EDCI combined with NHS in MES aqueous buffer (pH=5.5) (Figure 17). The linkage between CS-A,C and collagen increased the water-binding capacity of the biomaterial up to 65%. When implanted in rats, this biomaterial modulated tissue response by promoting angiogenesis and reducing foreign body reactions.[94] Hydrogels obtained by cross-linking CS-C with gelatin were proposed for the controlled delivery of cationic antibacterial proteins, since the incorporation of CS-C in gelatine increased the protein loading capacity and contemporarily extended its release time. [92] A CS-C-gelatin-HA tri-copolymer was also prepared, again by carbodiimide chemistry. [95] It was investigated *in vivo* as a biomimetic scaffold of natural cartilage tissues for the treatment of articular defects [96] and as a biomatrix for wound healing [97]. Furthermore, it was proposed by *in vitro* tests as a bioactive scaffold for regenerating human nucleus pulposus. [98]

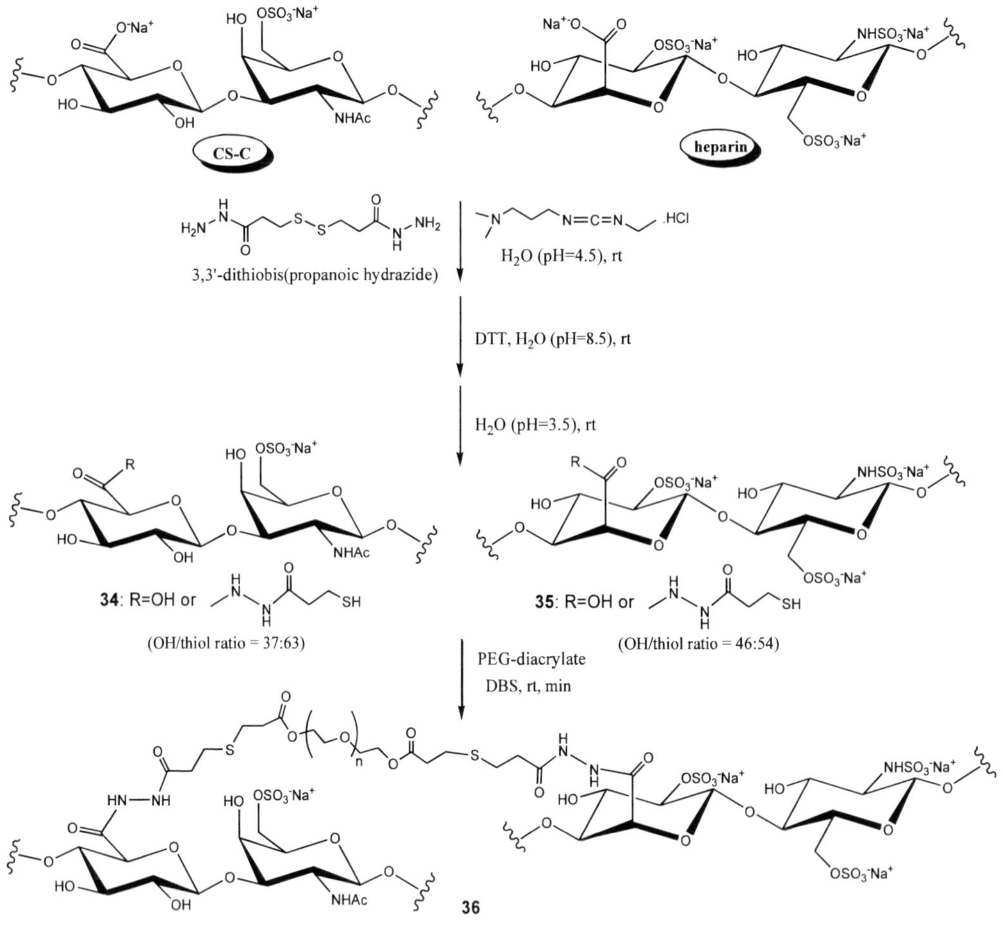

Figure 16. CS-C-heparin cross-linking through thiol-ene coupling.

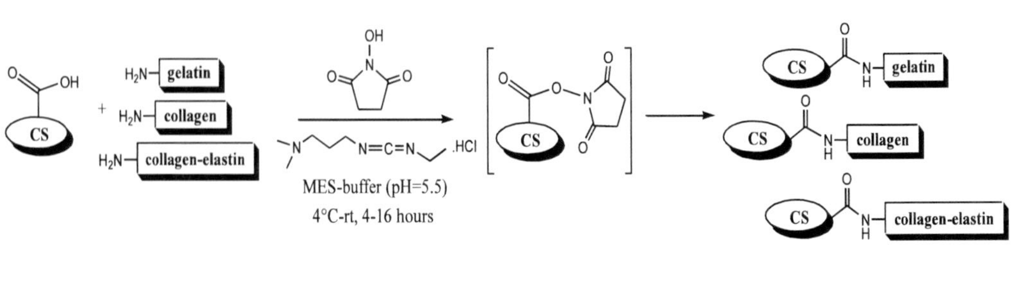

Figure 17. CS-protein cross-linking.

The linkage of CS polysaccharides to non-carbohydrate molecules was accomplished also through linkages involving CS hydroxyl functions. Chlorin e6, a fluorescent emitter carrying a carboxylic acid function, was coupled to CS-A in two steps: firstly, a non-quantitative acetylation of the polysaccharide with acetic anhydride and pyridine in formamide at rt was performed, thus affording DMSO-soluble polymer derivative **37**, [99] that was in turn reacted with chlorine e6 in the presence of DCC and DMAP (Figure 18). The same strategy was repeated with a similar fluorescent molecule such as zinc(II) tetracarboxyphthalocyanine. The obtained fluorescent CS derivatives **38** and **39** were proposed as nanodrugs for photodynamic therapy. [100, 101]

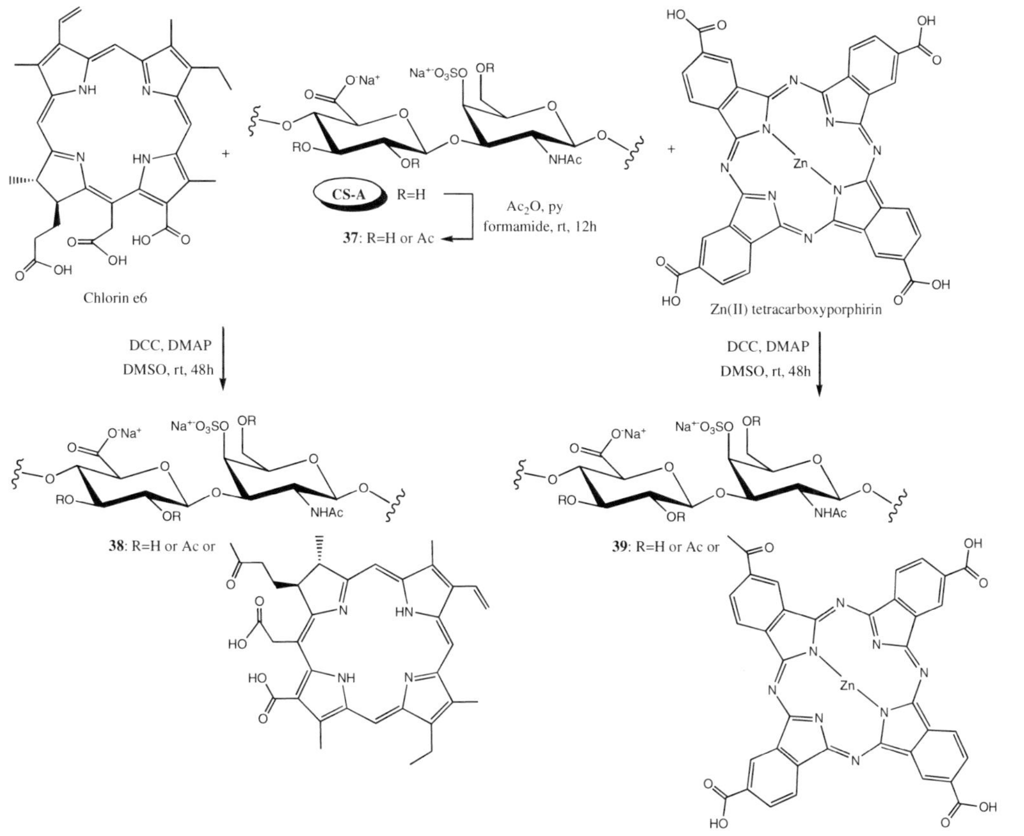

Figure 18. Synthesis of CS-A conjugates for photodynamic therapy.

Hydroxyl reactivity was also used for grafting CS-A onto poly(L-lactide) chains. The grafting was obtained through a ring opening polymerization of L-lactide by the hydroxyl functions of CS-A in DMSO at 140°C for 3 hours in the presence of stannous octoate as catalyst (Figure 19). [102] The obtained amphiphilic grafted copolymer **40** formed films for chondrocyte encapsulation useful in cartilage tissue engineering applications, [103] as well as nanoparticles for drug delivery. [104]

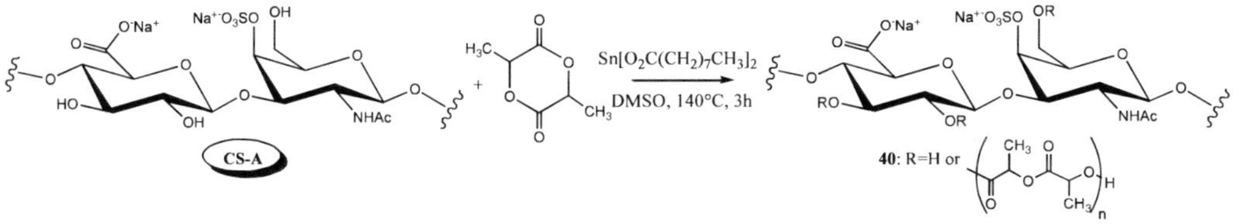

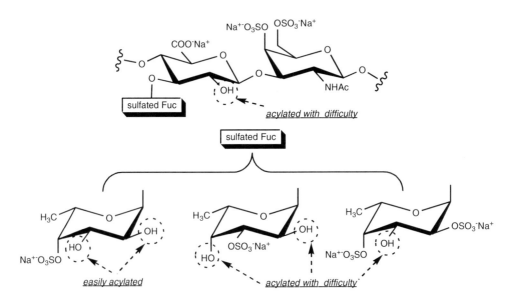

Figure 19. Synthesis of CS-A- poly(L-lactide) grafted copolymer.

The chemical and chemoenzymatic manipulation of fucosylated CS polysaccharides is an almost virgin research field. However, in order to understand the relationships between fucosylated CSs structure and their anticoagulant activity, some reactions have been performed. Since fucose is a 6-deoxyhexose, its glycosidic linkage is more acid-labile than that formed by GlcA or GalNAc. Therefore, a mild acid hydrolysis of fucosylated CS from sea cucumber *Ludwigothurea grisea* was conducted with aqueous 150 mM sulfuric acid at 100°C for 30 min, allowing a large, but non complete, release of sulfated fucose branches together with a much smaller cleavage of the chondroitin backbone interglycosidic bonds. [105] Interestingly, the partially defucosylated polysaccharide showed no anticoagulant properties, thus demonstrating that sulfated fucose branches account for the antithrombotic activity of fucosylated CSs. [106] An alternative mild breakage of fucosylated CS from sea cucumber *Pearsonothuria graeffei* was performed by irradiation with γ-rays from a ^{60}Co source in water solution, thus obtaining a partial depolymerization by cleavage of the glycosidic bonds involving selectively some GlcA units. The anticoagulant activity of the obtained fragments reduced with decreasing molecular weights. [107]

Figure 20. Acylation of fucosylated CS hydroxyls from *Thelenata ananas*.

Very recently, the *O*-acylation of the tetrabutylammonium salt of fucosylated CS from sea cucumber *Thelenata ananas* was carried out with acetic, propionic or succinic anhydride in the presence of butylamine and DMAP in DMF at 40-60°C for 24-48 hours. Acyl groups were preferentially introduced at positions 2 and 3 of Fuc4S units, whereas a difficulty in acylating the hydroxyls at position 3 of Fuc2,4S units, at positions 2 and 4 of Fuc3S residues, and at position 2 of GlcA ones was observed (Figure 20). However, a 95% substitution degree could be achieved through a propionylation reaction conducted at 60°C for 48 hours. The acylation of fucosylated CS did not affect its anticoagulant activity. [108]

Conclusion

This chapter is aimed to provide an overview of the chemical and chemoenzymatic transformations performed on natural CS and chondroitin polysaccharides.

In the first part, known methods to modify their sulfation patterns have been presented, with attention both on selective sulfation/desulfation reactions performed on natural CSs and on multistep protection/deprotection strategies aimed to the regioselective sulfation of microbial sourced chondroitin. In the future, the development of novel protection patterns and/or new regioselective sulfation/desulfation reactions is expected in order to enlarge further the family of semi-synthetic CS polysaccharides with biologically relevant sulfation profiles.

In the second part of the chapter a survey of the chemical transformations on CSs not directed to the modification of the sulfation pattern have been reported. Major attention was focused on the preparation of CS cross-linked hydrogel structures, that show interesting biomedical potentialities especially for tissue engineering and controlled drug delivery applications.

In a near future, an increasing attention will be very probably devoted also to the chemical and/or chemoenzymatic manipulation of fucosylated CS species, on which almost no transformations have been reported yet, in spite of their very promising anticoagulant activity.

References

[1]　N. Volpi, *Chondroitin Sulfate: Structure, Role and Pharmacological Activity*, Academic Press, San Diego (2006).

[2]　R.P. Vieira, B. Mulloy and P.A.S. Mourão, *J. Biol. Chem. 266*, 13530 (1991).

[3]　S. Chen, C. Xue, L. Yin, Q. Tang, G. Yu and W. Chai, *Carbohydr. Polym. 83*, 688 (2011).

[4]　C.I. Gama, S.E. Tully, N. Sotogaku, P.M. Clark, M. Rawat, N. Vaidehi, W.A. Goddard III, A. Nishi and L.C. Hsieh-Wilson, *Nat. Chem. Biol. 2*, 467 (2006).

[5]　J.-Y. Reginster, F. Heraud, B. Zegels and O. Bruyere, *Mini-Rev. Med. Chem. 7*, 1051 (2007).

[6]　S. Yamada and K. Sugahara, *Curr. Drug Discov. Technol. 5*, 289 (2008).

[7]　R.J.C. Fonseca, and P.A.S. Mourão, *Thromb. Haemostasis 96*, 822 (2006).

[8]　S. Moll, and H.R. Roberts, *Semin. Hematol. 39*, 145 (2002).

[9]　J. Tamura, *Trends Glycosci. Glycotechnol. 13*, 65 (2001).

[10]　N. Karst and R.J. Linhardt, *Curr. Med. Chem. 10*, 1993 (2003).

[11]　A. Vibert, J.-C. Jacquinet and C. Lopin-Bon, *J. Carbohydr. Chem. 30*, 393 (2011).

[12] E. Bedini and M. Parrilli, *Carbohydr. Res. 356*, 75 (2012).

[13] V.L. Campo, D.F. Kawano, D.B. da Silva Jr. and I. Carvalho, *Carbohydr. Polym. 77*, 167 (2009).

[14] S.N. Pawar and K.J. Edgar, *Biomaterials 33*, 3279 (2012).

[15] M.L. Wolfrom and B.O. Juliano, *J. Am. Chem. Soc. 82*, 2588 (1960).

[16] K. Nagasawa and Y. Inoue, *Chem. Pharm. Bull. 19*, 2617 (1971).

[17] C. Bartolucci, L. Cellai, M.A. Iannelli, D. Lamba, L. Liverani, G. Mascellani and E. Perola, *Carbohydr. Res. 276*, 401 (1995).

[18] B. Casu, A. Naggi and G. Torri, in B.O. Fraser-Reid, K. Tatsuta and J. Thiem, *Glycoscience: chemistry and chemical biology*, Vol. 3, pp.1895-1903, Springer, Berlin Heidelberg (2001).

[19] T. Maruyama, T. Toida, T. Imanari, G. Yu and R.J. Linhardt, *Carbohydr. Res. 306*, 35 (1998).

[20] A. Greinacher, J. Michels, M. Schäfer, V. Keifel and C. Mueller-Eckhardt, *Br. J. Haematol. 81*, 252 (1992).

[21] M. Guerrini, D. Beccati, Z. Shriver, A. Naggi, K. Viswanathan, A. Bisio, I. Capila, J.C. Lansing, S. Guglieri, B. Fraser, A. Al-Hakim, N.S. Gunay, Z. Zhang, L. Robinson, L. Buhse, M. Nasr, J. Woodcock, R. Langer, G. Venkataraman, R.J. Linhardt, B. Casu, G. Torri and R. Sasisekharan, *Nat. Biotechnol. 6*, 669 (2008).

[22] T.K. Kishimoto, K. Viswanathan, T. Ganguly, S. Elankumaran, S. Smith, K. Pelzer, J.C. Lansing, N. Sriranganathan, G. Zhao, Z. Galcheva-Gargova, A. Al-Hakim, G.S. Bailey, B. Fraser, S. Roy, T. Rogers-Cotrone, L. Buhse, M. Whary, J. Fox, M. Nasr, G. J. Dal Pan, Z. Shriver, R.S. Langer, G. Venkataraman, K.F. Austen, J. Woodcock and R. Sasisekharan, *New. Engl. J. Med. 358*, 2457 (2008).

[23] K. Nagasawa, H. Uchiyama and N. Wajima, *Carbohydr. Res. 158*, 183 (1986).

[24] K. Sugahara, Y. Tanaka, S. Yamada, N. Seno, H. Kitagawa, S.M. Haslam, H.R. Morris and A. Dell, *J. Biol. Chem. 271*, 26745 (1996).

[25] C. Cai, K. Solakyildirim, B. Yang, J.M. Beaudet, A. Weyers, R.J. Linhardt and F. Zhang, *Carbohydr. Polym. 87*, 822 (2012).

[26] M.L. Rodriguez, B. Jann and K. Jann, *Eur. J. Biochem. 177*, 117 (1988).

[27] M. Manzoni, S. Bergomi, F. Molinari and V. Cavazzoni, *Biotechnol. Lett. 18*, 383 (1996).

[28] E. Valoti, N. Miraglia, D. Bianchi, M. Valetti and P. Bazza, *PCT Int. Appl.* No. WO2012159655, Nov 29, 2012.

[29] V.D. Nadkarni, T. Toida, C.L. Van Gorp, R.L. Schubert, J.M. Weiler, K.P. Hansen, E.E.O. Caldwell and R.J. Linhardt, *Carbohydr. Res. 290*, 87 (1996).

[30] Y. Ito and O. Habuchi, *J. Biol. Chem. 275*, 34728 (2000).

[31] O. Habuchi, R. Moroi and S. Ohtake, *Anal. Biochem. 310*, 129 (2002).

[32] S. Nadanaka and K. Sugahara, *Glycobiology 7*, 253 (1997).

[33] T. Yamaguchi, S. Ohtake, K. Kimata and O. Habuchi, *Glycobiology 17*, 1365 (2007).

[34] M. Kobayashi, G. Sugumaran, J. Liu, N.W. Shworak, J.E. Silbert and R.D. Rosenberg, *J. Biol. Chem. 274*, 10474 (1999).

[35] S. Ohtake, K. Kimata and O. Habuchi, *J. Biol. Chem. 278*, 38443 (2003).

[36] X. Zhou, K. Chandarajoti, T.Q. Pham, R. Liu and J. Liu, *Glycobiology 21*, 771 (2011).

[37] Y. Xu, S. Masuko, M. Takieddin, H. Xu, R. Liu, J. Jing, S.A. Mousa, R.J. Linhardt and J. Liu, *Science 334*, 498 (2011).

[38] M. Masayoshi, R. Takano, K. Kamei-Hayashi and S. Hara, *Carbohydr. Res. 241*, 209 (1993).

[39] T. Toida, A. Suzuki, K. Nakajima, A. Chaidedgumjorn and T. Imanari, *Glycoconj. J. 17*, 393 (2000).

[40] A.I. Usov, K.S. Adamyants, L.I. Miroshnikova, A.A. Shaposhnikova and N.K. Kochetkov, *Carbohydr. Res. 18*, 336 (1971).

[41] Y. Inoue and K. Nagasawa, *Carbohydr. Res. 46*, 87 (1976).

[42] K. Nagasawa, Y. Inoue and T. Kamata, *Carbohydr. Res. 58*, 47 (1977).

[43] A. Malleron, A. Benjdia, O. Berteau and C. Le Narvor, *Carbohydr. Res. 353*, 96 (2012).

[44] C. Schiraldi, D. Cimini and M. De Rosa, *Appl. Microbiol. Biotechnol. 87*, 1209 (2010).

[45] P.L. DeAngelis, *Appl. Microbiol. Biotechnol. 94*, 295 (2012).

[46] P.L. DeAngelis, N.S. Gunay, T. Toida, W.Mao and R. J. Linhardt, *Carbohydr. Res. 337*, 1547 (2002).

[47] O.F. Restaino, D. Cimini, M. De Rosa, A. Catapano, M. De Rosa and C. Schiraldi, *Microb. Cell Fact. 10*, 10 (2011).

[48] C. Schiraldi, A. Alfano, D. Cimini, M. De Rosa, A. Panariello, O.F. Restaino and M. De Rosa, *Biotechnol. Prog. 28*, 1012 (2012).

[49] D. Cimini, O.F. Restaino, A. Catapano, M. De Rosa and C. Schiraldi, *Appl. Microbiol. Biotechnol. 85*, 1779 (2010).

[50] O.F. Restaino, D. Cimini, M. De Rosa, C. De Castro, M. Parrilli and C. Schiraldi, *Electrophoresis 30*, 3877 (2009).

[51] G. Zoppetti and P. Oreste, *United States Patent* No. 6,777,398 B2, Aug 17, 2004.

[52] M. Adinolfi, G. Barone, L. Guariniello and A. Iadonisi, *Tetrahedron Lett. 40*, 8439 (1999).

[53] E. Bedini, C. De Castro, M. De Rosa, A. Di Nola, A. Iadonisi, O.F. Restaino, C. Schiraldi and M. Parrilli, *Angew. Chem. Int. Ed. 50*, 6160 (2011).

[54] E. Bedini, M. De Rosa, C. De Castro, A. Di Nola, M. Parrilli, O.F. Restaino and C. Schiraldi, *PCT Int. Appl.* No. WO201262917, May 18, 2012.

[55] S. Bertini, A. Bisio, G. Torri, D. Bensi and M. Terbojevich, *Biomacromolecules 6*, 168 (2005).

[56] A. La Gatta, M. De Rosa, I. Marzaioli, T. Busico and C. Schiraldi, *Anal. Biochem. 404*, 21 (2010).

[57] A.O. Adebowale, D.S. Cox, Z. Liang and N.D. Eddington, *J. Am. Nutraceutical Assoc. 3*, 37 (2000).

[58] M. McCoy, *Chem. Eng. News 78* (14), 20 (2000).

[59] D. Bianchi, M. Valetti, P. Bazza, N. Miraglia and E. Valoti, *PCT Int. Appl.* No. WO2012152872, Nov 15, 2012.

[60] E. Bedini, C. De Castro, M. De Rosa, A. Di Nola, O.F. Restaino, C. Schiraldi and M. Parrilli, *Chem. Eur. J. 18*, 2123 (2012).

[61] E. Bedini, M. De Rosa, C. De Castro, A. Di Nola, A. Iadonisi, A. La Gatta, M. Parrilli and C. Schiraldi, *PCT Int. Appl.* No. WO2012130753, Oct 4, 2012.

[62] A. Kinoshita, S. Yamada, S.M. Haslam, H.R. Morris, A. Dell and K. Sugahara, *J. Biol. Chem. 272*, 19656 (1997).

[63] A. Kumar Shetty, T. Kobayashi, S. Mizumoto, M. Narumi, Y. Kudo, S. Yamada and K. Sugahara, *Carbohydr. Res. 344*, 1526 (2009).

[64] T. Mikami and K. Sugahara, *Trends Glycosci. Glycotechnol. 18*, 165 (2006).

[65] S.S. Deepa, Y. Umehara, S. Higashiyama, N. Itoh and K. Sugahara, *J. Biol. Chem. 277*, 43707 (2002).

[66] L. Cui, J.L. Cohen, C.K. Chu, P.R. Wich, P.H. Kierestead and J.M.J. Fréchet, *J. Am. Chem. Soc. 134*, 15840 (2012).

[67] E. Bedini, C. De Castro and M. Parrilli, unpublished data.

[68] I.Y. Ponedel'kina, E.S. Lukina and V.N. Odinokov, *Russ. J. Bioorg. Chem. 34*, 1 (2008).

[69] J. Schiller, J. Becher, S. Möller, K. Nimptsch, T. Riemer and M. Schnabelrauch, *Mini-Rev. Org. Chem. 7*, 290 (2010).

[70] S.V. Madhunapantula, R.N. Achur, V.P. Bhavanandan and D.C. Gowda, *Glycoconj. J. 24*, 465 (2007).

[71] I. Danishefsky and E. Siskovic, *Carbohydr. Res. 16*, 199 (1971).

[72] Y. Inoue and K. Nagasawa, *Carbohydr. Res. 111*, 113 (1982).

[73] C.Y. Pumphrey, A.M. Theus, S. Li, R.S. Parrish and R.D. Sanderson, *Cancer Res. 62*, 3722 (2002).

[74] A.D. Baldwin and K.L. Kiick, *Biomaterials 94*, 128 (2010).

[75] S. Van Vlierberghe, P. Dubruel and E. Schacht, *Biomacromolecules 12*, 1387 (2011).

[76] K.R. Kirker, Y. Luo, J.H. Nielson, J. Shelby and G.D. Prestwich, *Biomaterials 23*, 3661 (2002).

[77] A. Sintov, N. Di-Capua and A. Rubinstein, *Biomaterials 16*, 473 (1995).

[78] M.F. Tsai, Y.L. Chiang, L.F. Wang, G.W. Huang, G.W. and P.C. Wu, *J. Biomater. Sci. Polym. Ed. 16*, 1319 (2005).

[79] S.-C. Wang, B.-H. Chen, L.-F. Wang and J.-S. Chen, *Int. J. Pharm. 329*, 103 (2007).

[80] R. Jin, B. Lou and C. Lin, *Polym. Int. 62*, 353 (2013).

[81] S.J. Bryant, K.A. Davis-Arehart, N. Luo, R. Shoemaker, J.A. Arthur and K.S. Anseth, *Macromolecules 37*, 6726 (2004).

[82] Q. Li, D. Wang and J.H. Elisseeff, *Macromolecules 36*, 2556 (2003).

[83] Q. Li, C.G. Williams, D.D.N. Sun, J. Wang, K. Leong and J.H. Elisseeff, *J. Biomed. Mat. Res. A 68*, 28 (2004).

[84] D. Wang, S. Varghese, B. Sharma, I. Strehin, S. Fermanian, J. Gorham, D.H. Fairbrother, B. Cascio and J.H. Elisseeff, *Nat. Mater. 6*, 385 (2007).

[85] S. Varghese, N.S. Hwang, A.C. Canver, P. Theprungsirikul, D.W. Lin and J.H. Elisseeff, *Matrix Biol. 27*, 12 (2008).

[86] S.J. Bryant, J.A. Arthur and K.S. Anseth, *Acta Biomater. 1*, 243 (2005).

[87] T.C. Suekama, J. Hu, T. Kurokawa, J.P. Gong and S.H. Gehrke, *ACS Macro Lett. 2*, 137 (2013).

[88] T. Matsuda, M.J. Moghaddam and K. Sakurai, *United States Patent* No. 5,462,976, Oct 31, 1995.

[89] J.M.G. Reyes, S. Herretes, A. Pirouzmanesh, D. Wang, J.H. Elisseeff, A. Jun, P.J. McDonnell, R.S. Chuck and A. Behrens, *Invest. Ophthalmol. Vis. Sci. 46*, 1247 (2005).

[90] S. Cai, Y. Liu, X.Z. Shu and G.D. Prestwich, *Biomaterials 26*, 6054 (2005).

[91] J.S. Pieper, A. Oosterhof, P.J. Dijkstra and J.H. Veerkamp, *Biomaterials 20*, 847 (1999).

[92] A.J. Kuipers, G.H.M. Engbers, T.K.L. Meyvis, S.S.C. de Smedt, J. Demeester, J. Krijgsveld, S.A.J. Zaat, J. Dankert and J. Feijen, *Macromolecules 33*, 3705 (2000).

[93] W.F. Daamen, H.T.B. van Moerkerk, T. Hafmans, L. Buttafoco, A.A. Poot, J.H. Veerkamp and T.H. van Kuppevelt, *Biomaterials 24*, 4001 (2003).

[94] J.S. Pieper, P.B. van Wachem, M.J.A. van Luyn, L.A. Brouwer, T. Hafmans, J.H. Veerkamp, T.H. van Kuppevelt, *Biomaterials 21*, 1689 (2000).

[95] C.-H. Chang, H.-C. Liu, C.-C. Lin, C.-H. Chou and F.H. Lin, *Biomaterials 24*, 4853 (2003).

[96] C.-H. Chang, T.-F. Kuo, C.-C. Lin, C.-H. Chou, K.-H. Chen, F.-H. Lin and H.-C. Liu, *Biomaterials 27*, 1876 (2006).

[97] T.-W. Wang, J.-S. Sun, H.-C. Wu, Y.-H. Tsuang, W.-H. Wang and F.-H. Lin, *Biomaterials 27*, 5689 (2006).

[98] S.-H. Yang, P.-Q. Chen, Y.-F. Chen and F.-H. Lin, *Artif. Organs 29*, 806 (2005).

[99] W. Park, S. Park and K. Na, *Colloids Surf. B 79*, 501 (2010).

[100] F. Li and K. Na, *Biomacromolecules 12*, 1724 (2011).

[101] S.Y. Baek and K. Na, *J. Porphyrins Phthalocyanines 17*, 125 (2013).

[102] C.-T. Lee, C.-P. Huang and Y.-D. Lee, *Biomacromolecules 7*, 1179 (2006).

[103] C.-T. Lee, C.-P. Huang and Y.-D. Lee, *Biomacromolecules 7*, 2200 (2006).

[104] C.-T. Lee, C.-P. Huang and Y.-D. Lee, *Biomol. Eng. 24*, 131 (2007).

[105] P.A.S. Mourão, M.S. Pereira, M.G. Pavão, B. Mulloy, D.M. Tollefsen, M.-C. Mowinckel and U. Abildgaard, *J. Biol. Chem. 271*, 23973 (1996).

[106] P.A.S. Mourão, M.A.M. Guimarães, B. Mulloy, S. Thomas and E. Gray, *Br. J. Haematol. 101*, 647 (1998).

[107] N. Wu, X. Ye, X. Guo, N. Liao, X. Yin, Y. Hu, Y. Sun, D. Liu and S. Chen, *Carbohydr. Polym. 93*, 604 (2013).

[108] N. Gao, M. Wu, S. Liu, W. Lian, Z. Li and J. Zhao, *Mar. Drugs 10*, 1647 (2012).

In: Chondroitin Sulfate
Editor: Vitor H. Pomin

ISBN: 978-1-62808-490-0
© 2013 Nova Science Publishers, Inc.

Chapter 2

Novel Glycosaminoglycan Glycotechnology: Efficient Synthesis and Elongation Procedure of Chondroitin Sulfate Oligosaccharides

Masanori Yamaguchi[1]* and Masahiko Endo[2]
[1]Department of Organic Chemistry, Faculty of Education,
Wakayama University, Wakayama, Japan
[2]Department of Glycobiochemistry, Hirosaki University Graduate School of Medicine,
Hirosaki, Japan

Abstract

The constructions of chondroitin sulfate oligosaccharides using the chemoenzymatic procedures were investigated. Enzymatically prepared alkyne-containing chondroitin sulfate repeating disaccharide and ligated to the azide polyethylene glycol by click chemistry. Then, utilizing the pegylated disaccharide as an acceptor for the transglycosylation reaction of bovine testicular hyaluronidase, chondroitin sulfate oligosaccharides were successfully constructed on the polyethylene glycol. These synthesized chondroitin sulfate oligosaccharides will be clarify novel biological activities, and various medicinal treatment applications can be expected. We believe the present method will contribute to the development glycosaminoglycan glycobiology and technology.

Abbreviations

BTH, bovine testicular hyaluronidase;
ChS, chondroitin sulfate;

---

* E-mail address: masayama@center.wakayama-u.ac.jp,

ESI-MS, electrospray ionization mass spectrometry;
GAG, glycosaminoglycan;
GalNAc, N-acetylgalactosamine;
GlcA, glucuronic acid;
HPLC, high-performance liquid chromatography;
PEG, polyethylene glycol;
RP, reverse phase;
SEC, size exclusion chromatography;
TFA, trifluoroacetic acid.

Introduction

Chondroitin sulfate (ChS) is a glycosaminoglycan (GAG) having repeating disaccharide units [GlcAβ(1-3)GalNAc 4-O-sulfate or 6-O-sulfate]. It exists in tissues of many mammalian species and is widely distributed in the cell surface and extracellular matrix. It exists abundantly, especially in the cartilage of the joint and relates to the support of the structure. It is one of the most negatively charged elements in the organism because the sulfate and carboxyl group are contained.

ChS is highly variable because the position and degree of sulfation differ on the same chain. Furthermore, ChS has various important biological roles in cell migration, recognition, and morphogenesis [1]. ChS has many types of structural domains that are known to participate in specific physiological functions. Recently, greater attention has been directed towards the functions of ChS in the brain, optic nerves and chondrocytes [2, 3]. However the structure details that relate bioactivities have not been completely clarified. If these detailed bioactive sites (i.e., the composition of oligosaccharides) are clarified, the medical treatment applications of the ChS become possible more efficiently.

The elucidated bioactive sites of GAG tend to consist of below ten saccharides, [4, 5, 6, 7] and require the glycotechnology which can synthesize these scale oligosaccharides. There are several methods to obtain GAG oligosaccharides artificially.

First, in the chemical synthesis, many synthetic steps are needed to synthesize the repeating disaccharide unit (e.g., GlcAβ(1-3)GalNAc 4-O-sulfate) [8].

Second, the enzymatic synthesis utilizing glycosyltransferase is a possible efficient procedure if the glycosyltransferase and sugar nucleotides are well supplied [9]. In the present technique, however, it is difficult to supply them for synthetic requirements. Compared with these methods, utilizing the glycosidase (bovine testicular hyaluronidase: BTH), which catalyzes transglycosylation reaction as a reverse reaction of hydrolysis, was one of the effective synthetic methods [10]. Hyaluronidase, its glycosyl donor GAG (i.e., hyaluronic acid, ChS and dermatan sulfate) and its glycosyl acceptor pyridylaminated oligosaccharide can be supplied easily. In addition, the method can produce various GAG oligosaccharides by changing its glycosyl donors [11].

In this chapter, we describe enzymatic preparation of alkyne-containing ChS-disaccharide utilizing the transglycosylation activity of BTH and chemically ligated it with polyethylele glycol (PEG). Furthermore, we demonstrate the construction of the ChS oligosaccharide by using the pegylated disaccharide as an acceptor for the transglycosylation reaction.

Results and Discussion

Synthetic Strategy

We have tried to introduce the ChS-disaccharide into PEG. It is advantageous to use PEG as a core material, because its safety for medical treatment has been confirmed. Furthermore, pegylated ChS oligosaccharides are indicating a resistance of degradation and can extend the biological half-life of ChS oligosaccharides [12].

However, in our previous research, PEG was not a suitable acceptor for the transglycosylation reaction utilizing BTH (Unpublished data). Though to solve these problems, we have utilized a chemical ligation reaction (Scheme 1).

In order to do this, we employed two key compounds, alkyne-containing ChS-disaccharide and azido group-containing PEG. The alkyne-containing ChS-disaccharide prepared using propargyl alcohol as an acceptor for transglycosylation reaction. The azido group-containing PEG which was prepared by chemically introduced 4-azidobenzoic acid to PEG methyl ether [13]. The ligation reaction for ChS-disaccharide and PEG utilized click chemistry to afford the target pegylated ChS-disaccharide. The conditions of click chemistry afford superior regioselectivity, high tolerance of other functionalities, and almost quantitative transformation under mild conditions [13-18] (Scheme 1).

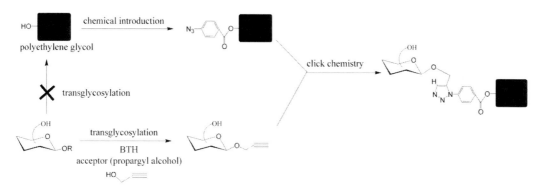

Scheme 1. Synthetic strategy of pegylated oligosaccharides.

Synthesis of alkyne-containing Disaccharide

The source of ChS was proteoglycan which drives from salmon nasal cartilage. The proteoglycan was exhaustive digested with actinase E and obtained chondroitin sulfate peptide **1** (ChS-peptide). The ChS-peptide **1** was enzymatically converted into alkyne-containing disaccharide **2** utilizing the transglycosylation reaction of BTH. Namely, we employed **1** as a source of disaccharide donor, propargyl alcohol as an acceptor for the reaction. The released disaccharide was translated to the propargyl alcohol which presence high density in the reaction buffer (Scheme 2). The resulting products were then subject to HPLC (polyamine II column) and then, desalted by the sephadex G-25 column and analyzed by ESI-MS spectrometry in the negative ion mode (Figure 1).

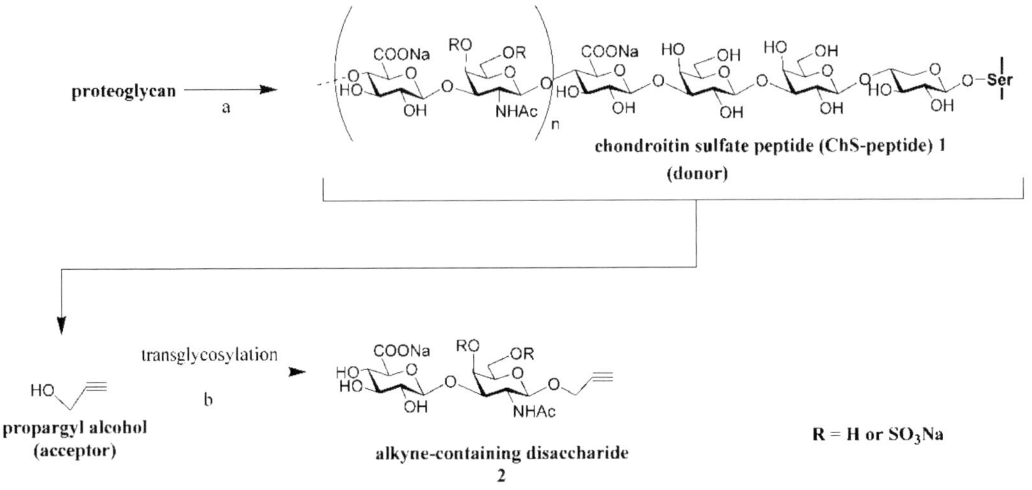

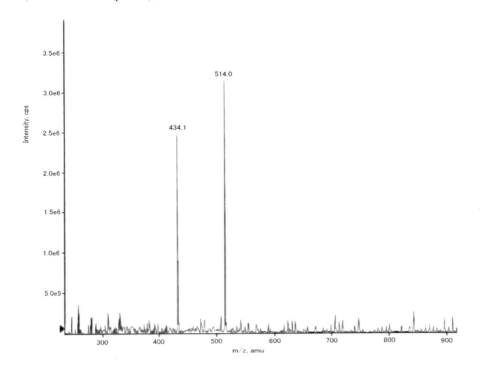

Scheme 2. Enzymatic preparation of alkyne-containing disaccharide **2**.
(a) actinase E, 0.1 M Tris-HCl buffer (pH 8.0) containing 10 mM $CaCl_2$, 40°C, 48 h., (b) BTH, 125 m M, Tris-HCl buffer (pH 7.0), 37°C, 24 h.

Figure 1. ESI-MS spectrum of alkyne-containing disaccharide **2**.

Synthesis of Pegylated Disaccharide

The click chemical reaction which ligates disaccharide **2** and PEG **3** was carried out under mild conditions (room temperature, 3 h) using 10 mM $CuSO_4$ with 10 mM sodium ascorbate as the in situ reducing agent to generate the Cu (I) species [16] (Scheme 3).

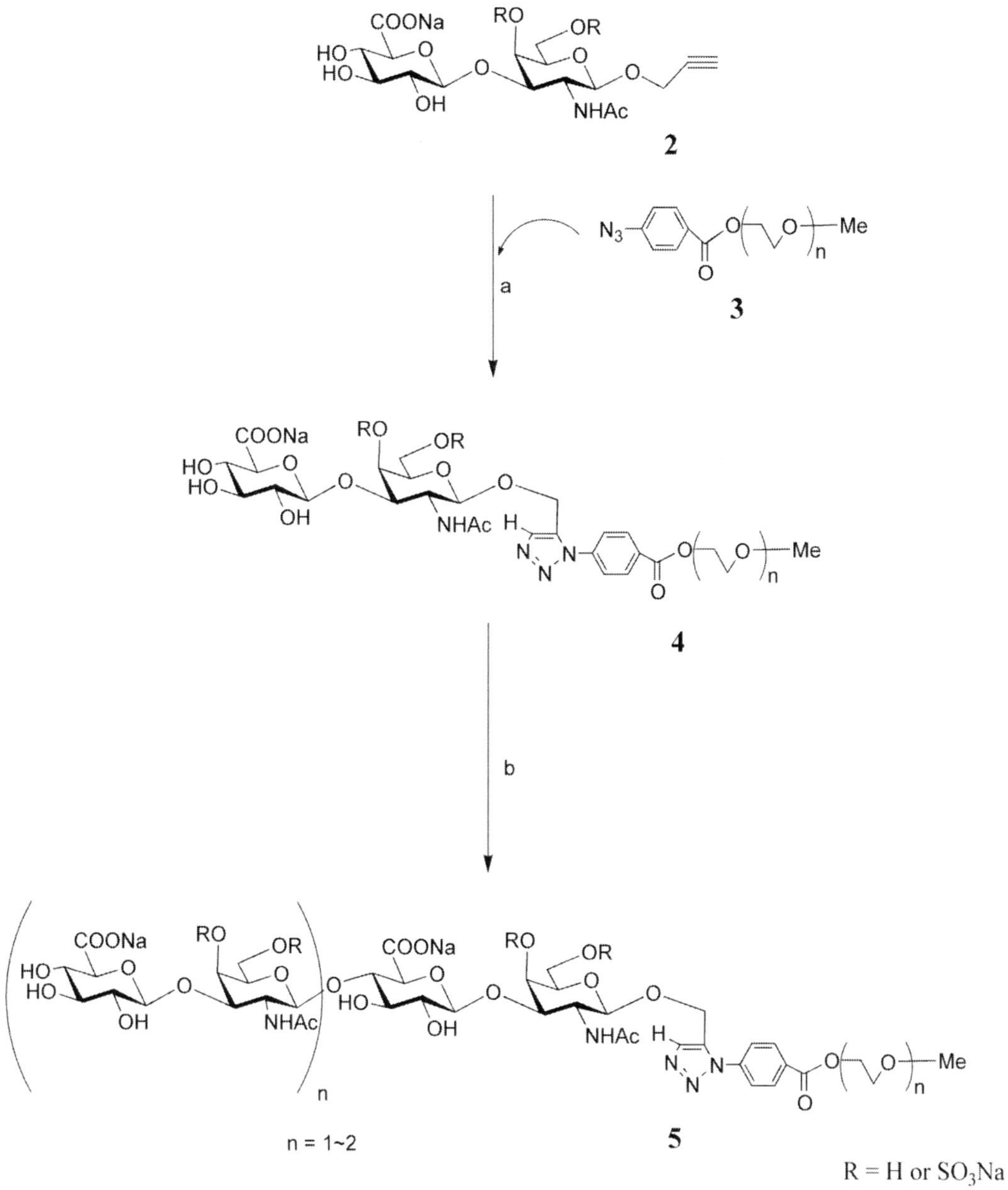

Scheme 3. Synthesis of pegylated ChS oligosaccharides.
(a) 10 mM CuSO$_4$, 10 mM sodium ascorbate, 37°C, 24 h, 95 %., (b) BTH, ChS-peptide **1**, 125 mM Tris-HCl buffer (pH 7.0), 37°C, 24 h.

The resulting product was subject to HPLC (TSK-gel ODS-100V; RP-column). The peak of PEG **3** disappeared completely and a new peak appeared at an early time, resulting from the disaccharide **2** bound to the PEG **3**. Judging from these results, the yield of peglated desaccharide **4** based on **3** was almost quantitative (Figure 2).

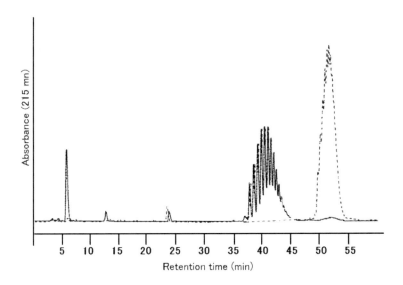

Figure 2. HPLC profiles of compound **3** and pegylated disaccharide **4**.
Compound **3** was shown dotted line and **4** was shown solid line.

Furthermore, in the MALDI-TOF-MS analysis, pegylated disaccharide peaks (the average molecular weight was m/z 1234.20) were observed (Figure 3).

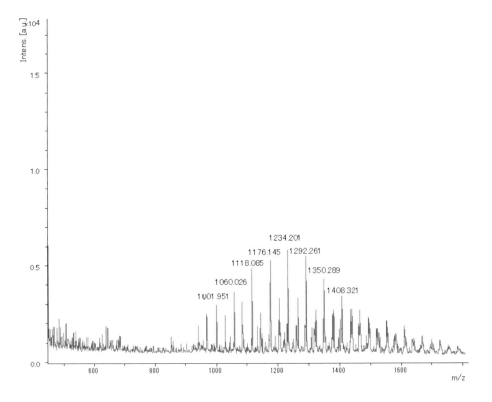

Figure 3. MALDI-TOF-MS spectrum of pegylated disaccharide **4**.

Enzymatic Elongation of Pegylated ChS Oligosaccharides

We employed the ChS-peptide **1** as a source of disaccharide donor, pegylated-disaccharide **4** as an acceptor for the reaction (Scheme 3). The resulting products were purified by C18-Sep-Pac cartridge column, and then subject to MALDI-TOF-MS analysis. The pegylated-tetrasaccharide and pegylated-hexasaccharide peaks were observed respectively (Figure 4). These results indicated that pegylated-disaccharide could be a suitable acceptor and then expand the GAG oligosaccharide synthesis utilizing the transglycosylation reaction of BTH.

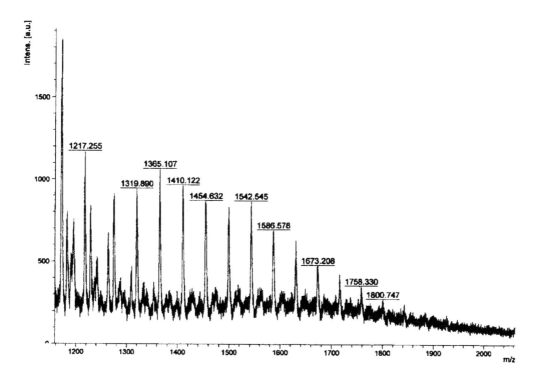

Figure 4. MALDI-TOF-MS spectrum of pegylated ChS oligosaccharides.

Conclusion

In our previous study, we utilized pyridylaminated GAG hexasaccharide as an only acceptor for the transglycosylation reaction of BTH and provided significant GAG oligosaccharides [10, 11, 19-22].

We have demonstrated for the first time that an alkyne-containing disaccharide can prepare a utilizing transglycosylation reaction of BTH. The disaccharide can be easily ligated with azido group-containing compounds, employing a click chemical reaction. In this chapter, the ligation of the disaccharide and PEG was verified.

Then, utilizing the pegylated disaccharide as an acceptor for the transglycosylation reaction of BTH, we have enabled the elongation reaction of ChS oligosaccharides on the PEG. The elongation of ChS oligosaccharides provided the nontoxic negative charge part into the PEG. These polymers must be good candidate for the pharmaceutical applications such as drug delivery system [23].

Furthermore, the synthesized alkyne-containing ChS disaccharide can be used for the study of cluster glycoside effect [24]. For example, azido group-containing dendrimer can be suitable core structure for the disaccharide. Each material can be easily ligated between azides and alkynes, and construct the carbohydrate decorated dendrimers.

In addition, in the case of using only the oligosaccharides, the PEG part could easily loose from the oligosaccharides under alkaline conditions.

The present method makes it possible to create further diverse GAG oligosaccharides and expands both the application of glycoengineering and the study of glycosaminoglycans.

Experimental Section

General Methods

Proteoglycan was purchased from Glycosmo Int. Co. (Aomori, Japan). Actinase E was purchased from Kaken Pharmaceutical Co. (Tokyo, Japan). Bovine testicular hyaluronidase (Type 1-S) was purchased from Sigma-Aldrich (St. Louis, MO). Sephadex G-25 was purchased from GE Healthcare Bio-Sciences (Uppsala, Sweden). All other chemicals were obtained from commercial sources.

HPLC: A high-performance liquid chromatography (Hitachi L-6200, Hitachi Co., Tokyo, Japan) connected to a UV-detector (Hitachi L-4200, Hitachi Co.) was used.

Analysis of ChS-peptide 1 was carried out with a size filtration chromatography Shodex OH pack SB-804 HQ (300 x 8.0 mm, Showa Denko Co., Kawasaki, Japan), which was eluted with 0.2 M NaCl at a flow rate of 1 mL/min and column temperature of 40°C. The eluates were monitored by UV absorbance at 215 nm.

Analysis of disaccharides 2 was carried out with a Polyamine II column (4.6 x 250 mm; YMC Co., Tokyo, Japan). The eluates were monitored by UV absorbance at 215 nm. The elution conditions were as follows. Eluent A, 16 mM NaH_2PO_4 and eluent B, 1 M NaH_2PO_4. The column was equilibrated with eluent A, and the ratio of eluent B to eluent A was increased linearly to 100 % over a 90-min period at a flow rate of 1.0 mL/min at 40°C.

Analyses of 3 and 4 were carried out using reverse-phase chromatography ODS 100V (4.6 x 150 mm; TOSOH Co., Tokyo, Japan). The eluates were monitored by UV absorbance at 215 nm. The elution conditions were as follows. Eluent A, H_2O containing 0.14 % TFA and eluent B, MeCN containing 0.14 % TFA. The column was equilibrated with eluent A, and the ratio of eluent B to eluent A was increased linearly to 55 % over a 60-min period at a flow rate of 1.0 mL/min at 40°C.

A mass spectrum of alkyne-containing disaccharide 2 was obtained on an API-III triple-quadrupole mass spectrometer (Sciex, Thornhill, Ontario, Canada). The samples were dissolved in 0.1 % formic acid containing acetonitrile (50 : 50) and injected at 3 µL/min with a micro-HPLC syringe pump.

MALDI-TOF mas spectra of pegylated saccharides 4 and 5 were recorded on a BRUKER Daltonics Autoflex III MDLDI-TOF Mass spectrometer instrument using a 2,5-dihydroxybenzoic acid matrix.

Preparation of ChS-peptide 1

ChS-peptide **1** was prepared from proteoglycan (100 mg) derived from salmon nasal cartilage. The procedure was as follows: the proteoglycan was digested with actinase E (10 mg) in 100 mM Tris-HCl buffer (pH 8.0) containing 10 mM $CaCl_2$ at 40°C in a total volume of 4 mL. The reaction mixture was incubated for 48 h at 40°C, and the reaction was terminated by immersion in a boiling water bath for 3 min. After centrifugation, the resulting supernatants were passed through a C18-Sep-Pack cartridge column to remove soluble hydrophobic components. The resulting eluate was cooled to 0°C, and 4 volumes of NaCl-saturated ethanol (16 mL) were added. The resulting precipitate was ChS-peptide **1** (54 mg).

SEC-HPLC: t_R = 9.36 min. The average molecular weight of **1** was estimated to be approximately 25,000 using the calibration curve derived from chondroitin sulfate chain standards of known molecular weight.

Preparation of Alkyne-containing Disaccharide 2

ChS-peptide **1**, (20 µL; 10 wt. % H_2O solution) as a donor and propargyl alcohol (50 µL) as an acceptor, and 1.0 NFU of BTH dissolved in 50 µL of 125 mM Tris-HCl buffer (pH 7.0) were incubated at 37°C for 24 h. After lyophilization to remove the excess acceptor, and then the residue was dissolved in H_2O (100 µL), the solution was passed through a C18-Sep-Pac cartridge and eluted with H_2O (2 mL) to remove the hydrophobic components resulting from the enzyme reaction, followed by lyophilization.

The residue was again dissolved in 30 µL of deionized water, and the solution was subjected to HPLC (Polyamine II column). Then, the fraction corresponding to **2** was desalted by Sephadex G-25 column chromatography (4 x 120 cm) with an eluent of H_2O : ethanol = 9 : 1 to give compound **2**.

HPLC (Polyamine II column): t_R = 21.44 min.
ESI-MS calcd. for $C_{17}H_{25}NO_{15}S$ [M- H]⁻ 514.09, found 514.0 [M- H]⁻, 434.1 [M-SO_3H]⁻.

Preparation of Pegylated Disaccharide 4

To a solution of **2** (1.5 mg, 2.91µmol) in H_2O (50 µL) were added **3** (1.62 mg, 2.33µmol) in DMSO (10 µL), $CuSO_4$ (15 µL; 10 mM) andsodium ascorbate (15 µL; 10 mM). The reaction mixture was vortexed and allowed to react at 40°C for 24 h under a N_2 atmosphere. Column chromatography (H_2O : EtOH = 9 : 1) of the residue on Sephadex G-25 gave the crude target molecule, and this was purified using a C18-Sep-Pac cartridge (MeOH : H_2O = 0 : 100 to 50 : 50) to afford **4** (2.68 mg, 95 %, based on N_3-PEG **3**).

HPLC (ODS 100V): t_R = 49.62-54.82 min. (Figure 2, dotted line).
MALDI-TOF-Mass analysis: m/z 1234 (average molecular weight).

Preparation of Pegylated ChS Oligosaccharides 5

The ChS-peptide **1**, (20 μL; 10 wt. % H_2O solution) as a donor, **4** (1 mg) as an acceptor, and 1.0 NFU of BTH dissolved in 50 μL of 125 mM Tris-HCl buffer (pH 7.0) were incubated at 37°C for 24 h. The reaction was terminated by immersion in a boiling water bath for 3 min and then filtrated. The filtrate was passed through C18-Sep-Pac cartridge (MeOH : H_2O = 0 : 100 to 50 :50) to afford **5**.

MALDI-TOF-Mass analysis: m/z 1500-1900 (synthesized pegylated tetrasaccharide and hexasaccharide peaks were observed in this mas range) (Figure 4).

Acknowledgments

We dedicate this chaptor to the late Prof. Keiichi Takagaki. We thank Mr. Naohiro Hyashi, Otsuka Chemical Co., Ltd., for the MALDI-TOF mass analysis.

This work was supported by Japan Society for the Promotion of Science (Gant-in-Aid for Young Scientists (B) No. 21710230) and Scientific Research (C) No. 24510297).

References

[1]   Sugahara, K. Mikami, T. Uyama, T. Mizuguchi, S. Nomura, K. and Kitagawa, H. (2003). Recent advances in the structural biology of chondroitin sulfate and dermatan sulfate. *Curr. Opin. Struct. Biol.,* 13, 612-620.

[2]   Iida, J. Pei, D. Kang, T. Simpson, M. A. Herlyn, M. Furcht, L. T. and McCarthy, J. B. (2001). Melanoma Chondroitin Sulfate Proteoglycan Regulates Matrix Metalloproteinase-dependent Human Melanoma Invasion into Type I Collagen. *J. Biol. Chem.,* 276, 18786-18794.

[3]   Maeda, N. He, J. Yajima, Y. Mikami, T. Sugahara, K. and Yabe, T. (2003). Heterogeneity of the Chondroitin Sulfate Portion of Phosphacan/6B4 Proteoglycan Regulates Its Binding Affinity for Pleiotrophin/Heparin Binding Growth-associated Molecule. *J. Biol. Chem.,* 278, 35805-35811.

[4]   Lyon, M. Deakin, A. J. Rahmoune, H. Fernig, G. D. Nakamura, T. and Gallagher, T. J. (1998). Hepatocyte Growth Factor/Scatter Factor Binds with High Affinity to Dermatan Sulfate. *J. Biol. Chem.,* 273, 271-278.

[5]   Kreuger, J. Salmivirta, M. Sturiale, L. Gallego, G. G. and Lindahl, U. (2001). Sequence Analysis of Heparan Sulfate Epitopes with Graded Affinities for Fibroblast Growth Factors 1 and 2. *J. Biol. Chem.,* 276, 30744-30752.

[6]   Taylor, R. K. Rudisill, A. J. and Gallo, L. R. (2005). Structural and Sequence Motifs in Dermatan Sulfate for Promoting Fibroblast Growth Factor-2 (FGF-2) and FGF-7 Activity. *J. Biol. Chem.,* 280, 5300-5306.

[7]   Bao, X. Muramatsu, T. and Sugahara, K. (2005). Demonstration of the Pleiotrophin-binding Oligosaccharide Sequences Isolated from Chondroitin Sulfate/Dermatan Sulfate Hybrid Chains of Embryonic Pig Brains. *J. Biol. Chem.,* 280, 35318-35328.

[8]   Jacquinet, J. C. Rochepeau-Jobron, L. and Combal, J. P. (1998). Multigram syntheses of the disaccharide repeating units of chondroitin 4- and 6-sulfates. *Carbohydr. Res.*, 314, 283-288.

[9]   Luca, D. C. Lansing, M. Martini, I. Crescenzi, F. Shen, G. J. O'Regan, M. and Wong, C. H. (1995). Enzymic Synthesis of Hyaluronic Acid with Regeneration of Sugar Nucleotides. *J. Am. Chem. Soc.*, 117, 5869–5870.

[10]   Saitoh, H. Takagaki, K. Majima, M. Nakamura, T. Matsuki, A. Kasai, M. Narita, H. and Endo, M. (1995). Enzymic reconstruction of glycosaminoglycan oligosaccharide chains using the transglycosylation reaction of bovine testicular hyaluronidase. *J. Biol. Chem.*, 270, 3741-3747.

[11]   Takagaki, K. Munakata, H. Majima, M. and Endo, M. (1999). Enzymatic reconstruction of a hybrid glycosaminoglycan containing 6-sulfated, 4-sulfated and unsulfated *N*-acetylgalactosamine. *Biochem. Biophys. Res. Commun.*, 258, 741-744.

[12]   Yamaguchi, M. New Horizon of Glycosaminoglycan Glycotechnology. Berhardt, L. V. (Eds.), ADVAVCES in MEDICINE and BIOLOGY (52). New York: Nova Science Publishers, Inc.; 2012; pp271-288.

[13]   Yamaguchi, M. Kojima, K. Hayashi, N. Kakizaki, I. Kon, A. and Takagaki, K. (2006). Efficient and widely applicable method of constructing neo-proteoglycan utilizing copper (I) catalyzed 1,3-dipolar cycloaddition. *Tetrahedron. Lett.*, 47, 7455-7458.

[14]   Kolb, C. H. and Sharpless, K. B. (2003). The growing impact of click chemistry on drug discovery. *D.D.T.*, 8, 1128-1137.

[15]   Lewis, W. G. Green, G. Grynszpan, F. Radic, Z. Carlier, P. R. Taylor, P. Finn, M. G. and Sharpless, K. B. (2002). Click Chemistry In Situ: Acetylcholinesterase as a Reaction Vessel for the Selective Assembly of a Femtomolar Inhibitor from an Array of Building Blocks. *Angew. Chem. Int. Ed.*, 41, 1053-1057.

[16]   Rostovtsev, V.V. Green, G. L. Fokin, V.V. and Sharpless, K. B. (2002). A Stepwise Huisgen Cycloaddition Process: Copper(I)-Catalyzed Regioselective "Ligation" of Azides and Terminal Alkynes. *Angew. Chem. Int. Ed.*, 41, 2596-2599.

[17]   Torn□e, C.W. Christensen, C. and Meldal, M. (2002). Peptidotriazoles on Solid Phase: [1,2,3]-Triazoles by Regiospecific Copper(I)-Catalyzed 1,3-Dipolar Cycloadditions of Terminal Alkynes to Azides. *J. Org. Chem.*, 67, 3057-3064.

[18]   Yamaguchi, M. Takagaki, K. Kojima, K. Hayashi, N. Chen, F. Kakizaki, I. Kon, A. and Endo, M. (2010). Novel proteoglycan glycotechnology: chemoenzymatic synthesis of chondroitin sulfate-containing molecules and its application. *Glycoconj. J.*, 27, 189-198.

[19]   Hase, S. Ikenaka, T. and Matsushima, Y. (1981). A highly sensitive method for analyses of sugar moieties of glycoproteins by fluorescence labeling. *J. Biochem.*, 90, 407-414.

[20]   Takagaki, K. Nakamura, T. Izumi, J. Saitoh, H. and Endo, M. (1994). Characterization of hydrolysis and transglycosylation by testicular hyaluronidase using ion-spray mass spectrometry. *Biochemistry.*, 33, 6505-6507.

[21]   Takagaki, K. Munakata, H. Kakizaki, I. Majima, M. and Endo, M. (2000). Enzymatic reconstruction of dermatan sulfate. *Biochem. Biophys. Res. Commun.*, 270, 588-593.

[22]   Yamaguchi, M. Kakizaki, I. and Endo, M. (2010). Novel glycosaminoglycan glycotechnology: Method for hybrid synthesis of glycosaminoglycan chains. *J. Carbohydr. Chem.*, 29, 315-331.

[23] Veronese, F. M. and Pasut, G. (2005). PEGylation, successful approach to drug delivery. *Drug Discovery Today.,* 10, 1451–1458.

[24] Mammen, M. Choi, Seok-Ki. and Whitesides, G. M. (1998). Polyvalent Interactions in Biological Systems: Implications for Design and Use of Multivalent Ligands and Inhibitors. *Angew. Chem. Int. Ed.,* 37, 2754-2794.

In: Chondroitin Sulfate
Editor: Vitor H. Pomin

ISBN: 978-1-62808-490-0
© 2013 Nova Science Publishers, Inc.

Chapter 3

Manufacturing Chondroitin Sulfate: From Animal Source Extraction to Biotechnological Production

Odile Francesca Restaino, Mario De Rosa,
Donatella Cimini and Chiara Schiraldi
Dept. of Experimental Medicine, Second University of Naples, Naples, Italy

Abstract

The world industrial production of chondroitin sulphate (CS) uses animal tissue sources as raw materials: CS is extracted with long and complex procedures that start with the recovery of CS from the cartilaginous tissues and continue with numerous steps of purifications for the complete removal of all the contaminants. Shark fins, bovine and chicken trachea or porcine muzzles are actually the most commonly used sources; but, according to the different origins, CS structure could vary in terms of molecular weight, type and grade of sulfation. Two different biotechnological approaches have been investigated so far to replace the traditional way of CS production. In the first case CS is obtained enzymatically by *in vitro* chain elongation using UDP-sugar precursors and biotechnologically produced synthase enzymes. In the other case CS is produced by using a biotechnological-chemical strategy consisting of three main steps: fermentative production of a chondroitin-like polysaccharide by capsulated bacteria, purification from the fermentation broth and then site specific chain sulfation. The extractive and the biotechnological process approaches resulted completely different from a productive point of view: in the "top-down-like" extractive process CS chains of specific sulfation patterns and chain lengths, according to the tissue of origin, are obtained after diverse steps of purification; in the "bottom-up-like" biotechnological approaches the processes could be designed to obtain structural tailored cut molecules. In this chapter the whole productive schemes are described, underlining the different nature of the starting materials and comparing the diverse structural transformations occurring during both the extractive and biotechnological processes up to obtain CS as a final product.

Introduction

Chondroitin sulfate (CS) is a negatively charged complex polysaccharide belonging to the class of the glycosaminoglycans (GAG), found in nature as one of the main constituent of the extracellular matrix of the animal tissues. CS is made of repeating disaccharide units of β(1→4) D-glucuronic acid (GlcA) β(1→3) N-acetyl-D-galactosamine (GalNAc). The disaccharides could be variously sulfated in different positions of the chain. Mono-sulfation can occur in 4 or 6 position of GalNAc (in this case the disaccharide are classified as CS-A and CS-C type, respectively); di-sulfation, instead, can take place in both 4 and 6 positions of the amino sugar (CS-E), or in only one of these positions and in position 2 of GlcA (2,4-sulfation in case of CS-B and 2,6-sulfation in case of CS-D) (Figure 1) [1, 2]. Non-sulfated disaccharides (CS-O) could also be present along the chain although they usually occurred in small percentages (lower than 8%) [3]. (Figure 1, Table 1). Type and grade of sulfation could vary within a single CS molecule, producing assorted structural motifs in the same polysaccharide. The relative percentages of the different disaccharide patterns along the chain and the prevalence of a specific motif is dependent on the species of origin, as well as on organ and tissue type, as revealed by structural analyses [1-5]. High contents of CS-A disaccharides were found, for example, in bovine cartilages while in shark ones the chain showed mainly 6-sulfated units (CS-C) [3-5] (Table 1). Animal derived CS shows also different molecular weight values in a range from 14 to 70 KDa, as determined by high performance size-exclusion chromatography [3, 5] (Table 1). The sulfation pattern variability and the different lengths of the polysaccharide chains determined also a wide structural heterogeneity in terms of both charge density and molecular weight distributions (Table 1), that influences the CS biological functions too. In the connective tissues CS is one of the main components of the extra cellular matrix present as proteoglycan (PG), bounded to a serine residue of a proteic core through a trisaccharide linking region made of two galactose units and a xylose one. Together with this structural role, CS, similarly to other GAGs, has also fundamental functions in physiological and pathological processes like cell growth and development, angiogenesis and cancer, acting as a binder of a wide variety of proteins, signalling molecules and ligands present in the extra cellular environment [2, 6]. It has demonstrated to bind the fibronectin [7] as well as the $\alpha_4\beta_1$ integrines of melanoma cells [8] and to act as a regulator of neuronal patterning in the retina [9]. CS-A and CS-B showed differential effects on monocyte and B-cell activation [10], CS-D oligosaccharides of shark cartilage origin demonstrated to have a neurite outgrowth promoting activity [11], while the CS-E disaccharide unit has been considered important for plasminogen activation [12]. The CS structural composition variety gives also rise to diverse pharmacological activities and different possibilities of applications [13]. CS type E has effect as anti-viral agent [14], chains containing different ratios of A and C or of A and E disaccharides are employed in tissue wound-healing processes [15] and as anti-malaria vaccines [16], respectively; while CS having A, C and E sulfation pattern types could help in the repair of central nervous system [17]. CS having A and C sulfation patterns and molecular weight in the range from 13 to 30 KDa is mainly commercialised as the active principle of anti-arthritis and anti-osteoarthritis drugs, used for the treatment of articular and joint pains [18-22], thanks to its good anti-inflammatory activity, that resulted comparable to the non steroidal anti-inflammatory drug one [23]. It acts also as symptomatic slow acting molecule [3, 24].

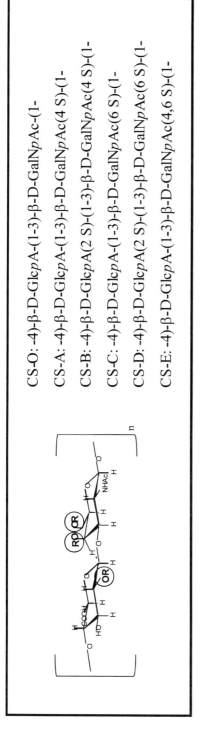

Figure 1. Disaccharide unit structures in CS chains.

CS-O: -4)-β-D-Glc*p*A-(1-3)-β-D-GalN*p*Ac-(1-

CS-A: -4)-β-D-Glc*p*A-(1-3)-β-D-GalN*p*Ac(4 S)-(1-

CS-B: -4)-β-D-Glc*p*A(2 S)-(1-3)-β-D-GalN*p*Ac(4 S)-(1-

CS-C: -4)-β-D-Glc*p*A-(1-3)-β-D-GalN*p*Ac(6 S)-(1-

CS-D: -4)-β-D-Glc*p*A(2 S)-(1-3)-β-D-GalN*p*Ac(6 S)-(1-

CS-E: -4)-β-D-Glc*p*A-(1-3)-β-D-GalN*p*Ac(4,6 S)-(1-

Table 1. Structural differences of CS of different origins

Origin	Structure and sulfation patterns	Mw (KDa)	Mn (KDa)	Polydispersity	Charge density
Bovine	6% CS-O, 61% CS-A, 33% CS-C	20-26	12-17	1.8-2.2	0.90-0.96
Porcine	6% CS-O, 80% CS-A, 14% CS-C	14-20	9-14	1.4-1.8	0.92-0.96
Chicken	8% CS-O, 72% CS-A, 20% CS-C	16-21	8-13	1.6-2.0	0.90-0.94
Shark	3% CS-O, 32% CS-A, 44% CS-C, 18% CS-D, 2% CS-E, 1% CS-B	30-70	25-40	1.0-2.0	0.45-0.90

Table 2. Some of the CS products sold on the market

Company	Product	Active Ingredient	Formulation	Application	Reference
BIOIBERICA	Condrosan®	Chondroitin sulfate	Hard Capsules [400 mg of CS]	Basic treatment of osteoarthritis, chondroprotective drug of slow action.	www.bioiberica.com
	Droglican®	Chondroitin sulfate and Glucosamine hydrocloride	Hard Capsules [200 mg of CS; 250 mg of GlcN·HCl]	Synthomatic treatment of osteoarthritis.	
	Condrovet®	Chondroitin sulfate	Tablets [500 mg of CS; 18 mg of Vitamin E; 30 mg of Manganese Sulfate]	Chondroprotective drug for dogs and cats with joint injuries and degenerative processes of the articular cartilage.	
FIDIA	CartiJoint®	Chondroitin sulfate and Glucosamine hydrocloride	Capsules	Supplement useful for joint diseases.	www.cartijoint.it
IBSA	Condrosulf®	Chondroitin sulfate sodium salt	Capsules [400 mg of CS]	In the treatment of osteoarthritis, this drug works as slow acting cartilage structure modifying agent.	www.ibsa-international.com
	Ialuril®	Hyaluronic acid and Chondroitin sulfate	Sterile solution [50 ml containing 800 mg of HA and 1 g of CS]	It is able to significantly reduce the production of pro-inflammatory cytokines and allow correct repair of the protective layer of the urothelial coating.	
SIGMA-TAU	AMEDIAL BF™	Chondroitin sulfate and Glucosamine hydrocloride	Powder [400 mg of CS; 500 mg of GlcN·HCl; 30 mg of hydrolised collagen and 350 mg of L-carnitine fumarate]	Dietary supplement.	www.sigma-tau.it

A "chondro-protective" effect has also been described: CS showed to induce cellular growth at bone and cartilage level and to slow down tissue degeneration by inhibiting degradative enzymes and promoting hyaluronic acid synthesis [25-28], thus being also defined as a structure modifying drug in osteoarthritis treatment [18]. CS resulted efficient if both intra-articular and orally administered [29]; as a matter of fact alone or in combination with glucosamine [30], CS is sold on the market as pills or capsules, as well as dietary supplement [31], and its oral administration resulted effective in the treatment of symptoms of osteo-arthritis, alleviating pain and improving the joint mobility in animals, like dogs [32] and horses [33], and in human beings [34]. When orally administered in dosages of 800-1200 mg/day, CS demonstrated to be highly tolerated and suitable for long treatment uses (3-6 months) [35, 36].

The actual market of the extractive CS, as raw material, is estimated to be around 600 metric tons, with a price ranging from 65 to 150 $ per kg, according to the purity grade. Table 2 shows some of the products containing CS that are nowadays sold on the market togheter with their applications.

The structure-function correlation has to be carefully taken in account when manufacturing GAGs; the pharmaceutical grade CS has to show specific composition as well as precise sulfation profiles and molecular weight according to the type of medical devices it has to be employed for. Thus manufacturing CS for drugs means mainly producing a pharmaceutical active molecule of defined structural characteristic and biological activity in a safe and economic way.

In this chapter different approaches to produce chondroitin sulfate (the extractive and the biotechnological ones) are described. The traditional extractive procedure is the one used nowadays for the current production of the CS sold on the market; the biotechnological approaches, instead, comprise different innovative procedures whose industrialisation is still in progress.

Chondroitin Sulfate Production by Extractive Processes

The commercial CS, employed as an orally administered anti-osteoarthtritis drug, is mainly produced by extraction and purification from animal cartilaginous tissues of shark fins, of bovine and chicken trachea or of pig muzzles [13]; but numerous other different species, like whales, salmons and zebra fishes have also been used as CS sources [37-43]. The extractive CS manufacturing process could be described with a "top-down-like" scheme, in which the molecule of interest is selected, recovered and finely purified from a very complex starting raw material matrix (Figure 2).

The cartilages are, first of all, pre-treated and cleaned with warm water (45°C) [44], residues of non connective tissues are, in case it is necessary, mechanically removed and then a long sequence of organic solvent washes (with acetone or ethanol) is used to eliminate fatty acids and lipids [45-46]; at that point the cartilage tissues resulted dried and could be eventually grinded to be more suitable for the next step of extraction. CS is extracted from the cartilages by breaking of the linkage with the protein core: to perform this step different solutions and alternative procedures have been studied so far; all of them tried to reach the cost effective as well as the purification standard targets necessary to satisfy the market requests and thus to assure highly safe drug products. To perform the extraction and to break the bound with the protein core, dried and granulated cartilage tissues are subjected to alkaline hydrolysis (0.1-0.5 M NaOH for 15-17 hours) and/or extensive proteolysis enzymatic digestion (Figure 2); in case of the enzymatic digestion, various procedures that use non-specific protease or papaine, alcalase or trypsine have been set up so far, according to the diverse tissues that had to be digested [37, 42-44, 46-48]. The enzymatic hydrolysis is generally performed under stirring conditions, in neutral pH buffers, at temperature values ranging from 50 to 65 °C, carried on for 6 to 20 hours, and usually followed by a final heating step for enzyme inactivation [42, 44, 46-48] (Figure 2). High ability of tissue solubilization, efficient withdrawal capacity, good product recovery and the non alteration of the CS structures are some characteristics necessary for an appropriate extraction process. Residual non-hydrolysed cartilage tissue pieces are then generally removed from the extracted solution by centrifugation, precipitation or even activated charcoal addition [43, 44, 48]. The procedure is not selective because other glycosaminoglycans could be extracted and remained in solution as well as other contaminants, like proteins and salts. CS could be recovered and further cleaned by selective precipitation with quaternary ammonium salts or sequential precipitation steps with organic solvents (40-70%), like ethanol or acetone [38, 40, 43, 44]. Recently also the use of ultra-filtration and dia-filtration membrane procedures have been reported for this step of purification [37]. Selection and separation of CS from other glycosaminoglycan contaminants could also be reached by fractionation, using increasing concentrations of organic solvents [44]. The precipitated material is generally re-dissolved in buffer or salt solution and then finely purified by using ion-exchange or size exclusion chromatography, eventually used in series [49-50]. The purified CS is thus finally recovered as white powder by solvent precipitation, exsiccated and eventually grinded (Figure 2). The overall CS yield from tissue extraction could vary and a range values of 25-30% has to be considered pretty good [42], but the various purification steps allowed to reach a purity grade of around 99% [40-42].

The quality of the product obtained is one of the main issue of the extractive procedures; besides the final molecule has to satisfy precise structural characteristics in terms of disaccharide compositions, sulfation pattern and molecular weight. The extractive procedures have to handle many safety, ecological and economic problems: sources are difficult to find and, in some cases, not sufficient to satisfy the market requests; the procedures are very long and time-consuming, while the use of large volumes of organic solvents is not environmental-friendly. Because legislation constrains in numerous countries are recently limiting the possibility to employ any animal derived molecules for pharmaceutical applications, alternatives ways of producing CS by using biotechnological approaches have gained great attention in the last decade.

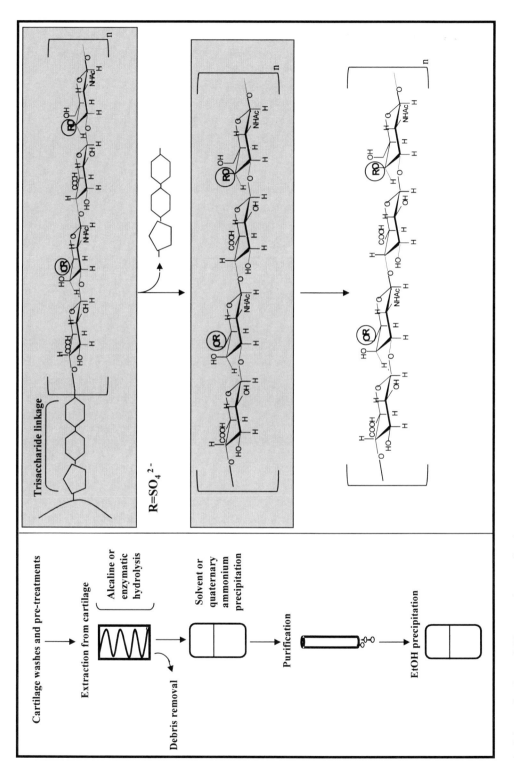

Figure 2. Schematic view of CS extractive production process.

Chondroitin Sulfate Production by Biotechnological Processes

Polysaccharides that are structurally similar to un-sulfated chondroitin are produced by both *Pasteurella multocida* type F and *Escherichia coli* O5:K4:H4 strains, as carbohydrate layers that surround their cell surfaces [51, 52]. The bacterial capsular polysaccharides (CPS), before being exported out-side the cells, are produced inside by specific synthase enzymes (polymerases) that act as glycosyl transferases and that elongate the chain by using UDP sugar precursors as building blocks [45]. From a biological point of view, these capsular polysaccharides (CPS) are used by bacteria as a protective barrier against environmental stressful conditions and as camouflages to avoid and elicit the host immune defence system [53]. But from a biotechnological point of view, these bacteria and/or their synthase enzymes constitute good microbial cell factories or potential enzymatic tools for the production of chondroitin-like polysaccharides. Two different approaches have been used so far for the biotechnological production of natural-like CS: *in vitro* biosynthesis and elongation of the CS-like chains by using purified or not purified bacterial synthase enzymes or CS structurally similar capsular polysaccharide production by using whole cells as producers in fermentation based strategies (Figure 3 and 4). In both cases the manufacturing strategy has a "bottom-up-like" formation scheme, starting the production of the CS chains directly from the building blocks (UDP-sugars) or from a structurally similar polysaccharide precursor. *Pasteurella multocida* type F synthase was used for the fist approach: the bacterial synthase enzyme was isolated, characterised, cloned and then used for *in vitro* production of chondroitin employing UDP-GlcA and UDP-GalNAc as precursors and a chondroitin-sulfated oligosaccharide as acceptor. (Figure 3) [51, 54]. The reaction occurred in Tris buffer at pH 7.2 and 30 °C. *Escherichia coli* K4 polymerase was employed, instead, in a similar way to obtain chondroitin exasaccharides [55].

In the second biotechnological approach, CS could be obtained directly by modification of the bacterial capsular polysaccharide chains, once produced by micro-organisms. In this case a possible biotechnological manufacturing scheme should include the capsular polysaccharide production by fermentation, the recovery and purification of the CPS and its final modification in order to have a sulfated natural-like chondroitin molecule (Figure 4). Following this scheme numerous results have been obtained by researchers in the last ten years, especially by using *E. coli* K4 as producer: this bacteria synthesizes a capsular polysaccharide (K4 CPS) whose disaccharide composition of the carbohydrate backbone is similar to the CS one, being made of D-glucuronic acid and N-acetyl-D-galactosamine β(1-3) and β(1-4) linked, as well; but the chain has also an extra side branching unit of fructose bound to the C-3 of the glucuronic residue (Figure 4). In this biotechnological manufacturing process the first step consists in the production of the capsular polysaccharide by fermentation; the main target that have to be reached in this phase is the optimisation of the culture conditions in order to have high cell density cultivations, high capsular polysaccharide production and high yield values, and thus good productivity standards (Table 3). The influence of physiological parameters, like pH and temperature, on the capsular polysaccharide production have been widely investigated as well as the influence of different types, concentrations and ratios of carbon and nitrogen sources in the media composition [56]; the studies demonstrated that the optimal conditions for growth (pH 7.5 and 37°C) resulted the best ones for CPS production too. Glucose or glycerol, tested as carbon sources in the media, resulted to be both able to sustain growth and the K4 CPS biosynthesis, although differences in terms of concentration of the produced polysaccharides were noted [56] (Table 3). Animal derived nitrogen sources, like casamino acids, were traditionally used to grow *E. coli* K4 strain [57], but new vegetable derived ones, like soya peptone, were recently preferred in the formulation of the medium for safety reasons in order to avoid any animal contaminations in a prospective of a possible industrial application [56]. Shake flask studies allowed to reach a K4 CPS concentration in the range of 100-120 mg/L on glycerol-based new formulated media [56], while a recent paper demonstrated that the supplementation in the medium, since the beginning of the growth, of the monosaccharides constituting the capsular polysaccharide resulted effective in further increase the K4 CPS production of 60% [58]. The development of strategies to increase the capsular polysaccharide production had included different solutions: from batch fermentations in 2 and 14 L scale reactors, that resulted in a 300 mg/L K4 CPS production [56, 57], to different types of fed-batch and microfiltration processes (Table 3). In the fed-batch ones, by supporting the growth with appropriate feeding profiles, a 5 fold increase of production was obtained, compared with the batch fermentation; in case of fermentations with microfiltration the feeding was associated with the removal from the medium of acetate, a growth inhibiting by-product of the metabolism, by using two appropriate microfiltration membranes inserted inside the vessel [59]. In this way high cell density cultivations were obtained and it was reached the maximum K4 CPS concentration, so far reported, by using the *E. coli* K4 wild type strain (4.7 g/L in 42-46 hours of fermentation) [59]. The creation of new over-producing mutant and recombinant strains of *E. coli* K4 has provided a further way to increase the K4 CPS production and it has opened the perspective to reach, in future, higher enhancements of capsular polysaccharide production by integration of the high cell density fermentation strategies and the use of molecular biology tools [60, 61] (Table 3). In an another case of molecular biology strategy, instead, *Pasteurella multocida* synthase was cloned and expressed in *Bacillus natto* bringing to a production of non-sulfated chondroitin of around 0.24 g/L in shake flasks [62] (Table 3). Because the K4 CPS is produced and then released in the medium, during the growth, as an extra-cellular product, the second step of the biotechnology process includes the recovery of the supernatant containing the capsular polysaccharide by centrifugation of the fermentation broth and with the removal of the bacteria biomass [63]. The supernatant contains the capsular polysaccharide but also numerous soluble proteins, amino-acids, nucleic acids, bacterial cell metabolic products and not utilised media components. But the main contaminant of the product resulted to be the lipopolysaccharide, the bacterial endotoxin produced by the bacteria during the growth and then released in the medium, as well as the K4 CPS [63]. Recovery of the polysaccharide from the supernatant was performed, in some cases, by taking advantage of the negative charge of the polysaccharide that was recuperated by a selective precipitation with cetylpyridinium chloride, a cationic quaternary ammonium compound. After that, the polysaccharide was re-suspended in NaCl solution and further purified by repeated precipitations with cold ethanol (4°C) that allowed the polysaccharide pureness to increase [52]. Membrane-based tangential flow systems (300-100 KDa), eventually associated with a protease digestion pre-treatments, were also used to purify, recover and concentrate the K4 CPS from the broth supernatant [57,63] (Figure 4). Applying a membrane based purification approach proteins and salts were easily removed [57, 63] and the recovery of the K4 CPS was around 74% [57]. A further improvement in the purification was reached integrating this protocol with a strategy that eliminated also the main contaminants, the lipopolysaccharides. As a matter of fact, because of their amphiphilic nature, the lipopolysaccharides are able to form, in presence of divalent cations, micelles of 300-1000 KDa or even vesicles of dimensions higher than 1000 KDa [64], which resulted in a difficult removal by ultrafiltration membranes. A mild acid hydrolysis reaction was used to chemically break the lipophilic portion of the endotoxin (lipid A); in this way the lipid A precipitates while the polysaccharide portion of the lipopolysaccharide remained in solution together with the K4 CPS and could be later removed by ultra-filtration, in an easier way [63]. Besides, in these chemical conditions the removal of the fructose residue of the K4 CPS chain also occurred, thus driving the process towards a polysaccharide chain whose carbohydrate backbone resulted similarly to the animal CS. A further final ultra filtration step (30-50 KDa) was then used to finally purify the solution from the polysaccharide part of the lipopolysaccharide and to concentrate the solution containing the K4 CPS; this purification scheme allowed to recover more than 80% of the initial K4 CPS concentration and to have a high purity grade (>90%). This downstream process was demonstrated to be also applicable to a 22 L scale, by using automated tangential flow purification systems [65]. For final recovery of the molecule cold ethanol precipitation has been extensively used [52, 57, 63] (Figure 4). Once purified, the chondroitin-like polysaccharide backbone has only to be modified by insertion of sulfate groups in specific chain positions (Figure 4). The bacterial cells, in fact, are not able to produce sulfated forms of the capsular polysaccharide chains and various chemical or enzymatic sulfation approaches have to be taken in account to integrate the fermentation production. Diverse chemical multi-reaction strategies, based on protection and de-protection of the carbohydrate chain, have been reported so far to specifically sulfate the microbial chondroitin-like chain [66, 67]. Bedini and co-workers reported the possibility to obtain chondroitin sulfate of microbial origin from K4 CPS; the structure of the molecule perfectly resembled, in terms of disaccharide composition and molecular weight, the commercial animal derived one [67]. (See also in this book *"Chemical and chemo-enzymatic manipulation of chondroitin sulfate polysaccharides"* by E. Bedini and M. Parrilli). The design of the CS biotechnological productive processes is nowadays still in progress and numerous problems have to be solved in order to obtain an identical CS homologue at reasonable prices and costs that could be competitive with the classical extractive procedure ones. One of the main issue of the biotechnological production is to drive the process to a final molecule that could be defined as natural-like, with similar composition of the animal derived CS, in terms of disaccharide composition, sulfation pattern and molecular weight. Structural identity is, actually, necessary to obtain similar pharmacological activity. But the biotechnological productive process could be designed properly in order to have structural tailored-cut molecules with specific chain lengths and sulfation patterns: the molecular weight of K4 CPS could be controlled, controlling the time and the conditions of the hydrolysis reaction during the purification process, while the sulfation patterns could be specifically designed by appropriate chemical reactions. New stricter regulatory constrains would push in future the pharmaceutical companies to shift the productive process towards biotechnological methods, but in order to be competitive with the CS extractive manufacturing procedure, the biotechnological processes should have comparable costs, should be reproducible and very easy to be performed. Thus the design of efficient, effective and highly productive fermentation protocols and/or the use of simple purification systems could be important factors to take into consideration in the scheming and the setting up of a productive process with industrial application potentials.

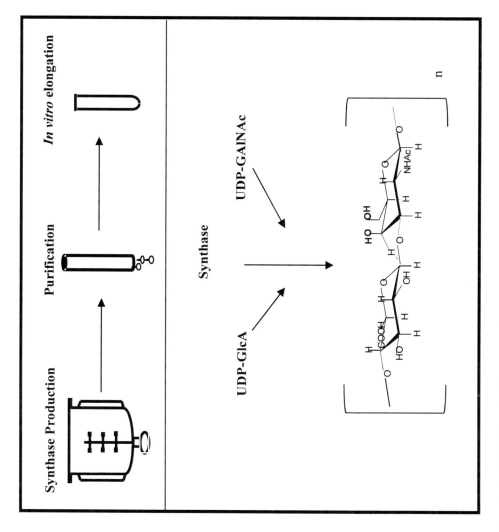

Figure 3. Schematic view of biotechnological CS production process based on in *vitro* elongation.

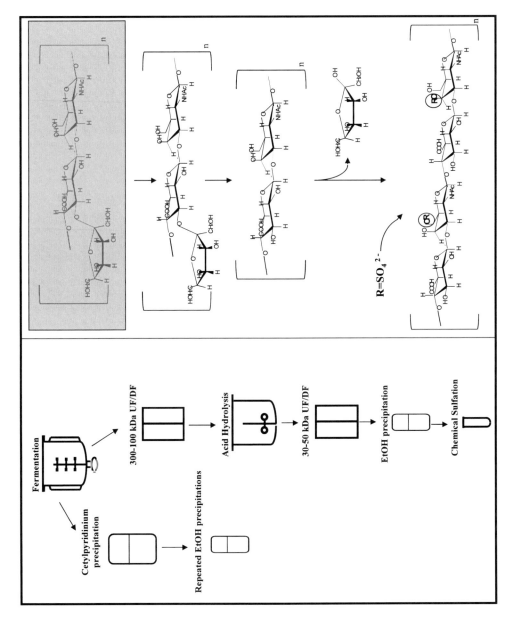

Figure 4. Schematic view of CS biotechnological production process based on fermentation technology.

Table 3. Biotechnological CS production process from bacterial capsular polysaccharides: fermentation step

Fermentation			E. coli O5:K4:H4	E. coli O5:K4:H4 VZ15	E. coli O5:K4:H4 BK4063	Bacillus natto
			K4 CPS	K4 CPS		Non-sulfated chondroitin
Shake flasks	0.1 L					0.24 g/L [62]
	0.2 L		0.047-0.180 g/L [56]			
Fermentor	Batch	2 L	0.20 g/L [56]	0.22 g/L [60]	0.25 g/L [61]	
		14 L	0.08 g/L [52] 0.20 g/L [57]		0.45 g/L [61]	
	Fed-batch	2 L	1.40 g/L [56]			
	Microfiltration	2 L	4.73 g/L [59]			
		22 L	3.0 g/L [65]			

Conclusion

Animal tissues of diverse origins and types are used as sources of CS of various sulfation patterns; according to the different structures, CS shows different biological activities and it has diverse fields of applications. The extractive procedures from animal tissue sources, that include several purifications steps, are nowadays commonly used to manufacture the CS as sold on the market. Time consuming protocols, difficulties in raising the animal raw materials and eco-unfriendly procedures are the main constrains of the CS extractive production that have pushed the researchers in the last few years to find new alternatives ways.

Two different biotechnological approaches have been investigated so far in order to obtain natural-like CS molecules: *in vitro* elongation of CS polysaccharide chain by using synthase enzymes and UDP-sugar precursors, or fermentation based strategies, that produce CS-like capsulare polysaccharide, followed by chemical sulfation steps. In both cases scale-up studies have still to be performed in order to demonstrate that these biotechnological processes are applicable to large industrial volumes, while economic analyses have to be carefully performed to investigate the possibility of their industrializations. But the biotechnological productions have numerous advantages compared to the extractive methods: raw materials are easier to find, the production is potentially unlimited, purification protocols are easily performed and CS molecules of determine structural characteristics could be obtained. Although further improvements in the biotechnological tools and sulfation strategies still have to be investigated, these first studies paved the way toward a real possibility of obtaining CS molecules of diverse and tailor-cut structures.

References

[1]   N. Volpi, *J. Pharmacy and Pharmacology*. 61, 1271-1280 (2009).
[2]   R. Raman, V. Sasisekharan and R. Sasisekharan., *Chemistry & Biology*. 12, 267-277 (2005).
[3]   N. Volpi, *Carbohydrate Polymers*. 55, 273-281 (2004).
[4]   N. Volpi, *J. Pharm. Sc.* 96(12), 3168-80 (2007).
[5]   E. P. Fuentes, V. B. Diaz, *Acta Farm. Bonaerense*. 17 (2), 135-142 (1998).
[6]   C. Malakawi, S. Mizumoto, N. Karamanos, K. Sugahara, *Connect. Tissue. Res.* 49, 199-139 (2008).
[7]   F. J. Barkalow, J. E. Schwarzbauer, *J. Biol. Chem.* 269, 3957-62 (1994).
[8]   J. Iida, M. L. Meijne, T. R. Jr Oegema, T. A. Yednock, N. L. Kovach et al., *J. Biol. Chem.* 273, 5955-62 (1998).
[9]   P. A. Brittis, D. R. Canning, J. Silver, *Science*. 255, 733-6 (1992).
[10]   J. Rachmilewitz, M. L. Tykocinski, *Blood*. 92, 223-9 (1998).
[11]   S. Nadanaka, A. Clement, K. Masayama, A. Faissner, K. Sugahara, *J. Biol. Chem.* 273, 3296-307 (1998).
[12]   T. Sakai, M. Kyogashima, Y. Kariya, T. Urano, Y. Takada, A. Takada, *Thromb. Res.* 100, 557-65 (2000).
[13]   C. Schiraldi, D. Cimini, M. De Rosa, *Appl. Microbiol. Biotechnol.* 87, 1209-1220 (2010).

[14] K. Bergefall, E. Trybala, M. Johansson, T. Uyama, S. Naito, S. Yamada, H. Kitagawa, K. Sugahara, T. Bergström, *J. Biol. Chem.* 283(37), 32193-32199 (2005).

[15] X. H. Zou, Y. K. Jiang, G. R. Zhang, H. M. Jin, T. M. Nguyen, H. W. Ouyang, *Acta Biomaterial.* 5(5), 1588-1595 (2008).

[16] A. Alkhalil, R. N. Achur, M. Valiyaveettil, C. F. Ockenhouse, D. C. Gowda, *J. Biol. Chem.* 277(11), 8882-8889 (2000).

[17] P. E. Fraser, A. A. Darabie, J. A. Mc Laurin, *J. Biol. Chem.* 273(9), 6412-6419 (2001).

[18] F. Ronca, L. Palmieri, P. Panicucci and G. Ronca, *Osteoarthritis Cartilage.* 6, 14-21 (1998).

[19] B. A. Michel, P. Brühlmann, G. Stucki and D. Uebelhart, *IBSA satellite symposium-European congress of rheumatology (EULAR)*, (2002).

[20] G. Rovetta, *Drugs Exptl. Clin. Res.* VII, 53-71 (1991).

[21] A. Fioravanti, A. Franci, A. Anselmi, L. Fattorini, R. Marcolongo, *Drugs Exptl. Clin. Res.* VII, 41-4 (1991).

[22] B. Leeb, H. Schweizer, K. Montan, J. Smolen, *J. Rheumatol*, 27: 205-211 (2000).

[23] B. A. Michel, G. Stucki, D. Frey, F. De Vathaire et al., *Arthritis Rheum.* 52, 779-86 (2005).

[24] P. Morreale, R. Manopulo, M. Galati, L. Boccanera, G. Saponati, L. Bocchi, *J. Rheumatol.* 3, 1385-91 (1996).

[25] C. Belcher, R. Yaqub, F. Fawthrop, M. Bayliss, M. Doherty, *Ann. Rhem. Dis.* 56(5), 299-307 (1997).

[26] L. Bucsi, G. Poor, *Osteoarthrithis Cart.* 6, 31-6 (1998).

[27] M. F. McCarty, A. L. Russel, M. P. Seed, *Med. Hypotheses.* 54, 798-802 (2000).

[28] J-P. Bali, H. Cousse and E. Neuzil, *Seminars in arthritis and rheumatism.* 31, 58-68 (2001).

[29] S. Coaccioli, A. Allegra, M. Pennacchi, C. Mattioli, F. Ponteggia et al., *Int. J. Clin. Pharm. Res.* XVIII, 39-50 (1998).

[30] T. E. McAlindon, M. P. LaValley, J. P. Gulin, D. T. Felson, *JAMA.* 283(11), 1469-1475 (2000).

[31] S. Sakai, E. Otake, T. Toida, Y. Goda, *Chem. Pharm. Bull.* 55(2), 299-303 (2007).

[32] A. Adebowale, J. Du, Z. Liang, J. L. Leslie, N. D. Eddington, *Biopharm. Drug. Dispos.* 23, 217-225 (2002).

[33] J. Du, N. White, N.D. Eddington, *Biopharm. Drug. Dispos.* 25, 109-116 (2004).

[34] N. Volpi, *Osteoarthritis and Cartilage.* 10, 768-777 (2002).

[35] P. Bourgeois et al. *Osteoarthritis Cartilage.* 6: 25-30 (1998).

[36] D. Uebelhart et al. *Osteoarthritis Cartilage.* 6: 39-46 (1998).

[37] B. Lignot, V. Lahogue, P. Bourseau, *J. Biotechnol.* 103, 281-284 (2003).

[38] M. A. Murado, J. Franguas, M. I. Montemayor, J. A. Vásquez, M. P. González, *Biochem. Eng. J.* 49, 126-132 (2010).

[39] A. R. C. Souza, E. O. Kozlowski, V. R. Cerqueira, et al., *Glycoconj. J.* 24, 521-530 (2007).

[40] M. Takai, H. Kono, *US Patent Application.* 20030162744, (2003).

[41] H. Kono, M. Takai, *European Patent.* 1270599 A1, (2003).

[42] J. A. Vázquez, I. Rodríguez-Amado, M. I. Montemayor, J. Fraguas, P. González Mdel, M.A. Murado, *Mar. Drugs.* 11(3), 747-74 (2013).

[43] E. Tadashi, *US Patent Application.* 20060014256, (2006).

[44] N. Volpi, *Academic Press*, (2006).

[45] P. DeAngelis, *Appl. Microbiol. Biotechnol.* 94, 295-305 (2012).

[46] G. F. Medeiros, A. Mendes, R. A. B. Castro, E. C. Baú, H. B. Nader, C. P. Dietrich, *Biochim. Byophys. Acta.* 1475, 287-294 (2000).

[47] L. A. G. Rocha, R. C. L. Martins, C. C. Werneck , E. J. Feres-Filho, L. C. F. Silva, *J. Periodont. Res.* 35, 158-164 (2000).

[48] T. Nishigori, T. Takeda, T. Ohori, *JP Patent*, 2000273102-A (2000).

[49] D. A. Theocharis, N. Papageorgecopoulou, D. H. Vynios, et al., *J. Chromatogr. B.* 745, 297-309 (2001).

[50] R.C.L. Martins, C. C. Werneck, L. A. G. Rocha et al., *J. Renodon Res.* 38, 182-189 (2003).

[51] P. L. DeAngelis, A. J. Padgett-McCue, *J. Biol. Chem.* 275(31), 24124-24129 (2000).

[52] M-L. Rodriguez, B. Jann and K. Jann, *Eur. J. Biochem.* 177, 117-124 (1988).

[53] K. Jann and B. Jann, *Can. J. Microbiol.* 38, 705-710 (1992).

[54] P. L. DeAngelis, *US Patent Application.* 20030104601 (2003).

[55] N. Sugiugura, K. Koji, *US Patent Application.* 20090155851 (2009).

[56] D. Cimini, O. F. Restaino, A. Catapano, M. De Rosa, C. Schiraldi, *Appl. Microbiol. Biotechnol.* 85(6), 1779-87 (2010).

[57] M. Manzoni, S. Bergomi, F. Molinari, V. Cavazzoni, *Biotechnology letters.* 18, 383-386 (1996).

[58] O. F. Restaino, I. di Lauro, D. Cimini, E. Carlino, M. De Rosa, C. Schiraldi, *Appl. Microbiol. Biotechnol.* 97(4),1699-709 (2013).

[59] O. F. Restaino, D. Cimini, M. De Rosa, A. Catapano, M. De Rosa, C. Schiraldi, *Microbial cell fact.* 10, 10 (2011).

[60] A. Zanfardino, O. F. Restaino, E. Notomista, D. Cimini, C. Schiraldi, M. De Rosa, M. De Felice and M. Varcamonti, *Microbial cell fact.* 9, 34 (2010).

[61] D. Cimini, M. De Rosa, A. Viggiani, O. F. Restaino, E. Carlino, C. Schiraldi, *J. Biotechnology* 150, 324-331 (2010).

[62] Amano Enzyme USA, *PCT WO2009149155 A1* (2009).

[63] C. Schiraldi, I. L. Carcarino, A. Alfano, O. F. Restaino, A. Panariello, M. De Rosa, *Biotechnology Journal.* 6(4), 410-9 (2011).

[64] D. Petsch and F. B. Anspach, *J. Biotechnol.* 76, 97-119 (2000).

[65] C. Schiraldi, A. Alfano, D. Cimini, M. De Rosa, A. Panariello, O. F. Restaino, M. De Rosa, *Biotechnol. Prog.* 28(4), 1012-8 (2012).

[66] G. Zoppetti, F. Petrucci, P. Oreste, US *Patent* 6, 77, 398, (2004).

[67] E. Bedini, C. De Castro, M. De Rosa, A. Di Nola, A. Iadonisi, O. F. Restaino, C. Schiraldi, M. Parrilli, *Angew. Chem. Int. Ed. Eng.* 50 (27), 6160-3 (2011).

In: Chondroitin Sulfate
Editor: Vitor H. Pomin

ISBN: 978-1-62808-490-0
© 2013 Nova Science Publishers, Inc.

Chapter 4

Understanding Specificities in Enzymatic Digestions of Chondroitin Sulfates A and C by Monitoring Sulfation Patterns of the Produced Oligosaccharides

Vitor H. Pomin[*]

Program of Glycobiology, Institute of Medical Biochemistry, and University Hospital
Clementino Fraga Filho, Federal University of Rio de Janeiro, Rio de Janeiro, Brazil

Abstract

Enzymes like lyases and hydrolyses that degrade chondroitin sulfates are well-known to reproducibly release just certain oligosaccharide types in terms of their sulfation patterns. Here, we have characterized the disaccharides and hexasaccharides produced from enzymatic digestions of chondoritin sulfates A and C when treated with bacterial chondroitinases ABC and C and ovine testicular hyaluronidase. The structural characterization was based on nuclear magnetic resonance spectroscopy combined with mass spectrometry. These chemically well-defined oligosaccharides were obtained by a combination of size-exclusion chromatography and strong-anion exchange chromatography of the products generated from limited digestions of chondoritin sulfates A and C. The amounts of released products were measured and the endolytic versus exolytic activities were confirmed for each enzyme type. The catalytic directionality was also determined through MS experiments by using chemically modified products at their reducing terminus. Analysis based on the structures of the released products indicates the preferential enzymatic sites of cleavage in terms of sulfation patterns. In all, 15 chondroitin sulfate hexasaccharide structures have been produced and structurally characterized. These may serve as a useful library of chondroitin sulfates to be assayed in future biological or physicochemical assays.

[*] pominvh@bioqmed.ufrj.br.

Abbreviations

btCS-A, bovine tracheal chondroitin sulfate-A; CS, chondroitin sulfate; GAG, glycosaminoglycan; GalNAc, *N*-acetylgalactosamine; GlcA, glucuronic acid; gHSQC, gradient heteronuclear single quantum coherence; HPLC, high pressure liquid chromatography; MS, mass spectrometry; NMR, nuclear magnetic resonance; SAX, strong anion-exchange; scCS-C, shark cartilage chondroitin sulfate-C; SEC, size-exclusion chromatography; UF, unfractionated.

Introduction

Although lyases and hydrolases that degrades glycosaminoglycans (GAGs) have been used for decades (Dodgson, K. S. & Lloyd, A. G. 1958, Ototani, N. & Yosizawa, Z. 1979), some of their mechanisms are still unclear (Jandik, K. A., et al. 1994, Lunin, V. V., et al. 2004, Michel, G., et al. 2004, Rigden, D. J. & Jedrzejas, M. J. 2003, Shaya, D., et al. 2008, Zhang, Z. Q., et al. 2009), and in some cases apparently conflicting observations on specificity have been made (Hardingham, T. E., et al. 1994; Jandik, K. A., et al. 1994). Among many combinations of enzymes and chondoritin sulfate (CS) substrates are available for study (Ernst, S., et al. 1995), here we have chosen three commonly used commercially available CS degrading enzyme preparations, the CS lyases chondroitinase ABC from *Proteus vulgaris* and chondroitinase C from *Flavobacterium heparinum*, and the hydrolase testicular hyaluronidase from sheep testes to assess their utility in oligosaccharidic production. We chose two CS standards for investigation, bovine tracheal CS-A (btCS-A, mostly 4-sulfated), and shark cartilage CS-C (scCS-C, predominantly 6-sulfated) (Pomin, V. H., et al. 2010). A comparison of yields and structures of the major disaccharide and hexasaccharide products from the six digestion combinations is, therefore, presented. After proper isolation by a combination of size-exclusion chromatography (SEC) and strong-anion exchange (SAX) chromatography, both coupled to high pressure liquid chromatography (HPLC) system, all oligosaccharide species were characterized by a combination of nuclear magnetic resonance (NMR) spectroscopy and mass spectrometry (MS).

Results and Discussion

Disaccharide Analysis of Near-Completely Digested btCS-A and scCS-C

In order to establish a standard for further analysis of disaccharides released under more limited digestion conditions, a nearly complete digestion of btCS-A and scCS-C was attempted (Figures 1A and 1B). After a weeklong digestion of btCS-A polymers (8-50 kDa) during which enzymes were replaced periodically, SAX-HPLC analysis showed disaccharide content to be 8% ΔC0S, 42% ΔC6S, and 50% ΔC4S (Figure 1C, Table 1). This is in reasonable agreement with previous works (Muthusamy, A., et al. 2004, Mucci, A., et al. 2000) (10% ΔC0S, 40% ΔC6S, and 50% ΔC4S).

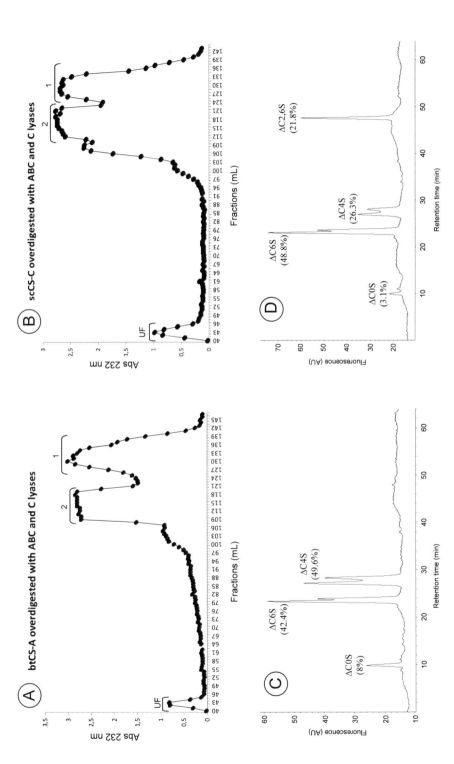

Figure 1. Liquid-chromatography analysis of homogeneous disaccharides of btCS-A (A and C), and scCS-C (B and D). Bio-Gel P10 chromatograms (SEC) from (A) btCS-A, and (B) scCS-C, both overdigested with ABC and C lyases, replaced periodically during one weeklong treatment. The digits 1 and 2 at the top of the peaks indicate the number of units, therefore, mono- and disaccharides, respectively. UF stands for unfractionated oligosaccharides whose MWs are above 20 KDa. (C and D) SAX-HPLC profiles of the disaccharides of each Bio-Gel P10 column. The percentage of each disaccharide type was estimated and they are represented between parentheses at the top of the peaks together with the respective structures.

Table 1. Yields of the disaccharides and the major hexasaccharides obtained from different digestion types within different time courses

Digestion		Disaccharides		Hexasaccharides	
Type	Time	Absolute yield [a]	Structure and relative yield [b]	Absolute yield [a]	Structure and relative yield [b]
near-complete digested btCS-A	7 days	~80 %	ΔC0S [c] (8 %); ΔC4S (50 %); ΔC6S (42 %)	< 1%	Not determined
near-complete digested scCS-C	7 days	~85 %	ΔC0S (3 %); ΔC4S (26 %); ΔC6S (49 %); ΔC2,6S (22 %)	< 1%	Not determined
ABC lyase + btCS-A	2 h and 30 min	~ 70 %	ΔC0S (7 %); ΔC4S (60 %); ΔC6S (33 %)	~ 3 %	ΔC6;6;4S-ol (20 %); ΔC6;4;4S-ol or ΔC4;6;4S-ol (35 %); ΔC4;4;4S-ol (46 %)
ABC lyase + scCS-C	2 h and 30 min	~ 70 %	ΔC0S (6 %); ΔC4S (37 %); ΔC6S (41 %); ΔC2,6S (16 %)	~ 3 %	ΔC2,6;0;4S (34 %); ΔC2,6;0;6S (33 %)
C lyase + btCS-A	2 days	~ 8 %	ΔC0S (12 %); ΔC4S (43 %); ΔC6S (45 %)	~ 10 %	ΔC6;6;6S-ol (8 %); ΔC4;6;6S-ol (20 %); ΔC4;4;4S-ol (57 %)
C lyase + scCS-C	2 days	~ 8 %	ΔC0S (14 %); ΔC4S (15 %); ΔC6S (68 %); ΔC2,6S (3 %)	~ 10 %	ΔC6;6;6S-ol (22 %); ΔC4;2,6;6S-ol (39 %)
hyaluronidase + btCS-A	2 days	< 1 %	Not determined	~ 15 %	C6;6;0S-ol (10 %); C6;4;0S-ol (8 %); C6;4;4S-ol (30 %); C4;4;4S-ol (19 %); C6;6;4S-ol (32 %)
hyaluronidase + scCS-C	2 days	< 1 %	Not determined	~ 10 %	C6;6;4S-ol (23 %); C6;4;4S-ol (18 %); C6;6;2,6S-ol (20 %); C6;2,6;6S-ol (19 %); C2,6;4;2,6S-ol (7 %)

[a] The absolute yield was estimated as the percentage of weight (mg of sample) recovered from the peaks 2 (disaccharides), and 6 (hexasaccharides) from the SEC (Bio-Gel P-10 column) of each digestion type. The values are relative to ~ 75 mg of loaded material into the column.

[b] The relative yield was determined as percentage of weight (mg of material) recovered as pure isomers fractionated by SAX-HPLC chromatography of the heterogeneous mixture of disaccharides or hexasaccharides from each digestion type. The values are compared to ~ 5 mg of material loaded into the column.

[c] In the structural codes, the comma (,) was used to separate hexoses, whereas semicolon (;) was used to separate disaccharide units. The digits 0, 4, and 6 denote respective positions of sulfation in the GalNAc units, whereas the 2 denotes 2-sulfation at uronic acid units. The -ol stands for reduced sugars (open rings at the reducing-ends).

HPLC disaccharide analysis of similarly digested scCS-C polymers (~10-50 kDa, Figure S2) showed disaccharide content to be 3% ΔC0S, 49% ΔC6S, 26% ΔC4S, and 22% ΔC2,6S

(Figure 1D, Table 1). Again this is in reasonable agreement with the literature (2% ΔC0S, 49% ΔC6S, 29% ΔC4S, 17% ΔC2,6S, 3% ΔC4,6S) (Mucci, A., et al. 2000, Sorrell, J. M., et al. 1993).

Limited chondroitinase ABC Digestion of btCS-A

SEC profiles of btCS-A digestion products from shorter periods of ABC lyase treatment are shown in Figure 2. MS has been used to determine the size of oligosaccharides eluted in representative peaks (data not shown), and the degree of polymerization is indicated above each peak in Figure 1. Disaccharides are the major products for short periods of digestion, consistent with the previously suggested presence of substantial exolytic cleavage activity (Hardingham, T. E., et al. 1994). HPLC analysis of disaccharide content of samples digested for 2.5 h (Figure 2 -Δ-) showed composition to be: 7% ΔC0S, 33% ΔC6S, and 60% ΔC4S (Table 1). In comparison to the extensively digested sample (Figure 1C), more ΔC4S disaccharide is clearly generated suggesting a preference for cleavage at a 4-sulfated GalNAc.

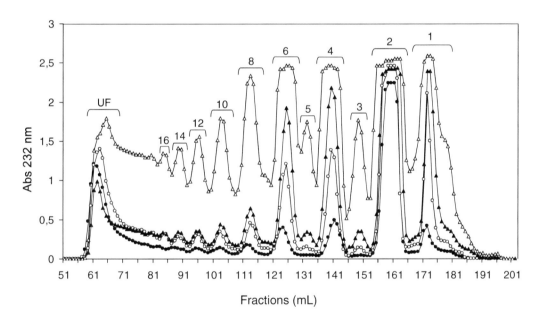

Figure 2. Size fractionation on Bio-Gel P-10 of the products from btCS-A digested with a commercial preparation of chondroitinase ABC from *P. vulgaris*. Data from different digestion times are shown: 10 min (-•-), 30 min (-○-), 1 h (-▲-), and 2.5 h (-Δ-). At the top of each peak the degree of polymerization is indicated. UF stands for unfractionated material.

Although dominant production of disaccharides in early periods of digestion is in full agreement with the expected high level of exolytic activity (Hardingham, T. E., et al. 1994), tetrasaccharides and hexasaccharides are significant at the initial periods as well (Figure 2 -•-, and -○-), and become progressively more abundant with longer digestions (Figure 2 -▲-, and -Δ-). Higher order oligosaccharides (longer than 6-mers) become gradually measurable as well. The commercial preparation of ABC lyase is in fact known to be a mixture of two enzymes suspected to differ in endolytic and exolytic activities, lyases I and II (Hamai, A., et al. 1997, Zhang, Z. Q., et al. 2009). Therefore it is reasonable to consider the production profile as a result of their combined and competing activities (Hamai, A., et al. 1997, Zhang, Z. Q., et al. 2009). As the time of digestion proceeds, the amount of high order oligosaccharides progressively decreases, likely due to continued exolytic action, until massive disaccharide amounts are formed as final products (Figure 1A).

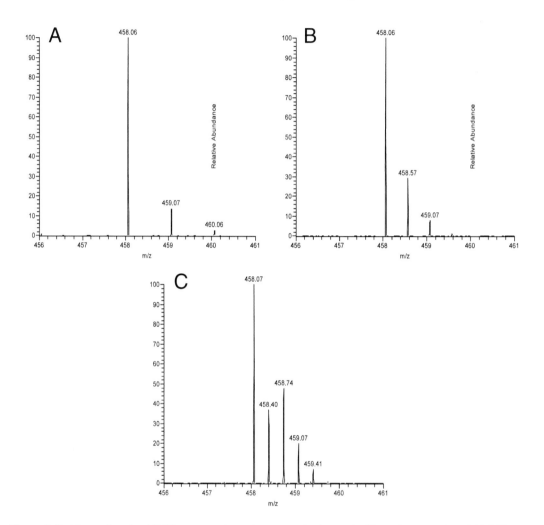

Figure 3. Evidence that the ABC lyase acts from the non-reducing end of its substrate. (A and C) MS spectra of disaccharides (A), tetramers (B), hexasaccharides (C) obtained from the 10 min ABC lyase digestion of a ~ 9kDa fragment that had been previously subjected to sodium borohydride reduction. This leads to an increase of a mass of 2 for fragments coming from the reducing end. Note that only the highest molecular fragment (hexasaccharide, panel C) contain masses characteristic of reduced terminals. While MS spectra of hexasaccharides (C) show the intensity of the peak M+2 (m/z= 458.74) to be somewhat higher than expected for the regular isotopomeric distribution of peaks M, M+1, and M+2, panels A and B for the disaccharides and tetrasaccharides show no evidence of enhance M+2 peaks and a reduced terminus.

There is a general consensus that the ABC lyase exolytic activity proceeds from the non-reducing end (Hardingham, T. E., et al. 1994). However, there have also been reports of related lyases proceeding from the reducing end (Michelacci, Y. M., et al. 1987). To assuage any concern about the directionality of exolytic cleavage we carried out an experiment in which the reducing end of a size selected fraction was marked by sodium borohydride reduction (increases mass by +2). Mass spectra of disaccharides and tetrasaccharides isolated after 10 min ABC lyase digestion showed no evidence of increased abundance of M+2 masses (Figure 3). This confirms exolytic action from the non-reducing end. The appearance of unreduced tetrasaccharides derived from the non-reducing end further supports the additional endolytic cleavage activity.

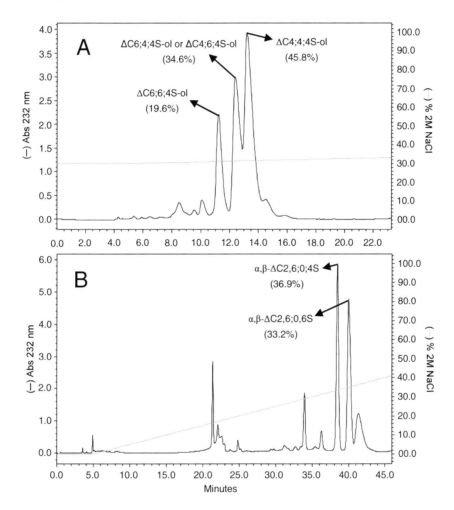

Figure 4. SAX-HPLC fractionation of unsaturated hexasaccharides from digestion of (A) btCS-A, and (B) scCS-C with a commercial preparation of chondroitinase ABC from *P. vulgaris*. Mixtures of hexasaccharides (reduced, and unreduced for btCS-A, and scCS-C, respectively) were obtained from peak 6 of their respective Bio-Gel P-10 chromatograms of 2.5 h digestions. The two fractionated isomers as characterized by NMR and MS spectroscopy were (A) ΔC6;6;4S-ol, and ΔC4;4;4S-ol for btCS-A, and (B) α,β-ΔC2,6;0;6S and α,β-ΔC2,6;0;4S for scCS-C. (A) The middle peak could be either ΔC6;4;4S-ol or ΔC4;6;4S-ol. The percentage of material in each peak is indicated in parentheses. The NaCL gradient is shown with the continuous light grey line.

The existence of sites less prone to exolytic activity may be reflected in the reducing end structure of some oligosaccharide products. The hexasaccharide fraction from limited ABC lyase digestion of unfractionated btCS-A was, therefore, further analyzed by separation on a SAX column followed by NMR and MS analysis. Prior to SAX-HPLC, the mixture of hexasaccharides (Figure 2, peak 6 -Δ-) was reduced via treatment with NaBH$_4$ to avoid possible complications from α-/β-anomeric mutarotation. This reaction was only used to facilitate structural characterization, and can be skipped when oligosaccharide production is the objective. Only three major peaks appeared in the SAX chromatogram (Figure 4A). Among the three fractions, only the two leading and trailing peaks gave ^{13}C-gradient heteronuclear single quantum coherence (gHSQC) spectra sufficiently free of contamination from species eluting at either side to allow structure determination (data not shown). The first peak was characterized as ΔC6;6;4S-ol. The last hexasaccharide from the SAX-HPLC was identified as the entirely 4-sulfated hexasaccharide (ΔC4;4;4S-ol).

The appearance of hexasaccharides with 6-sulfation at the non-reducing terminus and 4-sulfation at the reducing terminus are expected based on a lower preference for exolytic cleavage at 6-sulfated sites. Exolytic cleavage beginning at the non-reducing end would have been slow at this site allowing more time for endolytic cleavage at a downstream 4-sufated site. The high yield of a ΔC4;4;4S-ol oligosaccharide (Table 1) is likely a simple consequence of the higher percentage of 4-sulfation in the starting material.

Limited Chondroitinase ABC Digestion of scCS-C

The oligosaccharidic distribution using chondroitinase ABC to digest the atypical scCS-C substrate over a 2.5 h digestion period was observed similar to that seen for btCS-A at 1 h (Figure 2 -▲-). The slower progression of the digestion is consistent with a preference of the ABC lyase for 4-sulfation sites and the smaller percentage of 4-sulfation in the scCS-C substrate. scCS-C is 26 % 4-sulfated as opposed to 50 % in btCS-A (Figures 1C vs 1D, Table 1).

The presence of hexasaccharides, although comprising < 5% of the digested material after 2.5 h digestion (Table 1), are again consistent with significant endolytic activity of the commercial preparation of ABC lyase from P. vulgaris. Fractionation by SAX-HPLC of the unreduced hexasaccharides revealed two well-separated major peaks (Figure 4B); both were further characterized by ^{13}C-gHSQC spectra (data not shown). Positions of sulfate-related ^{1}H/^{13}C cross-peaks (data not shown) suggest the first fraction to be ΔC2,6;0;4S (Table 1), and the second fraction to be ΔC2,6;0;6S (Table 1).

The high representation of 2-sulfated GlcAs and non-sulfated GalNAcs in the hexasaccharide fraction is in sharp contrast to the lower amounts of disaccharides containing these sufation patterns under near-complete digestion conditions (22% and 3% respectively, Table 1). This sulfation pattern, ΔC2,6;0, may slow the exolytic action of the 4-sulfation-prefering ABC lyase allowing endolytic activity to produce hexasaccharides with an unexpectedly small number of isomers. 4-sulfation at the reducing end is more prevalent as expected based on preference for cleavage at a 4-sulfated site. The appearance of a hexasaccharide with 6-sulfation at this position likely reflects the abundance of these sites in the starting material.

Limited Chondroitinase C Digestion of scCS-C

Unlike the chondroitinase ABC preparation used, the chondroitinase C preparation appeared to be composed of a single relatively pure protein. The activity however was lower than that of chondroitinase ABC and hence longer digestion times were used (48 h on Figure 5 *vs* 2.5 h on Figure 2 -Δ-). Only the results after 2-day digestion are presented in Figure 5, and this plot is used to compare the size distribution results on digesting the preferred 6-sulfation-rich substrate, scCS-C, to the less preferred 4-sulfation-rich substrate, btCS-A. Interestingly, the distribution of oligosaccharide sizes appears similar for both substrates as confirmed by the quantitation of amounts of disaccharides and hexasaccharides presented in Table 1. This suggests a more 4-sulfation-dependent activity than commonly expected. The higher amounts of hexasaccharide and other oligosaccharides as compared to disaccharides for both digestions suggest a dominant endolytic activity for this single enzyme.

Disaccharide fractions after 2-day digestion of scCS-C showed 68% of the structures having a single 6-type sulfation (Table 1) while the starting material has ~ 49% (Figure 1D). Some 6-sulfation preference therefore exists.

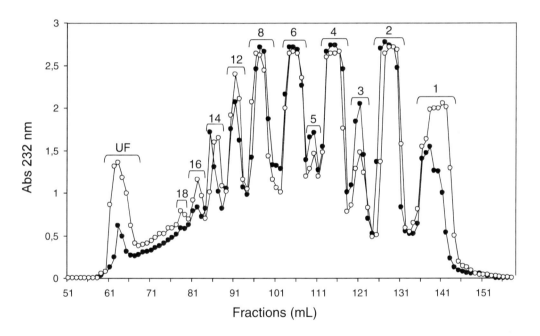

Figure 5. Size fractionation on Bio-Gel P-10 column of the products from 2-day digestions of scCS-C (-o-), and btCS-A (-●-) with a commercial preparation of chondroitinase C from *F. heparinum*. The degree of polymerization is given at the top of each peak. UF stands for unfractionated material.

The specificity of C lyase as seen in scCS-C digestions can be better assessed by examination of hexasaccharides isolated by SAX-HPLC (Figure 6A) combined with analysis by NMR and MS (data not shown). The large amount of hexasaccharide bearing 6-sulfated units at reducing ends, such as ΔC6;6;6S-ol and ΔC4;2,6;6S-ol (Table 1) would support specificity for cleavage at a 6-sulfated site, but may also be explained as a consequence of the preponderance of 6-sulfation in the starting material. A comparison with a C lyase digestion of btCS-A, as presented below, helps to differentiate these possibilities. The different numbers of sulfates in oligosaccharide products from scCS-C when 2-sulfation of the glucuronic acid occurs along with sulfation of the GalNAc is distinctive and facilitates the isolation of homogeneous hexasaccharides from this digestion type.

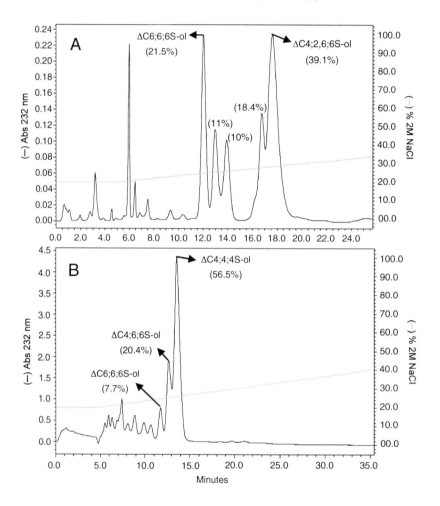

Figure 6. SAX-HPLC fractionation of reduced unsaturated hexasaccharides from 2-day digestions of (A) scCS-C, and (B) btCS-A with a commercial preparation of C lyase from *F. heparinum*. Both mixtures of hexasaccharides were obtained from peak 6 of their respective Bio-Gel P-10 chromatograms. The fractionated isomers are (A) ΔC6;6;6S-ol, and ΔC4;2,6;6S-ol for scCS-C, and (B) ΔC6;6;6S-ol, ΔC4;6;6S-ol, and ΔC4;4;4S-ol for btCS-A. The mean the percentage of material in each peak is given in parentheses. The NaCL gradient is shown with the continuous light grey line.

Limited Chondroitinase C Digestion of btCS-A

The slight preference of C lyase activity towards 6-sulfated regions was observed when the disaccharides, derived from the atypical substrate btCS-A were analyzed by SAX-HPLC (data not shown). Disaccharide analysis of products from 2-day incubation revealed nearly equivalent amounts of 4- and 6-sulfated disaccharides (43% and 45%) (Table 1), as compared to the excess of 4-sulfated disaccharides (50% vs 42%) seen on near-complete digestion of btCS-A (Figure 1C, Table 1).

As in the case of scCS-C, the amount of hexasaccharide is relatively high in btCS-A digestions showing substantial endolytic activity. Again a small number of isomers (three) was obtained from SAX-HPLC (Figure 6B) of the mixture of reduced hexasaccharides (peak 6 -Δ- in Figure 1). These were characterized by both ^{13}C-gHSQC NMR, and MS (data not shown), giving the following structures: ΔC6;6;6S-ol, ΔC4;6;6S-ol, and ΔC4;4;4S-ol (Table 1). The ~57 % occurrence of a ΔC4;4;4S-ol hexasaccharide was unexpectedly high (Table 1). Occurrence may have been elevated somewhat by the slight preference for cleavage at 6-sulfated sites, but it can also be a consequence of clustering of 4-sulfation in the starting material. The presence of the ΔC6;6;6S-ol hexasaccharide was likewise surprising, even though in small amounts. Random distributions of 6-sulfated sites in even a slightly 4-sulfate-rich sample would make occurrence of three in a row rare. Evidence supporting the occurrence of sulfation domains rather than random distribution in CS backbones does exist (Sorrell, J. M., et al. 1993). In any case, preference for cleavage in 6-sulfated regions over 4-sulfated regions is small when btCS-A is used as substrate for C lyase.

Hyaluronidase Digestion of btCS-A and scCS-C

It is clear from the above results that longer oligosaccharides are produced when endolytic activity dominates and production of certain products can be enhanced when reducing end processing is reduced by a less preferred sulfation pattern. It is therefore of interest to examine products from digestion with other enzymes for which endolytic activity naturally dominates. Commercial preparations of ovine hyaluronidase, a hydrolase named for its activity toward non-sulfated HA, is known to have such specificity (Takagaki, K., et al. 1994). Preference for cleavage at 4-sulfated or non-sulfated sites (Knudson, W. et al., 1984) should complement observations made using chondroitinase C where cleavage at 6-sulfated sites is slightly preferred. This hydrolase would also add saturated oligosaccharides to the growing library of unsaturated oligosaccharides produced by the lyases. Figure 7 presents gel-permeation results for digestions with hyaluronidase on both CS substrates. The small amounts of disaccharide and heavy distribution towards medium sized-oligosaccharides (ranging from 4- to 10-residues, Figure 7), support the predicted effects of high endolytic activity. Surprisingly, hyaluronidase appears to show some enhanced activity toward a 6-sulfation-rich substrate, as scCS-C appears to have been digested faster than btCS-A (Figure 7). The apparent acceleration of digestion may, however, reflect differences in accessibility due to secondary and tertiary structure as opposed to specificity at the cleavage site. Additional information can again be obtained by separation and characterization of hexasaccharide fractions.

Digestions of both btCS-A and scCS-C showed two well-separated groups of reduced hexasaccharides on SAX-HPLC (Figure 8). In the case of btCS-A, ^{13}C-gHSQC NMR, and MS spectra (data not shown) showed the first group to be C6;6;0S-ol, and C6;4;0S-ol, and the second group to be C6;6;4S-ol, C4;4;4S-ol, and C6;4;4S-ol (Figure 8A, Table 1). The groups of HPLC-peaks differ in the extent of sulfation. The hexasaccharides in the first group, with a non-sulfated GalNAc at the reducing end, were in fact anticipated based on the expected ability of hyaluronidase to cleave at non-sulfated sites (Knudson, W., et al. 1984). The relatively high percentage of hexasaccharides bearing 6-sulfation in both groups is consistent with the suggestion that 6-sulfated regions may be more accessible to the enzyme. It is noteworthy; however, that all hexasaccharides of the second group have 4-sufation at the reducing ends confirming a preference for cleavage between a 4-sulfated GalNAc and a GlcA (Knudson, W., et al. 1984).

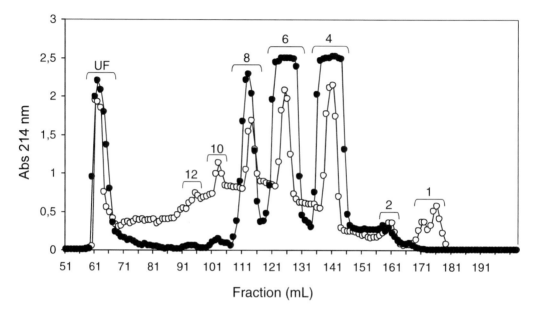

Figure 7. Size fractionation on Bio-Gel P-10 of the products from 2-day digestion of btCS-A (-○-), and scCS-C (-●-) with a commercial preparation of ovine hyaluronidase. The degree of polymerization is given at the top of each peak. UF stands for unfractionated material.

The major hexasaccharides from hyaluronidase digestion of scCS-C were characterized as follows: C6;6;4S-ol, C6;4;4S-ol, C6;6;2,6S-ol, C6;2,6;6S-ol and C2,6;4;2,6S-ol (Figures 8B). Curiously, these products do not contain any non-sulfated GalNAc units. However, the occurrence of non-sulfated GalNAc residues in these products is lower than in btCS-A (3%, Figure 1D). More prevalent are products eluting at higher salt concentrations containing 2,6-di-sulfated units. This shows some enhanced hyaluronidase activity for regions with 2,6-di-sulfated sites in scCS-C. Products from hyaluronidase digestion bearing 2-sulfation have been observed previously (Nadanaka, W., & Sugahara, K., 1997). Aside from some enhanced activity toward 2,6-sulfated regions, the high amount of hexasaccharides bearing C-type sulfation is consistent with the abundance in the starting material together with the suggested enzymatic accessibility to 6-sulfation-rich regions.

The occurrence of hexasaccharide products with 2 to 5 and potentially 6 sulfation sites (Figure 8) on digestion with hyaluronidase facilitates separation of discrete products on SAX-HPLC. Caution must be exercised, however, in assuming that hexasaccharide structures observed represent sequences abundant in native polymers. The transglycosidase activity of hyaluronidase can clearly generate sequences not present or abundant in its polymeric substrates (Takagaki, K., et al. 1994, 1999). However our observations are reproducible and remain relevant to the potential for defined product retrieval from both btCS-A and scCS-C.

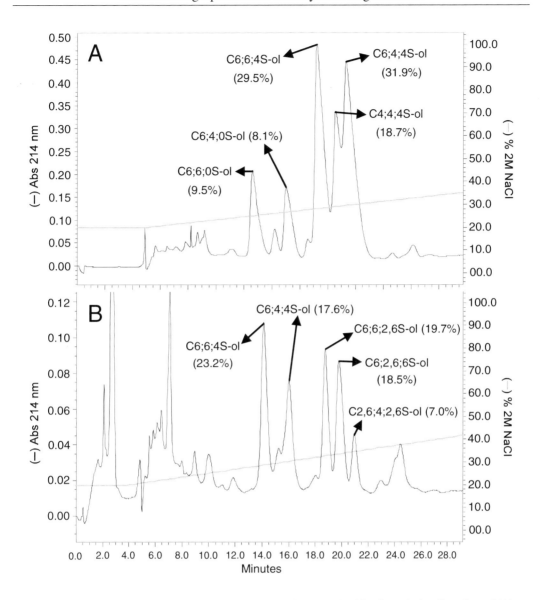

Figure 8. SAX-HPLC fractionation of reduced saturated hexasaccharides from 2-day digestion of (A) btCS-A, and (B) scCS-C with a commercial preparation of ovine hyaluronidase. The percentage of material in each peak is given in parentheses. The NaCL gradient is shown with the continuous light grey line.

Discussion

The current research was restricted to a study of the activity of just three commonly used commercial enzyme preparations, and their actions on just two readily available CS standards. However, comparative analysis of digestion products from the two differentially sulfated substrates provided some insight into the relationship of cleavage specificities of the enzyme preparations and the limited number of hexasaccharides produced. The hexasaccharide fractions were chosen for further characterization in this work due to a combination of potential biological interest and feasibility in HSQC-based structural determination. Endolytic activity contributes substantially to the production of the biologically interesting medium-sized products in digestions with C lyase and hyaluronidase, whereas, the substantial exolytic activity in ABC lyase preparations limit the production of larger oligosaccharides. However, for the small amounts of larger oligosaccharides produced, specificities for exolytic cleavage seem to contribute to production of limited numbers of isomers, possibly by enhancing opportunities for endolytic cleavage when regions of low exolytic activity are encountered. For example, the commercial preparation of ABC lyase from *P. vulgaris,* whose activity results from a competition between two enzymes (endolyase and exolyase), produced a very limited set of hexasaccharide structures, mostly with a non-reducing end 6-sulfated GalNAc or a 2,6;0S pattern penultimate to the reducing end (Table 1). Approximately 2 mg of the uncommon hexasaccharide, ΔC2,6;0;4S was prepared by treating 75 mg of scCS-C with ABC lyase. Based on our observations, preferences for exolytic cleavage by the commercially available chondroitinase ABC preparation would be 4S > 0S > 2,6S = 6S, with endolytic cleavage showing specificity toward 4-sulfated sites. Figure 9A summarizes these observations.

The commercial preparation of chondroitinase C from *F. heparinum* showed predominantly endolytic action. Only 8% disaccharides were produced with limited digestion as opposed to the 70% with limited ABC lyase digestion (Table 1), something that could obscure any effect of exolytic stalling on hexasaccharide product distributions. Analysis of the small amount of generated disaccharide products did unexpectedly show effective cleavage at 4-sulfated GalNAc units as well as 6-sulfated units. There is, in fact, only a slight elevation of 6-sulfation in disaccharides isolated after short digestions of btCS-A as compared to disaccharides produced on near-complete digestion. The 4,4,4 hexasaccharide isolated from a btCS-A digestion was also produced in large amounts (57%, Table 1) showing cleavage ability at a 4 sulfated site, but all other hexasaccharides from either btCS-A or scCS-C digestion have a 6-sulfated GalNAc unit located at their reducing ends. In addition, the SEC profiles of both substrates were observed to be similar (Figure 5). Hence, specificity for both 4- and 6-sulfated sites does exist, perhaps suggesting an AC designation to be more proper for this lyase. Specificities observed for this commercial preparation of chondroitinase C are summarized in Figure 9B.

As expected, the commercial hyaluronidase preparation from sheep testes exhibits major endolytic activity producing medium- (4- to 8-mers, Figure 7) and large-sized oligosaccharides (peaks UF in Figure 7) as primary products. As expected, it also displays a slightly enhanced ability to cleave after both 4-sulfated and non-sulfated GalNAc residues (Knudson, W. et al., 1984). For digestion of scCS-C there is an enhanced abundance of hexasaccharides that a carry 2- and 6-di-sulfated disaccharide units (Figure 8), indicating a possible preference for regions bearing additional sulfation on GlcAs as well. The number of hexasaccharide types is larger than that produced by the lyases studied here, but the number is still below statistical expectations. The occurrence of hexasaccharides with both less and more sulfation than one per GalNAc residue also facilitates separation of products by SAX in this case (Figure 8). The suspected specificities of the commercially available preparation of hyaluronidase are represented in Figure 9C.

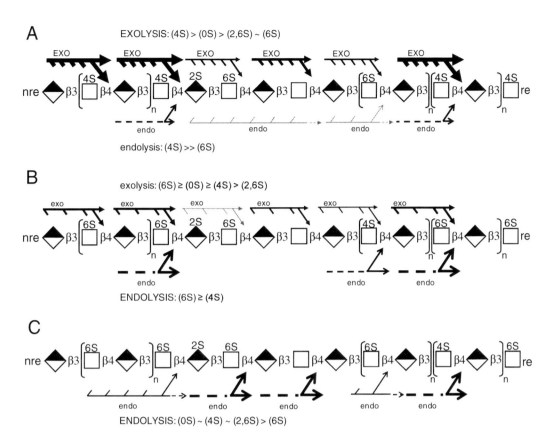

Figure 9. Schematic representation for the apparent preference for cleavage sites using readily available enzymatic preparations of (A) chondroitinase ABC, (B) chondroitinase C, and (C) hyaluronidase in digestions of typical CS substrates. In the panels A-C, the thickness of the arrows increases proportionally to preferential cleavage. Exo, and endo, stands for possible exolytic, and endolytic sites respectively. nre, and ne, stands for non-reducing end and reducing end respectively. Upper and lower cases denote stronger and weaker cleavage actions respectively. The white boxes and up-black diamonds represent GalNAc and GlcA units, respectively. The disaccharides inside brackets with Δ represent variation in chain lengths. The dashed lines represent possible extensions on the substrate chain that may be recognized by lyases/hydrolase. Lines with inclined traces represent substrate segments that regulate the enzymatic activity. The representation of CS backbones is hypothetical and does not reflect possible clustering of sulfation patterns as noted in the text. (A) Chondroitinase ABC showed mostly exolytic action regulated by sulfation positions as the following: (4S) > (0S) > (2,6S) = (6S). Its endolytic action is minor, but with 4-sulfation preference over 6-sulfation, also modulated by 6-sulfation or 2,6-di-sulfated units linked to non-sulfated disaccharides. (B) Chondroitinase C is a lyase with primarily endolytic action. There is a slight preference for 6-sulfation, but with specificity towards 4S-, and 0S-sites as well. (C) Hyaluronidase is a hydrolase with well-known endolytic activity. This hydrolase shows cleavage preferences towards non-sulfation, 4-sulfation and regions rich in 2,6-di-sulfation.

References

Dodgson, K. S., & Lloyd, A. G. (1958). Degradation of cartilage chondroitin sulphate by the chondroitinase of *Proteus vulgaris*. *Biochemical Journal*, 68, 88-94.

Ernst, S., Langer, R., Cooney, C. L., & Sasisekharan, R. (1995). Enzymatic degradation of glycosaminoglycans. *Critical Reviews in Biochemistry and Molecular Biology*, 30, 387-444.

Hamai, A., Hashimoto, N., Mochizuki, H., Kato, F., Makigushi, Y., Horie, K., & Suzuki, S. (1997). Two Distinct Chondroitin Sulfate ABC Lyases: an endoeliminase yielding tetrasaccharides and an exoeliminase preferentially acting on oligosaccharides. *Journal of Biological Chemistry*, 272, 9123-9130.

Hardingham, T. E., Fosang, A. J., Hey, N. J., Hazell, P. K., Kee, W. J., & Ewins, R. J. F. (1994). The sulfation pattern in chondroitin sulfate chains investigated by chondroitinase ABC and acil digestion and reactivity with monoclonal-antibodies. *Carbohydrate Research,* 255, 241-254.

Jandik, K. A., Gu, K. A., & Linhardt, R. J. (1994). Action pattern of polysaccharide lyases on glycosaminoglycans. *Glycobiology*, 4, 289-296.

Kudson, W., Gundlach, M. W., Schimid, T. M., & Conrad, H. E. (1984). Selective hydrolysis of chondroitin sulfates by hyaluronidase. *Biochemistry*, 23, 368-375.

Lunin, V. V., Li, Y. G., Linhardt, R. J., Miyazono, H., Kyogashima, M., Kaneko, T., Bell, A.W., & Cygler, M. (2004). High-resolution crystal structure of *Arthrobacter aurescens* chondroitin AC lyase: An enzyme-substrate complex defines the catalytic mechanism. *Journal of Molecular Biology*, 337, 367-386.

Michel, G., Pojasek, K., Li, Y. G., Sulea, T., Linhardt, R. J., Raman, R., Prabhakar, V., Sasisekharan, R., & Cygler, M. (2004). The structure of chondroitin B lyase complexed with glycosaminoglycan oligosaccharides unravels a calcium-dependent catalytic machinery. *Journal of Biological Chemistry*, 279, 32882-32896.

Michelacci, Y. M., Horton, D., & Poblacion, C. A. (1987). Isolation and characterization of an induced chondroitinase ABC from *Flavobacterium heparinum. Biochimica Et Biophysica Acta,* 923, 291-301.

Mucci, A., Schenetti, L., & Volpi, N. (2000). H-1 and C-13 nuclear magnetic resonance identification and characterization of components of chondroitin sulfates of various origin. *Carbohydrate Polymers*, 41, 37-45.

Muthusamy, A., Achur, R. N., Valiyaveettil, M., Madhunapantula, S. V., Kakizaki, I., Bhavanandan, V. P., & Gowda, C. D. (2004). Structural characterization of the bovine tracheal chondroitin sulfate chains and binding of Plasmodium falciparum-infected erythrocytes. *Glycobiology*, 14, 635-645.

Nadanaka, S., & Sugahara, K. (1997). The unusual tetrasaccharide sequence GlcA beta 1-3GalNAc(4-sulfate)beta 1-4GlcA(2-sulfate)beta 1-3GalNAc(6-sulfate) found in the hexasaccharides prepared by testicular hyaluronidase digestion of shark cartilage chondroitin sulfate D. *Glycobiology*, 7, 253-63.

Ototani, N., & Yosizawa, Z. (1979). Purification of chondroitinase-B and chondroitinase-C using glycosaminoglycan-bound AH-Sepharose-4B. *Carbohydrate Research*, 70, 295-306.

Pomin, V. H., Sharp, J. S., Li, X. Y., Wang, L. C, & Prestegard, J. H. (2010). Characterization of glycosaminoglycans by N-15 NMR spectroscopy and *in vivo* isotopic labeling. *Analytical Chemistry*, 82, 4078-4088.

Rigden, D. J., & Jedrzejas, M. J. (2003). Structures of *Streptococcus pneumoniae* hyaluronate lyase in complex with chondroitin and chondroitin sulfate disaccharides - Insights into specificity and mechanism of action. *Journal of Biological Chemistry*, 278, 50596-50606.

Shaya, D., Hahn, B. S., Bjerkan, T. M., Kim, W. S., Park, N. Y., Sim, J. S., Kim, Y.S., & Cygler, M. (2008). Composite active site of chondroitin lyase ABC accepting both epimers of uronic acid. *Glycobiology*, 18, 270-277.

Sorrell, J. M., Carrino, D. A., & Caplan, A.I. (1993). Structural domains in chondroitin sulfate identified by anti-chondroitin sulfate monoclonal-antibodies - Immunosequencing of chondroitin sulfates. *Matrix*, 13, 351-361.

Takagaki, K., Munakata, H., Majima, M., & Endo, M. (1999). Enzymatic reconstruction of a hybrid glycosaminoglycan containing 6-sulfated, 4-sulfated, and unsulfated N-acetylgalactosamine. *Biochemical and Biophysical Research Communications*, 258, 741-744.

Takagaki, K., Nakamura, T., Izumi, J., Saitoh, H., Endo, M., Kojima, K., Kato, I., & Majima, M. (1994). Characterization of hydrolysis and transglycosylation by testicular hyaluronidase using ion-spray mass-spectrometry. *Biochemistry*, 33, 6503-6507.

Warner, R. G., Hundt, C., Weiss, S., & Turnbull, J. E. (2002). Identification of the heparan sulfate binding sites in the cellular prion protein. *Journal of Biological Chemistry*, 277, 18421-18430.

Zhang, Z. Q., Park, Y., Kemp, M. M., Zhao, W. J., Im, A. R., Shaya, D., Cygler, M., Kim, Y. S., Linhardt, R. J. (2009). Liquid chromatography-mass spectrometry to study chondroitin lyase action pattern. *Analytical Biochemistry,* 385, 57-64.

In: Chondroitin Sulfate
Editor: Vitor H. Pomin

ISBN: 978-1-62808-490-0
© 2013 Nova Science Publishers, Inc.

Chapter 5

Chondroitin-6-Sulfate Degradation by *N*-Acetylgalactosamine-6-Sulfatase and Implications for Mucopolysaccharidosis IV A (MPS IV A)

Yadilette Rivera-Colón and Scott C. Garman[*]

Molecular and Cellular Biology Program,
Department of Biochemistry & Molecular Biology,
University of Massachusetts Amherst, Amherst, MA US

Abstract

Mucopolysaccharides such as keratan sulfate, dermatan sulfate, heparan sulfate, heparin, and chondroitin sulfate are heterogeneous sulfated polysaccharides. Chondroitin sulfate contains primarily alternating *N*-acetylgalactosamine (both sulfated and unsulfated) and glucuronic acid residues, and is most commonly found as chondroitin-6-sulfate and chondroitin-4-sulfate, which differ in the position of the sulfate group on the *N*-acetylgalactosamine residues. Mucopolysaccharides are degraded in the lysosome by the sequential action of multiple enzymes. For example, chondroitin-6-sulfate degradation occurs primarily due to the enzymes *N*-acetylgalactosamine-6-sulfatase (GALNS), β-hexosaminidase, and β-glucuronidase. This chapter focuses on the degradation of chondroitin sulfate by the human lysosomal enzyme GALNS, and on the relationship of GALNS to the lysosomal storage disease mucopolysaccharidosis IV A (also known as MPS IV A and Morquio A). Loss of activity of the GALNS enzyme leads to accumulation of chondroitin-6-sulfate and keratan sulfate, which then leads to development of disease. Substrate accumulation leads to a range of disease symptoms, including dysostosis multiplex, joint mobility, hearing, vision and cardiovascular impairment. There are no approved therapies for MPS IV A; however enzyme replacement therapy using recombinant GALNS glycoprotein is currently in Phase III clinical trials in the United States. To better understand the molecular basis for the disease, we recently determined the three-dimensional structure of GALNS by X-ray

[*] E-mail address: garman@biochem.umass.edu.

crystallography. The structure of GALNS shows a catalytic gem diol nucleophile derived from enzymatic modification of a cysteine side chain in the active site. GALNS contains a large indentation around the active site, with many basic amino acid residues allowing charged interactions with the negatively charged substrates chondroitin-6-sulfate and keratan sulfate. In order to understand the effect on the protein due to disease-causing mutations, 120 missense mutations were mapped onto the GALNS structure. Most of these mutations are buried in the core of the protein, suggesting that in the majority of MPS IV A patients, GALNS activity loss is due to misfolding of the protein. The active site of GALNS falls at the base of a deep trench; thus GALNS may be a suitable target for rational design of small molecule therapeutics.

Introduction

The extracellular matrix contains four principal mucopolysaccharides (chondroitin sulfate, dermatan sulfate, heparan sulfate, and keratan sulfate), which mediate interactions between cells [1, 2]. Chondroitin sulfate, like many other glycosaminoglycans (GAGs), requires an orchestrated sequence of enzymatic reactions to be degraded. Chondroitin sulfate contains alternating N-acetylgalactosamine and glucuronic acid residues, the former of which is sulfated at either the 6- (in chondroitin-6-sulfate) or 4- position (in chondroitin-4-sulfate). GAGs are broken down into monosaccharides in the lysosome by the sequential action of multiple enzymes. For example, the degradation of chondroitin-6-sulfate requires at least three enzymes: N-acetylgalactosamine-6-sulfatase (GALNS), β-hexosaminidase, and β-glucuronidase (Fig. 1).

Mucopolysaccharidoses (MPSs) are lysosomal storage disorders caused by defects in genes that encode lysosomal enzymes responsible for the degradation of mucopolysaccharides or GAGs [1]. For example, deficiency in the activity of the lysosomal GALNS enzyme causes chondroitin-6-sulfate and keratan sulfate to accumulate in the lysosomes, leading to the lysosomal storage disorder known as mucopolysaccharidosis IV A (MPS IV A) [3]. Like many lysosomal storage diseases, MPS IV A presents a range of symptoms, including severe bone dysplasia, short trunk dwarfism, hearing loss, dysostosis multiplex, fine corneal deposits, aortic valve disease and high levels of chondrotitin-6-sulfate and keratan sulfate in the urine of patients [4]. MPS IV A also can present as a milder disease, with less severe manifestations which vary from patient to patient. Most of these symptoms result from undegraded mucopolysaccharide accumulation in the lysosomes, while the rest are secondary defects due to altered cell morphology resulting from lysosomal storgage. There is no currently approved treatment for MPS IV A. However, enzyme replacement therapy is in Phase III clinical trials, where MPS IV A patients are given intravenous injections of recombinant GALNS, and mannose-6-phosphate receptors on the cell surface presumably deliver the recombinant GALNS glycoprotein to the lysosome [5]. Because lysosomal storage diseases such as MPS IV A are primarily monogenetic, the structure of human GALNS can serve as a tool to predict the severity of a mutation on the protein and give insight into genotype-phenotype correlations. In this way, lysosomal storage diseases represent an ideal test case for personalized medicine, where a patient's treatment is guided by his or her DNA sequence.

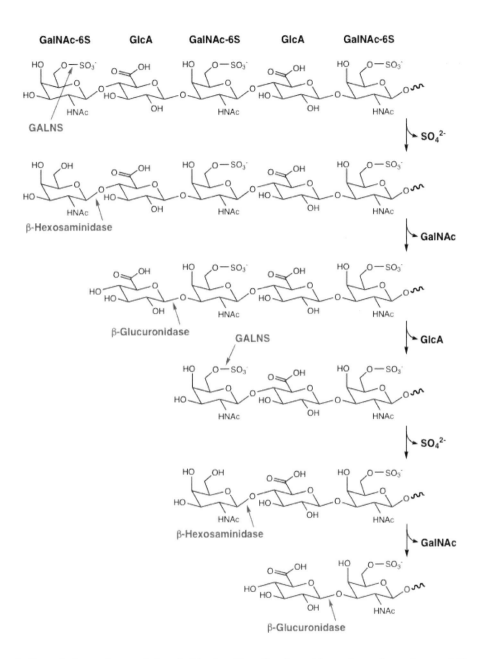

Figure 1. Degradation pathway of chondroitin-6-sulfate. Starting with an alternating polymer of *N*-acetylgalactosamine-6-sulfate (GalNAc-6S) and glucuronic acid (GlcA), three enzymes (in red) act sequentially on the non-reducing end of the polymer.

Structure of Human GALNS

The structure of human GALNS was determined by X-ray crystallography in 2012 [6]. The three-dimensional structure revealed a homodimeric protein with each monomer comprised of two globular domains and a C-terminal meander (Fig. 2). Domain 1 starts at the

N terminus and contains the active site, Domain 2 has a small antiparallel β-sheet and a long α-helix, and the polypeptide finishes with a C-terminal meander that packs against the first domain (Fig. 2). Domain 1 (residues 28–379) exhibits an α/β topology formed by a 10-stranded β-sheet flanked on either side by six α-helices. Domain 2 (residues 380–481) consists of four antiparallel β-strands perpendicular to a long α-helix. The C-terminal meander (residues 482–510) exits Domain 2 and then winds across the molecule, packing against Domain 1 and defining part of the active site pocket. The GALNS monomers assemble into a dimer with overall dimensions of approximately 55 x 55 x 85 Å.

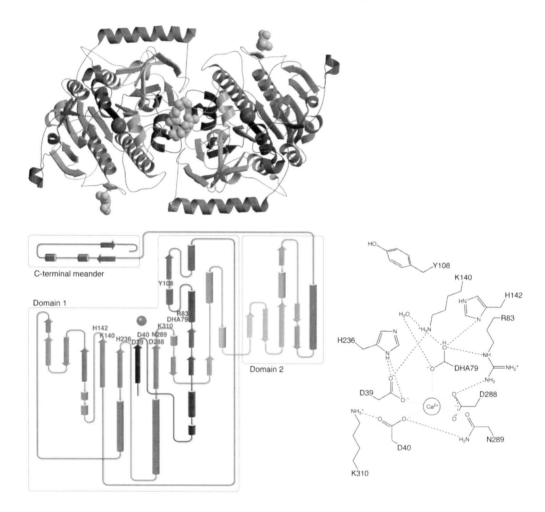

Figure 2. *Top*: Overview of the GALNS dimer. The protein is shown colored from blue at the N terminus to red at the C terminus, with Ca^{2+} represented by a magenta sphere and N-linked carbohydrate as green atoms. *Bottom left*: Topology diagram of the GALNS monomer. Secondary structural elements are colored as above, with domains boxed, and active site residues labeled in red. *Bottom right*: Active site residues and interactions in the active site.

The active site of GALNS lies at the base of a deep pocket in Domain 1. The active site contains a calcium ion bound to the side chains of five residues, one of which is the catalytic nucleophile. The C-terminal meander defines a portion of the GALNS active site (Figs. 2 and 3), however it is not conserved across the sulfatase family but is unique to GALNS among sulfatases with known structures. Compared to other related sulfatase structures, the GALNS amino-acid sequence identity is highest in Domain 1 (approximately 40%), is lower in Domain 2 (13-25%), and is undetectable in the C-terminal meander.

GALNS has two N-linked carbohydrates at positions 204 and 423; the latter rests close to the dimer interface and packs against the equivalent carbohydrate across the two-fold axis of the dimer (Fig. 2). GALNS has seven cysteine residues; six are involved in disulfide bonds (Cys308–Cys419, Cys489–Cys518, and Cys501–Cys507) and one is unpaired (164). The large interface between GALNS monomers buries over 3000 Å^2 of surface area in the dimer. The two active sites in the GALNS dimer are approximately 45 Å apart and point in orthogonal directions, suggesting that the two sites operate independently on substrates.

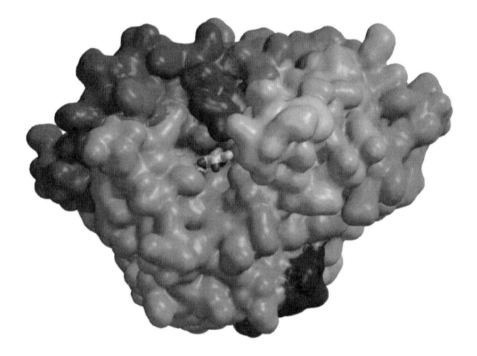

Figure 3. The GALNS monomer surface colored as in Fig. 2. The active site is marked by a GalNAc monosaccharide (a product of the catalytic reaction, shown as bonds), as determined by crystal structures of GALNS. The active site forms a deep pocket in the center of a monomer.

Catalytic Mechanism and Formylglycine Modification

The sulfatase family of enzymes (E.C. 3.1.6.X) can hydrolyze sulfate ester bonds from a variety of substrates [7]. Sulfatases require enzymatic modification of a cysteine side chain to generate a catalytic nucleophile. A cysteine (or occasionally a serine) is converted to a formylglycine aldehyde by the Formylglycine Generating Enzyme (FGE), which recognizes the consensus motif CXPXR [8, 9, 10, 11, 12, 13, 14]. Hydration of the formylglycine aldehyde leads to dihydroxyalanine (DHA), the active nucleophile [15, 16]. Both Ca^{2+} and Mg^{2+} can bind in the active sites of sulfatases [17, 18, 19]. Although Mg^{2+} binds at high concentrations [12], Ca^{2+} provides the maximal enzymatic activity [16, 20]. In the GALNS sulfatase, the gene encodes a cysteine at amino-acid residue 79, at the beginning of the sequence 79-CSPSR-83. FGE removes the cysteine thiol by oxidative desulfurization and converts the side chain into a formylglycine aldehyde.

The crystal structure of GALNS revealed a branched side chain at residue 79, consistent with the hydrated form of the formylglycine side chain in the resting state of the enzyme. The crystal structure suggests a catalytic mechanism of GALNS where substrate binds first, then DHA cleaves the substrate by nucleophilic attack on the sulfate, with His236 acting as a proton donor for the departing product (Fig. 4) [16]. The resulting covalent sulfoenzyme intermediate can then undergo intramolecular hydrolysis of the sulfate by abstraction of a proton from the gem diol by His142.

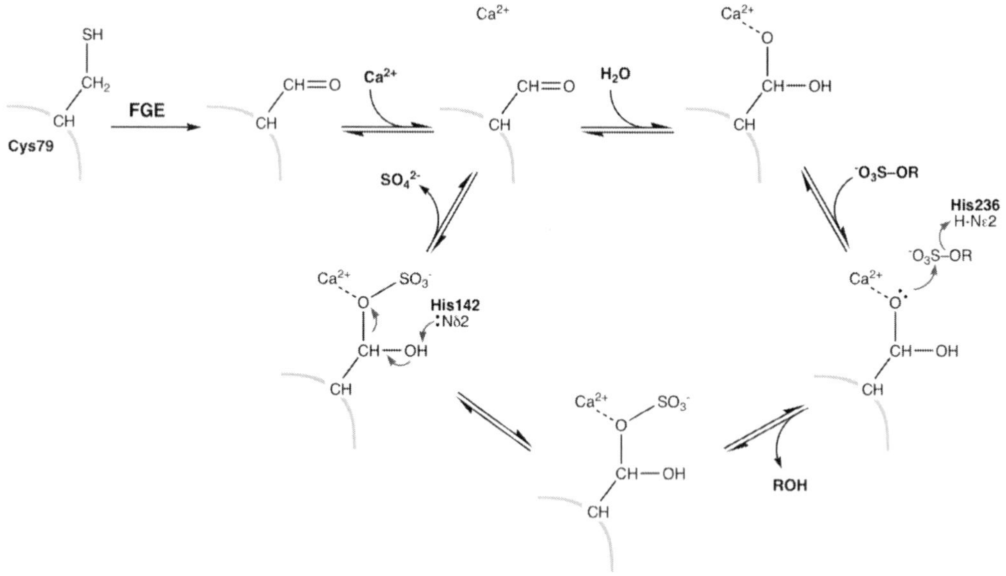

Figure 4. GALNS catalytic mechanism. Cys79 is enzymatically converted to a formylglycine aldehyde by the action of Formylglycine-Generating Enzyme (FGE). Ca^{2+} binding and hydration of the aldehyde lead to a gem diol nucleophile. Substrate binding and subsequent nucleophilic attack of the sulfate lead to a covalent sulfoenzyme intermediate, which then releases the sulfate and reverts to the aldehyde.

Active Site and Ligand Binding

In vitro, sulfatases are promiscuous and can hydrolyze synthetic substrates such as 4-methylumbelliferyl sulfate (4-MU-S), which shares only a sulfate group with the natural substrates. In humans, sulfatase activity is non-degenerate: a deficiency in any of the lysosomal sulfatases leads to disease, thus a given substrate requires a specific sulfatase and is not cleaved by a related sulfatase. GALNS discriminates viable substrate GAGs (for example, chondroitin-6-sulfate and keratan sulfate) from the multitude of other polysaccharides in the lysosome. The selection for substrate specificity occurs in the binding site pocket, containing 11 amino acids in the immediate vicinity of a Ca^{2+} ion: Asp39, Asp40, DHA79, Tyr108,

His142, Lys150, His236, Asp288, Asn289, Lys310 (Fig. 2). The calcium ion in the active site of GALNS is coordinated hexavalently by one oxygen each from Asp39, Asp40, DHA79, and Asn289 and two from Asp288. The basic residues around the active site result in a mostly positive electrostatic surface potential, suitable for binding polyanionic substrates such as chondroitin-6-sulfate (Figs. 2 and 5).

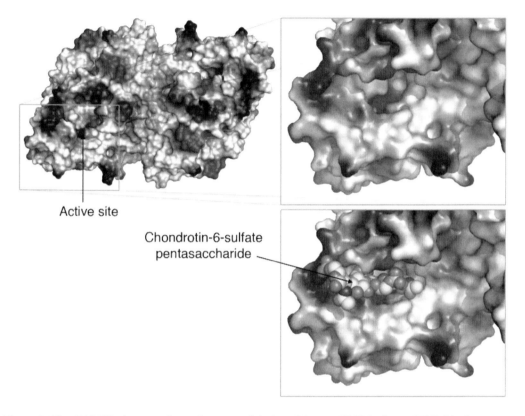

Active site

Chondrotin-6-sulfate
pentasaccharide

Figure 5. The GALNS electrostatic surface potential plotted from −57kT (red) to +57kT (blue) illustrates the positively charged areas around the active site. One active site is indicated by an arrow and is magnified in *upper right*. At *lower right*, a pentasaccharide fragment of chondroitin-6-sulfate has been modeled into the GALNS active site pocket, indicating both size and charge complementarity of the enzyme for the substrate.

The predicted isoelectric point of GALNS is 6.3 [21], and a map of the charge distribution on the surface of the dimer at neutral pH shows an overall high negative potential balanced by pockets of positive potential around the active site (Fig. 5). Chondroitin-6-sulfate, along with the other substrates for GALNS, is a highly negatively charged molecule; therefore positive patches around the active site increase the affinity for anionic substrates by electrostatic forces.

The mechanism of substrate binding to GALNS is of immense clinical interest; however heterogeneous polymers such as chondroitin-6-sulfate are not ideal for crystallographic experiments. In an effort to understand molecular recognition of substrates by GALNS, we soaked a catalytic product, the *N*-acetyl-galactosamine (GalNAc) monosaccharide into the crystals (Fig 3). The resulting enzyme:product complex reveals that the sugar binds in a non-productive orientation, with the sugar rotated slightly in the active site. The specificity of

GALNS for the larger chondrotin-6-sulfate and keratan sulfate polymers appears to derive from interactions between the multiple negative charges of sulfate groups on the substrates with the multiple positive charges in the active site vicinity. Addition of up to 1M galactose, another product of the reaction, does not inhibit GALNS in a 4-MU-S cleavage assay, suggesting that the sulfate portion of the substrate is much more important than the sugar component.

Mucopolysaccharidosis IV A Mutations

Currently, 187 disease-causing mutations have been identified in the *GALNS* gene [22, 23]. The *GALNS* mutations can be binned by category: nonsense (19), splicing defects (15), insertion/deletion (1), deletions (24), insertions (6) and two defined as complex mutations [22]. Sixty-four percent (120) of the *GALNS* mutations are missense mutations leading to a single amino acid substitution in the protein. For the purpose of this chapter we will focus on the mutations leading to small changes in the polypeptide sequence; we will not address the mutations that grossly perturb the polypeptide sequence (such as splice mutations and insertions/deletions leading to a frame shift), as they are unlikely to yield folded GALNS polypeptide. The predicted effects of the missense and nonsense mutations are listed in Table 1. Some recurrent mutations in the *GALNS* gene range from 1.8% to 8.9% frequency of all missense mutations in the MPS IV A population, and lead to the R386C, G301C, I113F, T312S, and M391V substitutions, all of which are likely to perturb the hydrophobic core of the protein.

Combining the crystal structure of GALNS with the mutations in the gene reported in the literature allows for analyzing the overall effect of mutations in disease. For example, 5% of the missense mutations lie in the active site, 65% affect the hydrophobic core of the protein, and 27% are solvent exposed (Table 1). The crystal structure provides for the first time the ability to correlate disease severity with genetic changes, by mapping the effects of mutations onto the three-dimensional structure of the protein.

MPS IV A patients can be divided in two phenotypes based upon stature: severe phenotype (125 cm or less) and mild phenotype (over 125 cm) [23]. In Figure 6, the mutations causing the different phenotypes in MPS IV A patients are mapped onto the three-dimensional structure of GALNS. Since most of the disease-causing mutations result in disruption of the hydrophobic core of the protein, we conclude that MPS IV A is primarily a protein-folding disease. Of the missense mutations in GALNS, 78% in Domain 1 reside in the core, while 53% in Domain 2 are in surface residues, suggesting that Domain 1, the conserved sulfatase domain, is required for folding while Domain 2 may be more involved in macromolecular interactions. Because GALNS is known to interact with other lysosomal proteins involved in the degradation of GAGs [43, 44], we propose that Domain 2 may be the site of these interactions.

Table 1. Predicted effect of disease-causing mutation on GALNS

Position	Amino acid substitution	Effect on structure of GALNS	Access. $(\text{Å}^2)^a$	Mutation Category	Ref.
1	M>V	In signal sequence		Processing	[24]
10	W>Stop	In signal sequence		Processing	[25]
15	L>M	In signal sequence		Processing	[26]
23	G>R	In signal sequence		Processing	[27]
36	L>P	Buried in middle of β-strand; Pro would kink strand	0	Buried	[24]
41	M>L	Little room for branched side chain	0.2	Buried	[23]
42	G>E	No room for side chain	0	Buried	[26]
47	G>R	No room for side chain	0	Buried	[27]
53	S>F	Polar region near dimer interface; little room for large side chain	3.8	Surface	[26]
60	D>N	Unknown	7.5	Surface	[28]
61	R>W	Solvent-exposed hydrophobic residue	17.0	Surface	[29]
66	G>R	No room for large side chain	0	Buried	[26]
69	F>V	Loss of hydrophobic packing	0	Buried	[24]
77	P>R	No room for large side chain	0	Buried	[30]
79	C>Y	Loss of nucleophile	1.3	Active Site	[31]
80	S>L	Buried in polar environment, possible disruption of formylglycine modification	0	Active Site	[25]
88	T>I	Loss of buried hydrogen bonding	0	Buried	[32]
90	R>W	Partially buried; no room for Trp	3.4	Buried	[33]
94	R>G	Loss of ion pair to Glu121	3.2	Buried	[26]
94	R>C	Loss of ion pair to Glu121	3.2	Buried	[23]
94	R>L	Loss of ion pair to Glu121	3.2	Buried	[20]
96	G>C	Gly-specific phi/psi angles	0.1	Buried	[26]
96	G>V	Gly-specific phi/psi angles	0.1	Buried	[23]
97	F>V	Loss of hydrophobic packing	0	Buried	[28]
107	A>T	No room for larger side chain	0	Buried	[29]
111	Q>Stop	Stop	0.7	-	[25]
111	Q>R	Loss of buried hydrogen bonding	0.7	Buried	[34]
113	I>F	Buried; no room for larger side chain	0	Buried	[23]
116	G>S	Buried; no room for larger side chain	0	Buried	[33]
125	P>L	Buried; no room for larger side chain	0	Buried	[23]
129	K>Stop	Stop	17.6	-	[27]
135	S>R	Buried; no room for larger side chain	0.2	Buried	[35]
138	V>A	Loss of hydrophobic packing	0	Buried	[26]
139	G>S	Gly-specific phi/psi angles	0.1	Buried	[24]
141	W>R	Buried in hydrophobic core; near active site	0	Buried	[36]
141	W>C	Buried in hydrophobic core; near active site	0	Buried	[37]
142	H>R	Active site residue	0.7	Active Site	[23]
148	Q>Stop	Stop	18.5	-	[23]
150	H>Y	Buried; little room for larger side chain	1.9	Buried	[24]
151	P>S	Buried in hydrophobic core	0.2	Buried	[26]
151	P>L	Buried in hydrophobic core	0.2	Buried	[25]
155	G>R	Gly-specific phi/psi angles	2.5	Surface	[23]
155	G>E	Gly-specific phi/psi angles	2.5	Surface	[26]
156	F>S	Buried in hydrophobic core	0	Buried	[29]
156	F>C	Buried in hydrophobic core	0	Buried	[20]

Table 1. (Continued)

Position	Amino acid substitution	Effect on structure of GALNS	Access. (Å^2)^a	Mutation Category	Ref.
159	W>C	Buried in hydrophobic core	0.2	Buried	[26]
162	S>F	Buried; no room for larger side chain	0.1	Buried	[23]
163	P>H	Buried; little room for larger side chain	0.6	Buried	[23]
164	N>T	Disruption of buried hydrogen bonds	0.8	Buried	[38]
166	H>Q	Disruption of buried ion pair with Asp233	0	Buried	[29]
167	F>V	Near active site; mutation may affect substrate recognition or protein binding	15.2	Surface	[31]
168	G>R	Gly-specific phi/psi angles	1.6	Buried	[26]
171	D>A	Unknown	16.7	Surface	[25]
179	P>S	Completely buried	0	Buried	[32]
179	P>H	Buried; little room for larger side chain	0	Buried	[36]
179	P>L	Buried; little room for larger side chain	0	Buried	[33]
185	E>G	Unknown	17.9	Surface	[26]
203	A>V	Buried; little room for branched side chain	0	Buried	[33]
204	N>K	Glycosylation site	6	Surface	[25]
211	Q>Stop	Stop	17.8	-	[25]
230	W>G	Loss of hydrophobic packing	0	Buried	[36]
230	W>Stop	Stop	0	-	[23]
233	D>N	Disruption of buried ion pair with His166	0.3	Buried	[26]
236	H>D	Active site	4.7	Active Site	[26]
239	V>F	Buried; no room for larger side chain	0	Buried	[23]
247	G>D	Unknown	18.0	Surface	[32]
253	R>W	Partially buried; little room for Trp	6.6	Surface	[33]
257	A>T	Buried; little room for branched side chain	0	Buried	[23]
259	R>Q	Unknown	9.8	Surface	[25]
260	E>D	Loss of buried hydrogen bonding	0	Buried	[27]
284	F>V	Loss of hydrophobic packing	0.2	Buried	[27]
287	S>L	Loss of buried hydrogen bonding	0	Buried	[29]
289	N>S	Active site, metal binding residue	0	Active Site	[23]
290	G>S	Little room for larger side chain; near active site	0	Buried	[25]
291	A>T	Buried; little room for larger side chain	0.4	Buried	[25]
291	A>D	Buried; little room for larger side chain	0.4	Buried	[27]
295	S>F	Partly buried; little room for larger side chain	3.5	Surface	[23]
301	G>C	Buried; little room for larger side chain	3.7	Buried	[25]
307	L>P	Buried in hydrophobic pocket	0.4	Buried	[26]
309	G>R	Buried; no room for larger side chain	0.2	Buried	[28]
310	K>N	Active site	4.5	Active Site	[32]
312	T>A	Loss of hydrophobic packing	0	Buried	[27]
312	T>S	Loss of hydrophobic packing	0	Buried	[26]
316	G>V	Buried; no room for larger side chain	0.1	Buried	[36]
318	M>R	Buried; little room for larger side chain	0	Buried	[27]
324	A>E	Buried in hydrophobic core	0	Buried	[26]
325	W>Stop	Stop	0	-	[39]
325	W>C	Buried in hydrophobic pocket	0	Buried	[28]
338	Q>Stop	Stop	0.2	-	[23]
340	G>D	Buried in hydrophobic pocket	0.4	Buried	[27]
341	S>R	Little room for larger side chain	0.8	Buried	[33]
343	M>L	Buried; little room for branched side chain	1.6	Buried	[40]

Position	Amino acid substitution	Effect on structure of GALNS	Access. (Å²)[a]	Mutation Category	Ref.
343	M>R	Buried; little room for larger side chain	1.6	Buried	[27]
344	D>N	Loss of buried ion pair with Arg380	0.1	Buried	[28]
344	D>E	Disruption of buried ion pair with Arg380	0.1	Buried	[32]
345	L>P	Little room for Pro side chain in helix	0.7	Buried	[32]
346	F>L	Loss of hydrophobic packing	0	Buried	[26]
351	A>V	Little room for branched side chain	5.6	Surface	[26]
352	L>P	Partly buried in hydrophobic pocket	2.0	Buried	[25]
357	P>L	Unknown	8.1	Surface	[23]
361	R>G	Loss of ion pair with Asp360	6.6	Surface	[32]
366	L>F	Unknown	7.1	Surface	[29]
369	L>P	Little room for Pro side chain	3.6	Surface	[23]
374	Q>Stop	Stop	17.0	-	[39]
376	R>Q	Unknown	16.6	Surface	[23]
380	R>T	Loss of buried ion pair with Asp344	1.2	Buried	[32]
380	R>S	Loss of buried ion pair with Asp344	1.2	Buried	[27]
386	R>C	Disruption of hydrophobic core	1.1	Buried	[32]
386	R>H	Disruption of hydrophobic core	1.1	Buried	[33]
388	D>N	Loss of ion pair with His103	5.1	Surface	[33]
391	M>V	Disruption of hydrophobic core	0	Buried	[41]
392	A>V	Little room for larger side chain	0	Buried	[23]
395	L>V	Unknown	4.1	Surface	[33]
395	L>P	Phi-psi angles not favored for Pro	4.1	Surface	[32]
398	H>D	Loss of ion pair with Glu460	2.5	Surface	[33]
401	H>Y	Loss of buried ion pair with Glu450	0.1	Buried	[29]
407	N>H	Disruption of buried hydrogen bonds	0.4	Buried	[28]
409	W>S	Unknown	7.5	Surface	[23]
421	G>E	Little room for larger side chain	2.3	Surface	[26]
422	Q>K	Disruption of hydrogen bonds	4.6	Surface	[26]
422	Q>Stop	Stop	4.6	-	[27]
450	E>V	Loss of buried ion pair with His401	0	Buried	[38]
452	F>I	Loss of hydrophobic packing	7.7	Surface	[42]
452	F>L	Loss of hydrophobic packing	7.7	Surface	[29]
470	S>P	Little room for Pro side chain in helix	24.3	Surface	[27]
473	Q>Stop	Stop	20.2	-	[26]
484	P>S	Unknown	4.1	Surface	[33]
487	N>S	Disruption of hydrogen bonds	6.9	Surface	[26]
488	V>M	Unknown	17.5	Surface	[28]
494	M>V	Little room for branched side chain	1.8	Buried	[25]

[a]Accessible surface area per side chain atom, measured in Å².

Understanding the structure, assembly and mechanisms of the enzymes in the degradation pathway of chondroitin sulfate can lead to new avenues for treatments for bone and cartilage diseases such as osteoarthritis, rheumatoid arthritis and many MPSs [45]. Chondroitin sulfate has been tested for efficacy as a treatment for arthritis patients [45, 46]. Additional structural information on GALNS binding to chondroitin sulfate can clarify the mechanism of action of GAGs as therapeutics.

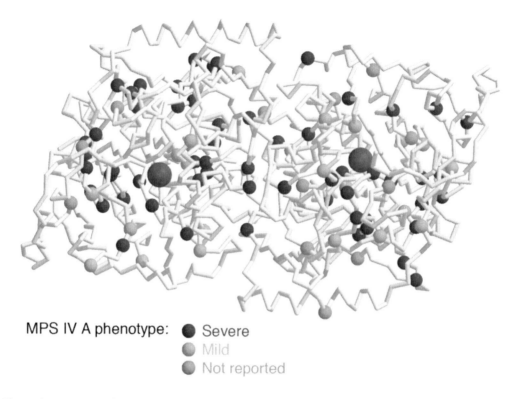

MPS IV A phenotype: ● Severe
                     ● Mild
                     ● Not reported

Figure 6. MPS IV A disease-causing mutations. Missense mutations are mapped onto the three dimensional structure of GALNS, along with their reported phenotype. The reported phenotype is indicated as severe (dark green), mild (light green) and not reported (yellow).

Conclusion

In conclusion, the structure of human GALNS has revealed the molecular basis for MPS IV A and the enzymatic mechanism of degradation of GAGs such as chondroitin sulfate. The active site of GALNS may be useful for rational drug design for compounds to stabilize the enzyme, leading to improved treatments for disease. The large fraction of MPS IV A mutations that map to the hydrophobic core of the GALNS protein suggest that the lysosomal storage disease is primarily a protein folding disease. The structure moves the disease toward personalized medicine, where the phenotype of a patient might be predicted (and therapeutic choices made) from understanding the effect of a mutation on the structure of the GALNS protein.

Acknowledgments

We gratefully acknowledge support from the National Institutes of Health (DK R01-76877 and T32 GM008515).

References

[1] M. F. Coutinho, L. Lacerda and S. Alves, "Glycosaminoaminoglycan storage disorders: a review," *Biochem Res Int,* Article ID 471325, 2012.

[2] J. Hernáiz and R. Linhardt, "Degradation of chondroitin sulfate and dermatan sulfate with chondroitin lyases," in *Proteoglycan Protocols*, Philadelphia, Humana Press, 2001, pp. 363-371.

[3] A. Dorfman, B. Arbogast and R. Matalon, "The enzymic defects in Morquio and Maroteaux-Lamy syndrome," *Adv Exp Med Biol,* vol. 68, pp. 261-276, 1976.

[4] E. Neufeld and J. Muenzer, "The mucopolysaccharidoses," in *In The Metabolic and Molecular Bases of Inherited Disease*, New York, McGraw-Hill, pp. 3421–3452, 2001.

[5] S. Tomatsu, A. Montaño, M. Gutierrez, J. Grubb, H. Oikawa, V. Dung et al., "Characterization and pharmacokinetic study of recombinant human *N*-acetylgalactosamine-6-sulfate sulfatase," *Mol Genet Metab,* vol. 91, pp. 69-78, 2007.

[6] Y. Rivera-Colón, E. Schutsky, A. Kita and S. Garman, "The structure of human GALNS reveals the molecular basis for mucopolysaccharidosis IV A," *J Mol Biol,* vol. 423, pp. 736-751, 2012.

[7] G. Parenti, G. Meroni and A. Ballabio, "The sulfatase gene family," *Curr Opin Genet Dev,* vol. 7, pp. 386-391, 1997.

[8] P. Bojarová and S. Williams, "Sulfotransferases, sulfatases and formylglycine-generating enzymes: A sulfation fascination," *Curr Opin Chem Biol,* vol. 12, pp. 573-581, 2008.

[9] M. Cosma, S. Pepe, I. Annunziata, R. Newbold, M. Grompe, G. Parenti et al., "The multiple sulfatase deficiency gene encodes an essential and limiting factor for the activity of sulfatases," *Cell,* vol. 113, pp. 445-456, 2003.

[10] T. Dierks, L. Schlotawa, M. Frese, K. Radhakrishnan, K. von Figura and B. Schmidt, "Molecular basis of multiple sulfatase deficiency, mucolipidosis II/III and Niemann–Pick C1 disease — lysosomal storage disorders caused by defects of non-lysosomal proteins," *Biochim Biophys Acta,* vol. 1793, pp. 710-725, 2009.

[11] I. Boltes, H. Czapinska, A. Kahnert, R. von Bülow, T. Dierks, B. Schmidt et al., "1.3 Å structure of arylsulfatase from *Pseudomonas aeruginosa* establishes the catalytic mechanism of sulfate ester cleavage in the sulfatase family," *Structure,* vol. 9, pp. 483-489, 2001.

[12] T. Dierks, B. Schmidt, L. Borissenko, J. Peng, A. Preusser, M. Mariappan et al., "Multiple sulfatase deficiency is caused by mutations in the gene encoding the human Cα-formylglycine generating enzyme," *Cell,* vol. 113, pp. 435-444, 2003.

[13] D. Roeser, A. Preusser-Kunze, B. Schmidt, K. Gasow, J. Wittmann, T. Dierks et al., "A general binding mechanism for all human sulfatases by the formylglycine-generating enzyme," *PNAS,* vol. 103, pp. 81-86, 2006.

[14] K. von Figura, B. Schmidt, T. Selmer and T. Dierks, "A novel protein modification generating an aldehyde group in sulfatases: its role in catalysis and disease," *Bioessays,* vol. 20, pp. 505-510, 1998.

[15] D. Ghosh, "Human sulfatases: a structural perspective to catalysis," *Cell Mol Life Sci,* vol. 64, pp. 2013-2022, 2007.

[16] S. Hanson, M. Best and C. Wong, "Sulfatases: structure, mechanism, biological activity, inhibition, and synthetic utility," *Angew Chem Int Ed Engl,* vol. 43, pp. 5736-5763, 2004.

[17] C. Bond, P. Clements, S. Ashby, C. Collyer, S. Harrop, J. Hopwood et al., "Structure of a human lysosomal sulfatase," *Structure,* vol. 5, pp. 277-289, 1997.

[18] F. Hernandez-Guzman, T. Higashiyama, W. Pangborn, Y. Osawa and D. Ghosh, "Structure of human estrone sulfatase suggests functional roles of membrane association," *J Biol Chem,* vol. 278, pp. 22989-22997, 2003.

[19] G. Lukatela, N. Krauss, K. Theis, T. Selmer, V. Gieselmann, K. von Figura et al., "Crystal structure of human arylsulfatase A: the aldehyde function and the metal ion at the active site suggest a novel mechanism for sulfate ester hydrolysis," *Biochemistry,* vol. 37, pp. 3654-3664, 1998.

[20] K. Sukegawa, H. Nakamura, Z. Kato, S. Tomatsu, A. Montaño, T. Fukao et al., "Biochemical and structural analysis of missense mutations in *N*-acetylgalactosamine-6-sulfate sulfatase causing mucopolysaccharidosis IVA phenotypes.," *Hum Mol Genet,* vol. 9, pp. 1283-1290, 2000.

[21] S. Tomatsu, A. Montaño, A. Ohashi, H. Oikawa, T. Oguma, V. Dung et al., "Enzyme replacement therapy in a murine model of Morquio A syndrome," *Hum Mol Genet,* vol. 17, pp. 815-824, 2008.

[22] "The Human Gene Mutation Database," [Online]. Available: http://www.hgmd.org. [Accessed 20 December 2012].

[23] S. Tomatsu, A. Montaño, T. Nishioka, M. Guiterrez, O. Pena, G. Tranda Firescu et al., "Mutation and polymorphism spectrum of the GALNS gene in mucopolysaccharidosis IVA (Morquio A)," *Hum Mutat,* vol. 26, pp. 500-512, 2005.

[24] S. Tomatsu, M. Filocamo, K. Orii, W. Sly, M. Gutierrez, T. Nishioka et al., "Mucopolysaccharidosis IVA (Morquio A): identification of novel common mutations in the *N*-acetylgalactosamine-6-sulfate sulfatase (GALNS) gene in Italian patients," *Hum Mutat,* vol. 24, pp. 187-188, 2004.

[25] Z. Wang, W. Zhang, Y. Wang, Y. Meng, L. Su, H. Shi et al., "Mucopolysaccharidosis IVA mutations in Chinese patients: 16 novel mutations," *J Hum Genet,* vol. 55, pp. 534-540, 2010.

[26] S. Bunge, W. Kleijer, A. Tylki-Szymanska, C. Steglich, M. Beck, S. Tomatsu et al., "Identification of 31 novel mutations in the N-acetylgalactosamine-6-sulfatase gene reveals excessive allelic heterogeneity among patients with Morquio A syndrome," *Hum Mutat,* vol. 10, pp. 223-232, 1997.

[27] T. Ogawa, S. Tomatsu, S. Fukuda, A. Yamagishi, G. Rezvi, K. Sukegawa et al., "Mucopolysaccharidosis IVA: screening and identification of mutations of the *N*-acetylgalactosamine-6-sulfate sulfatase gene," *Hum Mol Genet,* vol. 4, pp. 341-349, 1995.

[28] S. Tomatsu, T. Nishioka, A. Montaño, M. Gutierrez, O. Pena, K. Orii et al., "Mucopolysaccharidosis IVA: identification of mutations and methylation study in GALNS gene," *J Med Genet,* vol. 41, p. e98, 2004.

[29] N. Yamada, S. Fukuda, S. Tomatsu, V. Muller, J. Hopwood, J. Nelson et al., "Molecular heterogeneity in mucopolysaccharidosis IVA in Australia and Northern Ireland: nine novel mutations including T312S, a common allele that confers the mild phenotype," *Hum Mutat,* vol. 11, pp. 202-208, 1998.

[30] W. Qubbaj, A. Al-Aqeel, Z. Al-Hassnan, A. Al-Duraihim, K. Awartani, R. Al-Rejjal et al., "Preimplantation genetic diagnosis of Morquio disease," *Prenat Diagn,* vol. 10, pp. 900-903, 2008.

[31] Z. Kato, S. Fukuda, S. Tomatsu, H. Vega, T. Yasunaga, A. Yamagishi et al., "A novel common missense mutation G301C in the *N*-acetylgalactosamine-6-sulfate sulfatase gene in mucipolysaccharidosis IV A," *Hum Genet,* vol. 101, pp. 97-101, 1997.

[32] S. Tomatsu, T. Dieter, I. Schwartz, P. Sarmient, R. Giugliani, L. Barrera et al., "Identification of a common mutation in mucopolysaccharidosis IV A: a correlation among genotype, phenotype and keratan sulfate," *J Hum Genet,* vol. 49, pp. 490-494, 2004.

[33] S. Tomatsu, S. Fukuda, A. Cooper, J. Wraith, P. Ferreira, P. Di Natale et al., "Fourteen novel mucopolysaccharidosis IV A producing mutations in GALNS gene," *Hum Mutat,* vol. 10, pp. 368-375, 1997.

[34] M. Terzioglu, A. Tokatli, T. Coskun and S. Emre, "Molecular analysis of Turkish mucopolysaccharidosis IVA (Morquio A) patients: identification of novel mutations in the *N*-acetylgalactosamine-6-sulfate sulfatase (GALNS) gene," *Hum Mutat,* vol. 20, pp. 477-478, 2002.

[35] S. Fukuda, S. Tomatsu, M. Masue, K. Sukegawa, H. Iwata, T. Ogawa et al., "Mucopolysaccharidosis type IVA. N-acetylgalactosamine-6-sulfate sulfatase exonic point mutations in classical Morquio and mild cases," *J Clin Invest,* vol. 90, pp. 1049-1053, 1992.

[36] S. Tomatsu, S. Fukuda, A. Cooper, J. Wraith, G. Rezvi, A. Yamagishi et al., "Mucopolysaccharidosis type IVA: identification of six novel mutations among non-Japanese patients," *Hum Mol Genet,* vol. 4, pp. 741-743, 1995.

[37] A. Montaño, I. Kaitila, K. Sukegawa, S. Tomatsu, Z. Kato, H. Nakamura et al., "Mucopolysaccharidosis IVA: characterization of a common mutation found in Finnish patients with attenuated phenotype," *Hum Genet,* vol. 113, pp. 162-169, 2003.

[38] S. Laradi, T. Tukel, S. Khediri, J. Shabbeer, M. Erazo, L. Chkioua et al., "Mucopolysaccharidosis type IV: *N*-acetylgalactosamine-6-sulfatase mutations in Tunisian patients," *Mol Genet Metab,* vol. 87, pp. 213-218, 2006.

[39] S. Tomatsu, S. Fukuda, A. Cooper, J. Wraith, N. Yamada, K. Isogai et al., "Two new mutations, Q473X and N487S, in a Caucasian patient with mucopolysaccharidosis IVA (Morquio disease)," *Hum Mutat,* vol. 6, pp. 195-196, 1995.

[40] D. Cole, S. Fukuda, B. Gordon, J. Rip, A. LeCouteur, C. Rupar et al., "Heteroallelic missense mutations of the galactosamine-6-sulfate sulfatase (GALNS) gene in a mild form of Morquio disease (MPS IV A)," *Am J Med Genet,* vol. 63, pp. 558-565, 1996.

[41] S. Tomatsu, S. Fukuda, A. Cooper, J. Wraith, G. Rezvi, A. Yamagishi et al., "Mucopolysaccharidosis IVA: identification of a common missense mutation I113F in the *N*-Acetylgalactosamine-6-sulfate sulfatase gene," *Am J Hum Genet,* vol. 57, pp. 556-563, 1995.

[42] L. Carraresi, R. Parini, C. Filoni, A. Caciotti, G. Sersale, S. Tomatsu et al., "GALNS gene expression profiling in Morquio A patients' fibroblasts," *Clin Chim Acta,* vol. 397, pp. 72-76, 2008.

[43] A. Pshezhetsky and M. Ashmarina, "Lysosomal multienzyme complex: biochemistry, genetics, and molecular pathophysiology," *Prog Nucleic Acid Res Mol Biol,* vol. 69, pp. 81-114, 2001.

[44] A. Pshezhetsky and M. Potier, "Association of N-acetylgalactosamine-6-sulfate sulfatase with the multienzyme lysosomal complex of β-galactosidase, cathepsin A, and neuraminidase. Possible implication for intralysosomal catabolism of keratan sulfate," *J Biol Chem,* vol. 271, pp. 28359-28365, 1996.

[45] J. Monfort, J. Pelletier, N. Garcia-Giralt and J. Martel-Pelletier, "Biochemical basis of the effect of chondroitin sulphate on osteoarthritis articular tissues," *Ann Rheum Dis,* vol. 67, pp. 735-740, 2008.

[46] D. Uebelhart, "Clinical review of chondroitin sulfate in osteoarthritis," *Osteoarthritis Cartilage,* vol. 16, suppl 3, pp. s19-21, 2008.

In: Chondroitin Sulfate
Editor: Vitor H. Pomin

ISBN: 978-1-62808-490-0
© 2013 Nova Science Publishers, Inc.

Chapter 6

Pharmacoproteomics of Chondroitin Sulfate in Osteoarthritis Therapy

Valentina Calamia[1], Cristina Ruiz-Romero[1], Eulalia Montell[2],
Josep Vergés[2] and Francisco J. Blanco[1]

[1]Rheumatology Division, Proteomics Group-ProteoRed/ISCIII, INIBIC-CHU A Coruña,
A Coruña, Spain
[2]Pre-clinical R&D Area, Pharma Science Division, Bioibérica, Barcelona, Spain

Abstract

Chondroitin sulfate (CS) is a symptomatic slow-acting drug for osteoarthritis (OA) widely used for the treatment of this highly prevalent disease, which is mainly characterized by articular cartilage degradation. However, little is known about its mechanism of action and recent large-scale clinical trials have reported variable results on OA symptoms. Proteomic applications to pharmacological issues are termed pharmacoproteomics. In the field of OA research, quantitative proteomics technologies are demonstrating a very interesting power for studying the molecular effect of some drugs employed to treat OA patients, such as CS and glucosamine sulfate (GS). Herein, we present results on the modulations in the intracellular proteome and secretome of human articular cartilage cells treated with these drugs. An analysis of the effect of CS from different origin and purity using two complementary proteomic approaches (DIGE and SILAC) shows that three different CS compounds have diverse effects on the intracellular and extracellular human chondrocytes proteomes. Each of the studied compounds induced a characteristic protein profile in OA chondrocytes. CS from porcine origin displayed the widest effect, but increased cartilage oligomeric matrix protein and some catabolic or inflammatory factors like interstitial collagenase, stromelysin-1 and pentraxin-related protein. CS from bovine origin, on the other hand, increased a number of structural proteins, growth factors and extracellular matrix (ECM) proteins. Pharmacoproteomic approaches can also be useful to analyze the differences between simple and combined administration by proteomic analysis of normal human articular chondrocytes (HACs). A gel-based proteomic study using HACs stimulated with interleukin 1 beta (IL-1β) and treated with CS, alone or in combination with GS, shows a number of target proteins and points out the different mechanisms of action of these drugs. Regarding their predicted biological function, 35% of the proteins modulated by GS are involved in signal transduction pathways, 15% in redox and stress response, and 25% in protein synthesis and folding processes. Interestingly, CS affects mainly energy production (31%) and metabolic pathways (13%), decreasing the expression levels of ten proteins. Finally, an analysis of secretomes from normal chondrocytes stimulated with IL-1β, demonstrated how CS reduces inflammation directly, by decreasing the presence of several complement components (CFAB, C1S, CO3, and C1R) and also indirectly, by increasing proteins such as tumor necrosis factor-inducible gene 6 protein (TSG6). Moreover, a strong CS-dependent increase of an angiogenesis inhibitor, thrombospondin 1 (TSP-1), was found in this analysis. In summary, pharmacoproteomic studies of CS demonstrate that CS from porcine origin induces the activation of inflammatory and catabolic pathways, while bovine CS induces an anti-inflammatory and anabolic response. In addition, they unravel novel molecular evidences of the anti-angiogenic, anti-inflammatory, and anti-catabolic properties of CS in the presence of pro-inflammatory stimuli.

The overall goal of this review is to gather most of the available information about pharmacoproteomic studies of CS and also to discuss the clinical usefulness of proteomics and the perspectives for CS use in OA management.

Introduction

Osteoarthritis

Osteoarthritis (OA) is one of the most prevalent chronic diseases affecting more than 100 million individuals worldwide. Although its major features are progressive destruction of articular cartilage and extracellular matrix (ECM) breakdown [1], it is now accepted that OA is a global disease of the joint [2]. Synovial membrane, subchondral bone and periarticular soft tissues are involved in the onset and progression of the pathology (Figure 1), although chondrocytes are thought to play a primary role in mediating cartilage destruction [3]. These cells are essential in the control of matrix turnover through the production of structural proteins (like type II collagen and aggrecan) and enzymes (like metalloproteinases and aggrecanases), which are strictly necessary for the metabolism of the cartilage tissue. Therefore, human articular chondrocytes (HACs) primary culture is the technique most often used by researchers working on the pathogenesis of cartilage disorders, including OA.

Despite the increasing number of OA patients, due to the combination of an aged population and growing levels of obesity, treatments to manage this disease are limited to controlling pain and improving function and quality of life while limiting adverse events [4]. The drugs currently available are predominantly directed towards the symptomatic relief of pain and inflammation, but they do little to reduce joint destruction [5]. Unfortunately, effective therapies to regenerate damaged cartilage or to slow its degeneration have not been developed, leaving the only option of surgical interventions at advanced stages of the disease [6]. Early prevention of the structural damage still remains the key objective of new therapeutic approaches to treat OA. Until now, the pharmacological management of OA has been dominated by non-steroidal anti-inflammatory drugs (NSAIDs) and analgesics. However, multiple compounds, drugs and nutraceuticals have been investigated for their positive *in vitro* and/or *in vivo* effects [7-9]. Among them, symptomatic slow-acting drugs for osteoarthritis (SYSADOA) have been largely studied over the last decade. The use of chondroitin sulfate (CS) by OA patients, alone or in combination with glucosamine sulfate (GS), has been rising globally over the last decade. Both molecules are well recognized as SySADOA. Moreover, their application has an excellent safety profile, allowing long-term treatments [10-13]. Nevertheless, recent meta-analysis [14] and large-scale clinical trials [15] have demonstrated variable effects on OA symptoms. Although these reports were intended to resolve and clarify the clinical effectiveness of these supplements regarding OA [12, 14, 16-19], they leave doubts among the scientific community and fuel the controversy [20].

Chondroitin Sulfate in OA Therapy

CS has raised many interests over the past decades as a potential therapeutic drug against OA. More than three decades ago, it was proposed that CS supply could provide building blocks for the synthesis of new matrix components, since increasing CS concentration could act in favor of matrix regeneration and account for its beneficial effects as a therapeutic intervention to cartilage damage [21]. However, further data in the literature reveal that the mechanism of action of chondroitin sulfate is not limited to the fact that it is part of the aggrecan, one of the major structural proteoglycan found in the extracellular matrix of cartilage. *In vivo* studies in animal models and *in vitro* studies with human and animal articular cells suggest that the effects of CS result from a combination of numerous factors. CS has demonstrated the ability to diminish pro-inflammatory factors [22-25], to modify the chondrocyte death process [26], and to improve the anabolism/catabolism balance of extracellular cartilage matrix [10, 27]. It was also reported that CS could have an influence on the resorption process that takes place in the subchondral bone during OA [28]. CS was shown to have anti-oxidant properties [29]; it provides protection against hydrogen peroxide and superoxide anions by restoring endogenous anti-oxidants [30]. In addition, CS anti-angiogenic properties have been recently proven [31, 32].

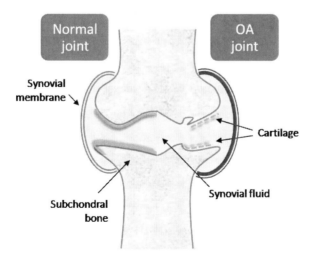

Figure 1. Schematic representation of normal (left) and OA (right) articular joint. Irreversible damages to joint structures are depicted: loss of articular cartilage, alterations in the subchondral bone, including osteophyte formation, and synovial inflammation.

CS is sold as over the counter dietary supplement in North America and is a prescription drug under the regulation of the European Medicine Agency (EMEA) in Europe. CS is part of the Osteoarthritis Research Society International (OARSI) recommendations for the management of knee OA [33, 34] and of the European League Against Rheumatism (EULAR) recommendations for the management of hip and knee OA [35, 36].

The Key Biochemical and Bioavailability Characteristics of CS for OA Treatment

CS is a natural sulfated glycosaminoglycan (GAG) present in the ECM surrounding cells, especially in the cartilage, skin, blood vessels, ligaments, tendons and brain, where it constitutes an essential component of proteoglycans (PGs). Chemically, CS is an unbranched polysaccharide formed by the (1→3) linkage of D-glucuronic acid to N-acetylgalactosamine, whose residues are sulfated either in position 4 (4-CS) or 6 (6-CS).

Some of its properties are due to its strong negative charge [37] capable to draw water into tissues and hydrates them [38]. The charge density values and the 4-sulfated/6-sulfated ratio are reliable parameters to determine the origin of the chondroitin sulfate contained in food supplement formulations. Regarding the different actions of CS isoforms, both C6S and C4S would exert an anti-arthritic action through mutual and individual mechanisms [39-42]. The sulfation pattern of chondroitin disaccharides from normal human articular cartilage varies with the age of the subject, the topography of the joint surface, and the zone of cartilage examined [43]. Measurements of 4- and 6-S disaccharides in joint fluids have been published as "markers" of proteoglycan metabolism [44]. Changes in chondroitin sulfation were also exploited in an attempt to differentiate between catabolic processes in inflammatory and noninflammatory arthritis [45] and most recently to differentiate between patients with different subsets of osteoarthritis [44]. Finally, the evaluation of the molecular mass parameters of chondroitin sulfate is a key factor related to pharmacological activity as degraded products are unable to produce comparable biological effects [46]. The sulfation heterogeneity which is responsible for great charge density variability as well as the number of disaccharide units forming the polymer are two key factors influencing biological and pharmacological activity of CS. As a consequence, sulfation grade and molecular mass parameters are of paramount importance for CS properties [47].

CS, like other natural macromolecules, has a complex structure that is known to change with the source tissue, organ and species [47]. CS from different sources contains disaccharides possessing sulfate groups in different positions and in different percentages within the polysaccharide chains [46]. Moreover, extraction and purification processes may introduce further modifications of the structural characteristics and properties, and may led to extracts more or less rich in chondroitin sulfate [46]. Additionally, CS is administered orally during therapy and bioavailability and pharmacokinetic parameters have been reported to change depending on its structural characteristics and origin [48, 49]. As a consequence, the low quality CS generally present in nutraceuticals would be unable to exert comparable pharmacological effects to those of the pharmaceutical-grade chondroitin sulfate.

Although the oral bioavailability of the drug is acceptable (15–24%), about 90% is depolymerised or degraded either in plasma or in the joints [11, 50]. Many *in vitro* studies have used high and variable concentrations of CS, ranging from 12.5 to 2000 µg/ml, but generally 200 µg/ml or lower. The relationship between *in vitro* pharmacological studies and what may be expected *in vivo* is therefore a matter that has still to be resolved for some target actions. This is particularly evident as, in general, only CS has been investigated for effects *in vitro* and virtually no information is available on the mixture of depolymerised or degradation products that are known to exist in inflamed joints [51]. Nonetheless, these *in vitro* investigations have provided insight into the likely actions of CS [11, 16, 29, 38, 50, 52-54]. Among the actions proposed from *in vitro* investigations (mainly using chondrocytes or cartilage explants of bovine or human origin) are: increased synthesis of proteoglycan and hyaluronic acid and aggrecan, blockade of proteoglycan degradation by interleukin-1 and other pro-inflammatory cytokines and metalloproteinases, prevention of oxyradical formation, reduction in chondrocyte signalling pathways (p38, MAPK and Erk1/2, nuclear factor κB (NFκB) for example, leading to the downstream gene-regulated production of cyclooxygenase-2, phospholipases, cytokines, metalloproteinases), control of apoptosis, and stress- or ageing-related changes in regeneration or repair [54]. Thus, as summarised in Figure 2, CS has inhibitory effects on multiple cartilage catabolic reactions whilst also enhancing anabolic processes.

Several *in vivo* studies in models of inflammatory joint destruction have confirmed and further established the anti-inflammatory effects of CS [11, 22, 50]. A particularly interesting recent finding has been that CS affects the expression of the receptor activator of NFκB ligand (RANKL) in relation to the expression of osteoprotegerin (a scavenger of RANKL) in such a way as to potentially control destructive processes in subchondral bone in OA [28]. Overall, the results of these investigations show that CS fulfills the biochemical requirements for being a biological response modifier at the level of biochemical evidence [51]. While evidence of the effects of degradation products *in vitro* is still required, the data show that CS itself has defined effects that are unique and influence the degradative processes in OA.

Proteomics in OA Research

Proteomics is a powerful technique for investigating protein expression profiles in biological systems and their modifications in response to stimuli or particular physiological or pathophysiological conditions. The basic scheme for proteomics relies on the separation of a large number of proteins and their identification by mass spectrometry (MS). The separation strategy is a critical step in proteomics, and may be accomplished using gel electrophoresis [55-61] or gel-free [31, 62-65] techniques usually including one or more chromatographic steps (Figure 3).

In OA research, proteomics has become a useful technology for gaining an understanding of the complex and unknown processes that participate in joint disease pathogenesis. In this field, our group exhibits a good track record employing quantitative proteomics technologies for improved diagnosis, prognosis and treatment of osteoarthritis. We started with the analysis of joint proteomes employing two-dimensional gel electrophoresis, as summarized in figure 4.

The first proteomic studies were carried out on cartilage cells (chondrocytes). Cartilage predominantly consists of water, with a high concentration of anionic macromolecules, including hyaluronan, aggrecan, and collagens, all of which build the extracellular matrix. Thus, the molecular composition of this tissue presents huge technical problems for proteomics studies. Therefore, the use of primary chondrocytes in culture represents a good alternative for the proteomic identification of OA targets. In normal conditions, these highly specialized cells are responsible for maintaining the structural and functional properties of the tissue [66]. This requires a delicate balance between the synthesis and degradation of the ECM components, which is controlled by the expression of anabolic and catabolic factors and their abundance in the tissue [67]. During OA, this balance is not maintained and dysregulation of chondrocyte metabolism leads to progressive degradation of the cartilage matrix. Indeed, chondrocytes isolated from OA cartilage show differing patterns of protein expression compared to healthy articular chondrocytes [60]. This alteration can be defined in terms of changes in protein expression levels inside the chondrocytes [60, 61, 68], and also on the proteins that are secreted by these cells into the surrounding tissue (the so- called "secretome") [62]. Alterations in the secretome can further disrupt the homeostasis of the ECM, potentially contributing to further cartilage loss [62].

Initially, two-dimensional gel electrophoresis (2-DE) and MS-based methods were employed to describe the cellular proteome of normal and osteoarthritic human chondrocytes in basal conditions [58-60], and also under proinflammatory cytokine (IL-1β) stimulation [56]. More recently, and due to the limitations of this technique regarding sensitivity and automatization, liquid chromatography coupled to tandem mass spectrometry (LC-MS/MS) techniques have begun to exercise their dominance in the OA research field [31, 63-65].

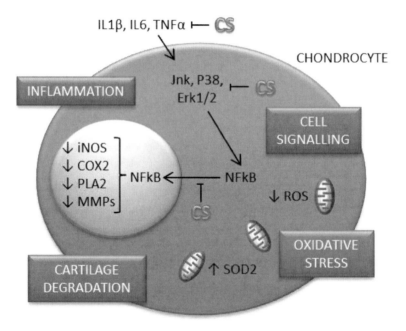

Figure 2. Schematic representation of chondroitin sulfate (CS) targets in OA chondrocytes as revealed by *in vitro* studies. CS primarily acts on cell signalling, inflammatory and catabolic pathways and on oxidative stress.

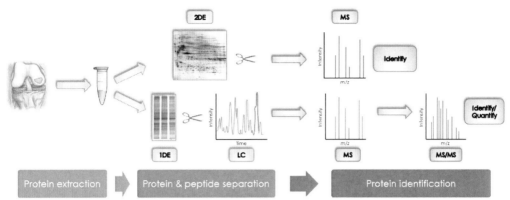

Figure 3. Gel-based and gel-free proteomic strategies in osteoarthritis research. These procedures are also termed MS-based proteomics because in both cases protein analysis and identification are carried out using mass spectrometry (MS). Similar to gel-based technique, chromatographic process may consist of one or more separation steps, including 1D gel electrophoresis. 1DE/2DE: monodimensional/bidimensional electrophoresis. LC: liquid chromatography. MS: mass spectrometry.

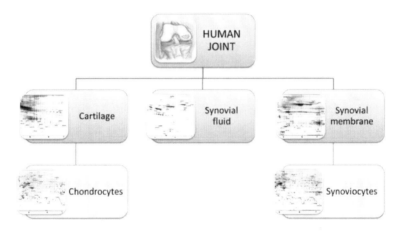

Figure 4. Different protein samples obtained from human joints for two-dimensional electrophoresis (2-DE) analysis.

Pharmacoproteomic Studies of CS for OA Therapy

Cartilage proteomics not only aims at elucidating pathophysiological mechanism underlying joint destruction but also at the identification of new drug targets for the treatment of OA. The application of proteomic technologies in the field of drug discovery development and assessment of drug administration is known as pharmacoproteomics. In the past few years, global proteomics profiling of drug treatment-induced changes in protein expression levels and/or post-translational modifications have started to become possible, mostly due to significant improvements in instrumentation. Therefore, proteomics strategies are being extensively applied by our group for the study of modes of action, side-effects and toxicity of anti-OA drugs. Ideally, tissues (cartilage, synovium, and subchondral bone), cell cultures (chondrocyte, synoviocytes, and osteoblast/osteoclast), and biological fluids (serum, plasma, and synovial fluid) can be used to study the drug's interaction with all components of the articular joint.

The pharmacoproteomics studies began with the analysis of cartilage cell cultures. Intracellular and extracellular proteome analyses of human articular chondrocytes treated with different exogenous CS, alone or in combination with GS, were performed by our group to more clearly define CS effects on cartilage biology. As the treatment efficacy of this compound appears to vary with the pathological severity of OA, we decided to use in some experiments an OA *in vitro* model consisting of normal human chondrocytes stimulated with interleukin 1 beta (IL-1β), a proinflammatory cytokine that acts as a mediator to drive the key pathways associated with OA pathogenesis [62].

Gel-Based Pharmacoproteomic Analyses of the Effect of CS on the Chondrocyte Intracellular Protein Profile

CS-mediated Changes in Chondrocytes Proteome

To date, several *in vitro* studies have shown how CS and GS could moderate some aspects of the deleterious response of chondrocytes to stimulation with IL-1β. In chondrocyte cultures, CS and GS diminish the IL-1β-mediated increase of metalloproteases [69, 70] the expression of phospholipase A2 [50, 71] and cyclooxygenase-2 [72] and the concentrations of prostaglandin E2 [73]. They also reduce the concentration of pro-inflammatory cytokines, such as tumor necrosis factor-α (TNF-α) and IL-1β, in joints, [74] and systemic and joint concentrations of nitric oxide [24] and reactive oxygen species (ROS) [75]. In 2010, we published the first pharmacoproteomic study aimed to unravel the molecular mechanisms driven by CS [76]. This study was focused on the investigation of the intracellular mechanisms modulated by CS and GS, which are the background for ulterior putative changes of ECM turnover. A classical gel-based proteomic study by two-dimensional gel electrophoresis (2-DE) was performed, whose schematic workflow is illustrated in Figure 5. Briefly, it consists in separating proteins by their isoelectric point and then by size (two dimensions) in a polyacrylamide gel, which is then stained with a fluorescent dye to visualize the protein spots [77]. Gel images are digitized for analysis and the interesting proteins are cut from the gel for its identification by mass spectrometry (MS) [78].

To assess the influence of CS alone or in combination with GS on the intracellular pathways of normal HACs stimulated with IL-1β, five different conditions were compared: cells before treatment (basal), IL-1β-treated cells (control), IL-1β + CS-treated cells, IL-1β + GS-treated cells and IL-1β + CS + GS-treated cells. 2-DE gels of each condition were obtained from three healthy donors (a representative image of them is shown in Figure 5). The 15 digitalized images of these gels were analyzed using dedicated software. After data normalization, 23 spots corresponding to 21 proteins were found to be altered with statistical significance by CS-treatment. These proteins are listed in Table 1. As shown in the Table, most of them are proteins related to metabolism (13%) and energy production (31%), and proteins related to glycolysis represent the largest functional group (we identified seven out of the ten enzymes that directly participate in this pathway). Remarkably, all except one (an enolase isoform) were decreased by CS. This suggests that, while IL-1β treatment tends to elevate glycolytic energy production [55, 56], it is then lowered by CS (which reduces five of these enzymes) and by the combination of both drugs (which reduces all seven glycolytic enzymes). Furthermore, the decrease of Neutral alpha-glucosidase AB (or glucosidase II, GANAB), and two other metabolism-related proteins (AK1C2 and UGDH), points also to a reduction of cellular metabolism.

When administered in combination with GS, the number of modulated proteins grows up to 28 (31 spots, see Table 1). Apart from energy production, they are mainly involved in protein synthesis and folding (PDIA1, PDIA3, GRP78), redox and stress responses (SOD2, HSPB1). Interestingly, only four proteins were found to be modulated by CS and GS (DPYL2, HSPB1, PGAM1, TAGL2) in combination but not by either of the drugs alone, whereas a quantitative synergistic effect of the combination was observed in a half of the altered proteins (Table 1). One of these proteins is the mitochondrial superoxide dismutase SOD2, which has substantial relevance in stress oxidative pathways and in cytokine-related diseases, such as OA [61, 79]. SOD2 was found to be increased by IL-1β [55, 56, 62], and decreased by CS and GS treatment, both at the transcriptional and protein levels (Real Time-PCR and Western Blotting). Thus, the influence of CS, alone or combined with GS, on oxidative stress is a possible mechanism of action for its protective effect on articular chondrocytes. The other biochemical pathways that may be altered when chondrocytes are treated with CS alone and/or in combination with GS are also indicated in Table 1.

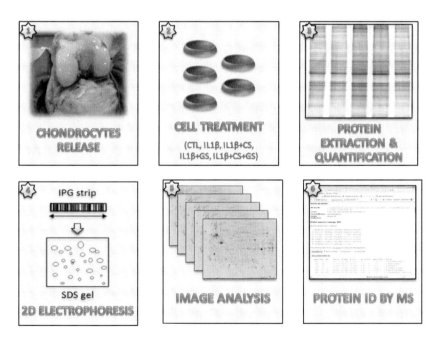

Figure 5. Schematic workflow of a gel-based (2DE) proteomic analysis of the effect of CS on human articular chondrocytes.

Finally, proteomic analysis of CS-treated HACs led to the identification of a number of putative target proteins, pointing out the wide-ranging effects of this drug, both in simple and combined administration (Figure 6). Until then, previous *in vitro* studies had shown similar results for both molecules mainly related to their anti-inflammatory effect. Employing a classical proteomic approach we highlighted, for the first time, the different intracellular pathways affected by CS or GS.

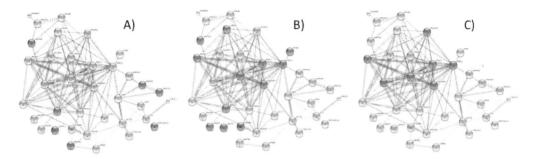

Figure 6. Protein-protein interaction network of chondrocytic CS-modulated intracellular proteins. The STRING database was searched for protein interaction analyses in order to elucidate the effect of CS, alone or in combination with GS, on normal chondrocytes stimulated with IL1β and OA chondrocytes. As shown in this Figure, almost all (27) of the altered proteins interact with each other to constitute a big network. These proteins are involved in three main GO biological processes: A) apoptosis, B) metabolism, and C) glycolysis.

Influence of CS Origin and Purity on its Effect on the Chondrocyte Proteome

It should be noted that CS employed in scientific studies is generally derived from animal sources by extraction and purification processes and is mainly obtained from bovine, porcine, chicken or marine cartilage. From these, bovine CS is the most often used *in vitro* and in clinical trials [80]. Although beneficial effects of orally administered CS in OA patients have been reported, caution should be exercised in the study or use of different CS formulations, as the species or tissue of origin could result in great differences in CS structural organization or disaccharide composition. In some cases the quality of the CS formulations (as those available as dietary supplements in some countries, such as the United States) is not strictly regulated, and this may affect the therapeutic outcome because of differences in molecular composition, tissue of origin, purity, and production/purification processes. Therefore, in our second pharmacoproteomic study, the best quantitative gel-based strategy to date (differential in-gel electrophoresis, DIGE), was followed to investigate deeper the diverse effects of three different CS compounds. The DIGE technique, is based on the fluorescent labelling of protein samples before mixing and running them on a 2D gel with a pool of all samples as an internal standard for quantification [81]. It permits the direct quantitative evaluation of changes, reduces inter-gel variation and false positives [82, 83], and results in highly reproducible data with biological significance.

To assess the influence of three different types of CS on the intracellular proteome of human OA chondrocytes, four different conditions were compared: cells before treatment (basal condition), CS1-treated cells (porcine origin, 90.4% purity), CS2-treated cells (bovine origin, 96.2% purity), and CS3-treated cells (bovine origin, 99.9% purity) [84]. All CS, originated from different manufacturers, were provided by Bioibérica S.A. (Barcelona, Spain). The samples were subjected to a six-plex 2-D DIGE analysis, and the gel images that were obtained were analyzed using SameSpots software, which allowed the detection of an average of 1500 protein spots on each image. The quantitative comparison between the effect of each CS compound and the basal condition (untreated OA chondrocytes) revealed the alteration of 28 spots in the gels, corresponding to 18 different proteins (Table 2). CS1 modulated 18 spots corresponding to 10 different proteins: 3 were decreased and 7 increased.

CS2 only decreased the expression of 1 protein, LEG3. Finally, CS3 modulated 9 spots corresponding to 7 different proteins: 4 were increased and 3 decreased (see Table 2).

Table 1. Chondrocyte intracellular proteins altered by CS, alone or in combination with GS, in IL1β-stimulated cells [55]

Cellular role	Protein name	Symbol	CS[‡]	CS+GS[‡]
Cell adhesion	Collagen alpha-1(VI) chain precursor	CO6A1	↓	↓
Cell cycle	Septin-2	SEPT2	↓	
Detoxification	Glutathione S-transferase P	GSTP1	↓	↓
	Superoxide dismutase mitochondrial	SODM		↓
Glycolysis	Fructose-bisphosphate aldolase A	ALDOA	↓	↓↓
	Alpha-enolase[*]	ENOA		↓
	Alpha-enolase[*]	ENOA	↑	↑
	Glyceraldehyde-3-phosphate dehydrogenase	G3P	↓	↓↓
	Pyruvate kinase isozymes M1/M2	KPYM	↓	↓↓
	Phosphoglycerate mutase 1	PGAM1		↓
	Phosphoglycerate kinase 1	PGK1	↓	↓
	Triosephosphate isomerase	TPIS	↓	↓↓
Metabolism	Aldo-keto reductase family 1 member C2	AK1C2	↓	↓↓
	Dihydropyrimidinase-related protein 2	DPYL2		↓
	Neutral alpha-glucosidase AB	GANAB	↓	
	UDP-glucose 6-dehydrogenase	UGDH	↓	↓
Respiration	ATP synthase subunit alpha, mitochondrial	ATPA	↓	↓↓
Protein synthesis & folding	78 kDa glucose-regulated protein precursor	GRP78		↑
	Heat shock cognate 71 kDa protein	HSP7C	↑	↑↑
	Protein disulfide-isomerase precursor	PDIA1	↑	↑↑
	Protein disulfide-isomerase A3 precursor[*]	PDIA3	↑	↑↑
	Protein disulfide-isomerase A3 precursor[*]	PDIA3	↑	↑↑
	T-complex protein 1 subunit gamma	TCPG	↓	↓↓
	Elongation factor 1-gamma	EF1G	↓	↓↓
Signal transduction	Annexin A1	ANXA1	↑	↑↑
	Annexin A5	ANXA5		↑
	Rho GDP-dissociation inhibitor 1	GDIR		↑
Stress response	Heat shock protein beta-1	HSPB1		↓
Cellular role	**Protein name**	**Symbol**	**CS‡**	**CS+GS‡**
Structural	Actin, cytoplasmic 1	ACTB		↓
	Gelsolin	GELS	↑	↑↑
	Transgelin-2	TAGL2		↓
Trafficking	Annexin A2[*]	ANXA2	↑	↑
	Annexin A2[*]	ANXA2	↑	↑

[‡]Average volume ratio vs IL-1β, quantified by PDQuest 7.3.1. software.
[*] Different isoforms. Double arrows indicate a synergistic effect.

The DIGE experiment thus allowed discriminating the diverse effects on chondrocytes of CS from different origin and purity. As observed in our first pharmacoproteomic analysis [55], in this study those proteins related to glycolysis and metabolism also represent the largest functional group modulated by CS in OA chondrocytes (Figure 6). Among them, a protein related to glycan metabolism, the neutral alpha-glucosidase AB (GANAB) is decreased by CS1 and CS3 treatment. GANAB is an ER-enzyme that has profound effects on the early events of glycoprotein metabolism and has been recently proposed as biomarker for detecting mild human knee osteoarthritis [85]. In this case, the results confirm those previously described [55], and demonstrate that GANAB is decreased by CS-treatment either in normal chondrocytes stimulated with IL1β and in OA chondrocytes. The effect of CS2 is more noticeable at the extracellular level (see next paragraph), whereas CS3 seems to affect mainly structural proteins, such as vimentin and caldesmon. As recently described, chondrocytes isolated from OA cartilage exhibit a disruption on the vimentin cytoskeleton [86]. Therefore, we hypothesized that CS3 could be effective in restoring a proper cytoskeleton network in OA-affected chondrocytes.

Table 2. List of chondrocyte intracellular proteins altered by three different CS compounds in OA cells [84]

Cellular role	Protein name	Symbol	CS1*	CS2*	CS3*
Cell adhesion	Vinculin	VINC	↓		
Glycolysis	Alpha-enolase	ENOA			↑
	Fructose-bisphosphate aldolase A[#]	ALDOA	↑		
	L-lactate dehydrogenase A chain	LDHA	↑		
	Pyruvate kinase isozymes M1/M2	KPYM	↑		
Inflammatory response	Galectin-3	LEG3		↓	
Metabolism	Glutamate dehydrogenase 1, mitochondrial	DHE3			↓
	Neutral alpha-glucosidase AB	GANAB	↓		
	Nicotinamide N-methyltransferase	NNMT	↑		
	Nicotinamide phosphoribosyltransferase	NAMPT	↑		
Protein synthesis & degradation	Proteasome subunit beta type-1	PSB1			↓
	Heat shock cognate 71 kDa protein	HSP7C			↑
	GTP-binding nuclear protein Ran	RAN	↑		
Redox regulation	Peroxiredoxin-4	PRDX4			↓
	Superoxide dismutase [Mn], mitochondrial[#]	SODM	↑		
Structural	Caldesmon[#]	CALD1			↑
	Lamin-A/C[#]	LMNA	↓		
	Vimentin	VIME			↑

[#]Different isoforms. *Average normalized volumes automatically recorded by the SameSpots software.

Pharmacoproteomic Analyses of the Effect of CS on the Profile of Chondrocyte Secreted Proteins (Secretome)

Once the utility of proteomics for analyzing the intracellular targets of this drug was proved, we decided to move on the analysis of the subset of chondrocyte extracellular proteins that are essential for cartilage ECM synthesis and turnover processes. The formation and organization of the cartilage ECM network depend on interactions of a number of molecules, mainly proteins, secreted by the resident cells (chondrocytes and synoviocytes) or carried by the bloodstream to the synovial joint. ECM is not only the scaffold for the anchorage of cartilage cells, the chondrocytes, but also confers articular cartilage some of its unique characteristics like load-bearing capability and compressive resistance. It is primarily composed of collagens and proteoglycans, which are invariably associated with other components, especially growth factors, cytokines, proteases, and protease inhibitors. Together, they comprise the cartilage extracellular environment and are pivotal for various disease processes, such as OA.

To date, only few studies had specifically targeted cartilage extracellular environment [87-89]. Moreover, most proteomics studies use whole cellular lysates, which are rich in cellular proteins that inevitably mask the identification of the less abundant proteins of the ECM. Thus, the composition of the cartilage ECM and its associated proteins remains poorly defined. Although HACs supernatants lack the complexity of the intact cartilage ECM, chondrocyte secretome may represent an attractive sub-proteome for understanding those mechanisms responsible of matrix remodelling, elucidating those pathophysiological pathways underlying cartilage degeneration during the OA process and also for the discovery of candidate OA biomarkers.

To avoid the limitations inherent to gel-based studies, and aiming to increase the dynamic range for more accurate protein quantification, an alternative quantitative proteomics method was developed in our laboratory. This strategy is based on stable isotope labelling with amino acids in cell culture (SILAC) for the quantitative analysis of chondrocytes proteome and secretome [62]. For the first time a complete labeling of the whole chondrocytes proteome (intracellular and extracellular proteins) was achieved, while maintaining their characteristic phenotype. This novel approach was useful for differential proteomic studies, including pharmacoproteomic analyses. The objective in SILAC experiments is to quantify the different protein abundance between two proteomes by the molecular weight of the light or heavy amino acids that are used during the growth of the two cell populations [90, 91]. During the cell culture, incorporation of the heavy amino acid into a peptide led to a known mass shift (easily detectable by mass spectrometry) compared with the peptide that contains the light version of the amino acid, but to no other chemical changes, thus allowing heavy and light samples to be mixed prior to LC-MS analysis. Then, protein quantification can be performed by calculating the protein abundance as ratios of the areas of the MS peaks of labeled *versus* unlabeled peptides. Figure 7 describes a typical SILAC proteomic workflow.

In this second part of the chapter we will focus on the results obtained with this novel methodology applied to the secretome analysis of CS-treated HACs. As for the intracellular proteome analysis, this study was carried out both in normal chondrocytes stimulated with IL-1β and in OA chondrocytes treated with the three different CS compounds.

CS-mediated Changes in the Chondrocytes Secretome

Employing this methodology, we first studied the secretome of primary HACs under IL-1β stimulation [62]. Then, we employed this model to generate a quantitative profile of chondrocytes extracellular protein changes driven by CS, always in presence of the same proinflammatory stimulus, in order to provide novel molecular evidences of CS effects [31].

Briefly, supernatants from IL1β-stimulated chondrocytes, with or without CS treatment, were collected after 48 hours of incubation. Then, equal amounts of proteins from the experimental conditions to be compared (treated or untreated with CS, both in the presence of the cytokine) were combined and the mixed samples were digested with trypsin, separated by liquid chromatography (LC) and subsequently analyzed by mass spectrometry (MALDI-MS/MS). This procedure resulted in the identification and quantification of 75 proteins present in the culture media of IL1β-treated cells with statistical confidence. Eighteen of them presented a significant alteration of their levels due to the pharmacological treatment (relative protein abundance calculated as average SILAC ratios in CS-treated versus untreated cells), which are shown in Table 3. They are involved in several processes, like cartilage ECM structural organization (including non-collagenous proteins and proteoglycans), ECM remodelling (including proteases and their inhibitors), immune response and angiogenesis. Figure 8 shows the interactions found by informatics analysis between the proteins belonging to the diverse functional groups. Interestingly, we detected a global decrease of immunity-related proteins, degradative enzymes (such as MMP1, MMP2, and MMP3), and some ECM structural proteins (such as fibronectin and chitinase-3-like protein 1) in CS-treated cells.

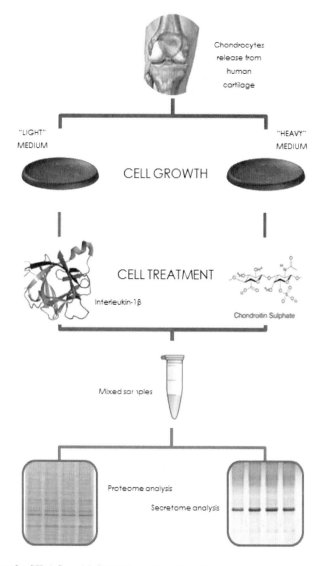

Figure 7. Workflow of a SILAC and LC-MS-based proteomics experiment.

Table 3. Chondrocyte extracellular proteins identified by SILAC and liquid chromatography-mass spectrometry (LC-MS) analysis whose secretion is modulated by CS treatment on IL1β-stimulated cells [31]

	Function	**Protein name**	**Symbol**
Decreased	Angiogenesis	Lactadherin	MFGM
		72 kDa type IV collagenase	MMP2
	Cell adhesion	Fibronectin	FINC
	Cell growth	Target of Nesh-SH3	TARSH
	ECM remodelling	Interstitial collagenase	MMP1
		Stromelysin-1	MMP3
	ECM structure	Chitinase-3-like protein 1	CH3L1
	Immunity	Complement factor B	CFAB
		Complement C1s subcomponent	C1S
		Complement C3	CO3
		Complement C1r subcomponent	C1R
		Clusterin	CLUS
Increased	Angiogenesis	Thrombospondin-1	TSP1
	Cell adhesion	Tumor necrosis factor-inducible gene 6 protein	TSG6
	Cell growth	Glia-derived nexin	SERPINE2
	ECM structure	Proteoglycan 4	PRG4
	Immunity	Beta-2-microglobulin	B2MG
	Redox	Sulfhydryl oxidase 1	QSOX1

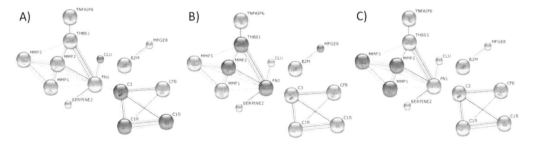

Figure 8. Protein-protein interaction network of ECM proteins whose secretion by chondrocytes is modulated with CS. The STRING database was searched for protein interaction analyses in order to elucidate the effect of CS on normal chondrocytes stimulated with IL1β. As shown in this Figure, almost all (14) of the altered proteins interact with each other to constitute a big network. These proteins are involved in three main GO biological processes: A) complement activation, B) collagen metabolic process, C) and angiogenesis.

We showed in this study how CS could reduce inflammation directly, by decreasing the presence of several complement components (see Table 3) and also indirectly, by increasing proteins such as tumor necrosis factor α-induced protein (TSG6). The mechanism driven by TSG6 leads to a decrease in proMMPs activation, which directly correlates with the decline in MMP1 and MMP3 levels observed in CS-treated chondrocytes even in the presence of acute inflammation (represented in our case by a high level of IL1β). These results point to the increase of TSG6 as a putative mediator of the reduction in proMMPs activation, suggesting an important role of this mechanism for the anti-catabolic effect of CS. Among those extracellular proteins described as decreased by IL1β [62] which were now increased by CS, we found thrombospondin 1 (TSP1), a potent angiogenesis inhibitor. In IL1β-stimulated chondrocytes, TSP1 presented a ratio IL1β/basal = 0, indicating a cytokine-dependent dramatic decrease of its release from these cells [62]. CS is capable to counteract the IL1β suppressive effect on TSP1 in normal chondrocytes, but also increases its secretion in OA cells without cytokine stimulation [31]. Furthermore, the selective inhibition of angiogenesis was also confirmed by the decrease of lactadherin, a protein which promotes the VEGF-dependent neo-vascularization [92], demonstrating a novel mechanism of action of CS in accordance with recent results obtained in synoviocytes [93].

Influence of CS Origin and Purity on Its Effect on the Chondrocyte Secretome

Once chondrocyte secretome emerged as an attractive starting point for the discovery of new OA drug targets, data from DIGE experiment (above reviewed) were complemented by analyzing secretomes from OA CS-treated chondrocytes employing the SILAC technique [84]. The same types of CS, previously used in the DIGE experiment, were tested: CS1 (porcine, purity 90.4%), CS2 (bovine, purity 96.2%), and CS3 (bovine, purity 99.9%).

Supernatants from SILAC-labeled chondrocytes, untreated and treated with CS, were collected after 48 hours of stimulation and analyzed by LC-MS/MS as reported above [94]. This procedure resulted in the identification and quantification of 96 proteins present in the culture media of CS1-treated condition, 95 proteins present in the culture media of CS2-treated condition, and 106 proteins present in the culture media of CS3-treated condition. A database search was performed to analyze the predicted subcellular localization of the proteins identified by this approach. As expected, most of them were cartilage ECM proteins, or proteins with well-established matrix functions. We were able to quantify in a relative way most of the identified proteins by comparing their SILAC ratios. Globally, 32 of these proteins exhibited a significant quantitative modulation of their secretion due to the pharmacological treatment. As indicated in Table 4, each of the studied compounds alters in a specific way the profile of proteins secreted by OA chondrocytes.

This study demonstrated how CS1 remarkably up-regulates catabolic pathways, by increasing the expression of degradative enzymes such as metalloproteases (MMP1 and MMP3) and reducing structural molecules such as collagens (COL12A1, COL15A1) and proteoglycans (HPLN1). In addition, CS1 also increased the secretion of inflammatory mediator such as pentraxin-related protein (PTX3). On the other hand, most of the proteins altered by bovine CS are growth factors: CS2 modulated proteins belonging to the IGF and the TGF-β families, while CS3 increased the connective tissue growth factor (CTGF), which promotes chondrocytes proliferation and differentiation [95]. CS3 also increased some extracellular matrix components, like prolargin (PRELP), and COL15A1. Contrary to porcine CS (CS1) that clearly evokes a catabolic and pro-inflammatory response in OA chondrocytes, those from bovine origin (CS2 and CS3) seem to induce mainly an anabolic response in OA chondrocytes increasing a number of structural proteins, growth factors and ECM proteins.

Altogether, the studies performed on the chondrocyte secretome samples highlight the usefulness of these type of approaches to specifically analyze the *in vitro* effects of CS on cartilage proteins involved in ECM synthesis and turnover, as they favor the identification of this subset of proteins (Figure 9).

Table 4. Chondrocyte extracellular proteins identified by SILAC and LC-MS analysis, whose secretion is modulated by three different CS treatments in OA chondrocytes [84]

Function	Protein name	Symbol	CS1*	CS2*	CS3*
Angiogenesis	Annexin A2	ANXA2		↓	
	Plasminogen activator inhibitor 1	SERPINE1			↑
	Thrombospondin-1	THBS1	↑	↑	
Ca^{2+} homeostasis	Nucleobindin-1	NUCB1			↑
Cell adhesion	Fibronectin	FN1	↑		
	Fibulin-1	FBLN1	↑		
	Periostin	POSTN		↓	
	Tenascin	TNC	↑	↓	
Cell growth & differentiation	Connective tissue growth factor	CTGF			↑
	Follistatin-related protein 1	FSTL1		↑	
	Glia-derived nexin	SERPINE2	↑		
	Insulin-like growth factor-binding protein 2	IGFBP2	↑	↑	
	Insulin-like growth factor-binding protein 3	IGFBP3		↑	
	Insulin-like growth factor-binding protein 7	IGFBP7	↑	↑	↑
	Transforming growth factor-beta-induced protein ig-h3	TGFBI	↓	↓	
Cell structure	Actin, cytoplasmic 2	ACTG1	↓	↓	↑
	Vimentin	VIM			↑
ECM remodelling	Cathepsin D	CTSD	↓		
	Interstitial collagenase	MMP1	↑		
	Metalloproteinase inhibitor 1	TIMP1	↑		
	Stromelysin-1	MMP3	↑		
ECM structure	Cartilage oligomeric matrix protein	COMP	↑		
	Chitinase-3-like protein 2	CHI3L2	↑		
	Collagen alpha-1(I) chain	COL1A1	↑		
	Collagen alpha-1(III) chain	COL3A1	↑		
	Collagen alpha-1(XII) chain	COL12A1	↓	↓	
	Collagen alpha-1(XV) chain	COL15A1	↓	↓	↑
	Collagen alpha-3(VI) chain	COL6A3		↓	
	Hyaluronan and proteoglycan link protein 1	HAPLN1	↓		
	Prolargin	PRELP			↑
	Serpin H1	SERPINH1			↓
Inflammation	Pentraxin-related protein	PTX3	↑		

* Average SILAC ratios (n = 3) that represent the relative protein abundance in CS-treated *versus* untreated cells.

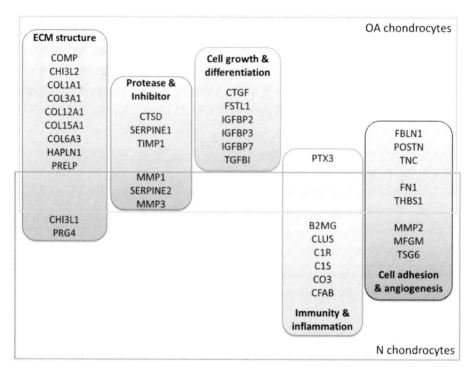

Figure 9. Functional distribution of secreted proteins that were identified as altered by CS either in OA chondrocytes, in normal chondrocytes stimulated by IL-1β, or in both conditions. Protein abbreviations, as in Tables 3 and 4.

Conclusion

Chondroitin sulfate is used as a drug or nutraceutical to treat osteoarthritis. In this chapter, we review the pharmacoproteomic studies carried out on human cartilage cells treated with different types of chondroitin sulfate compounds and formulations, in order to clarify its mechanism of action. Possible modulations of the intracellular and extracellular proteomes of CS-treated human articular chondrocytes, by proteomics means, have been summarized. We also present a coherent set of results obtained by quantitative proteomics experiments, providing clear examples of the usefulness of several complementary proteomic approaches (2DE, DIGE and SILAC) for anti-OA drug screening.

This chapter also demonstrates how proteomics has contributed to the description of a number of novel target proteins of CS, both in simple and combined administration with GS. The wide-ranging effects of these drugs on fundamental aspects of chondrocyte metabolism are pointed out, as well as their different mechanism of action. However, in most cases, both molecules modified chondrocyte proteome synergistically. Although our findings supported the efficacy of combining CS and GS, extrapolation of the *in vitro* data to the *in vivo* situation should be done with great caution. We also provide a comprehensive quantitative analysis of the effects of CS in IL1β-stimulated chondrocytes secretome, as well as novel molecular evidences of its anti-angiogenic, anti-inflammatory, and anti-catabolic properties. Proteins modulated by this drug are potential new targets for OA treatment (e.g. THBS1) (Figure 9).

These findings might provide a rationale for targeting angiogenesis as a disease-modifying therapy for osteoarthritis.

Furthermore, the potential application of proteomics techniques for pharmacological analyses is also to identify efficacy markers for monitoring different OA treatments. In this sense, the results obtained by the DIGE and SILAC experiments suggest that the variable effects of three different chondroitin sulfate compounds may be dependent on their origin and purity and emphasizes the importance of employing CS compounds of pharmaceutical grade in the therapy of OA. Taken together, these results underline the need of stricter regulations regarding CS quality control. These should be introduced to guarantee the manufacture of high quality products for nutraceutical utilization, and to protect customers from low-quality, ineffective and potentially dangerous products. As mentioned before, these data may be useful when translating back to a different efficacy profile *in vivo*, taking into account the limitations of the *in vitro* studies.

Finally, as clearly evidenced in this chapter, pharmacoproteomics has already contributed significantly to the identification of novel CS-targets in OA and the in-depth analysis of its mechanisms of action. The results obtained can be exploited in the near future for monitoring therapeutic effectiveness in clinical samples. However, despite recent technological improvements in MS-methods, the pharmacological applications of proteomics (pharmacoproteomics) are still not fully exploited. In our opinion, this interdisciplinary approach should be used more broadly because, in contrast to traditional drug discovery, it integrates the study of drug mode of action, side effects (including toxicity) and the discovery of new drug targets in a single experiment.

References

[1]   Aigner, T; McKenna, L. Molecular pathology and pathobiology of osteoarthritic cartilage. *Cell Mol Life Sci.*, 2002 Jan; 59(1), 5-18.

[2]   Martel-Pelletier, J; Lajeunesse, D; Pelletier, J. Etiopathogenesis of osteoarthritis. *A Textbook of Rheumatology.* 15th edn. ed. Baltimore: Lippincott, Williams & Wilkins;: In: Koopman WJ, Moreland LW, Eds. Arthritis & Allied Conditions., 2005.

[3]   Goldring, MB. The role of the chondrocyte in osteoarthritis. *Arthritis Rheum.*, 2000 Sep; 43(9), 1916-1926.

[4]   Berenbaum, F. New horizons and perspectives in the treatment of osteoarthritis. *Arthritis Res Ther.*, 2008; 10 Suppl 2, S1.

[5]   Alcaraz, MJ; Megías, J; García-Arnandis, I; Clérigues, V; Guillén, MI. New molecular targets for the treatment of osteoarthritis. *Biochem Pharmacol.*, 2010 Jul; 80(1), 13-21.

[6]   Iliopoulos, D; Gkretsi, V; Tsezou, A. Proteomics of osteoarthritic chondrocytes and cartilage. *Expert Rev Proteomics.*, 2010 Oct; 7(5), 749-760.

[7]   Bruyère, O; Burlet, N; Delmas, PD; Rizzoli, R; Cooper, C; Reginster, JY. Evaluation of symptomatic slow-acting drugs in osteoarthritis using the GRADE system. *BMC Musculoskelet Disord.*, 2008; 9, 165.

[8]   Henrotin, Y; Lambert, C; Couchourel, D; Ripoll, C; Chiotelli, E. Nutraceuticals, do they represent a new era in the management of osteoarthritis? - a narrative review from the lessons taken with five products. *Osteoarthritis Cartilage.*, 2011 Jan; 19(1), 1-21.

[9]   Matsuno, H; Nakamura, H; Katayama, K; Hayashi, S; Kano, S; Yudoh, K; et al. Effects of an oral administration of glucosamine-chondroitin-quercetin glucoside on the synovial fluid properties in patients with osteoarthritis and rheumatoid arthritis. *Biosci Biotechnol Biochem.*, 2009 Feb; 73(2), 288-292.

[10] Imada, K; Oka, H; Kawasaki, D; Miura, N; Sato, T; Ito, A. Anti-arthritic action mechanisms of natural chondroitin sulfate in human articular chondrocytes and synovial fibroblasts. *Biol Pharm Bull.*, 2010; 33(3), 410-414.

[11] Monfort, J; Pelletier, JP; Garcia-Giralt, N; Martel-Pelletier, J. Biochemical basis of the effect of chondroitin sulphate on osteoarthritis articular tissues. *Ann Rheum Dis.*, 2008 Jun; 67(6), 735-740.

[12] Kahan, A; Uebelhart, D; De Vathaire, F; Delmas, PD; Reginster, JY. Long-term effects of chondroitins 4 and 6 sulfate on knee osteoarthritis, the study on osteoarthritis progression prevention, a two-year, randomized, double-blind, placebo-controlled trial. *Arthritis Rheum.*, 2009 Feb; 60(2), 524-533.

[13] Sawitzke, AD; Shi, H; Finco, MF; Dunlop, DD; Harris, CL; Singer, NG; et al. Clinical efficacy and safety of glucosamine, chondroitin sulphate, their combination, celecoxib or placebo taken to treat osteoarthritis of the knee, 2-year results from GAIT. *Ann Rheum Dis.*, 2010 Aug; 69(8), 1459-1464.

[14] McAlindon, TE; LaValley, MP; Gulin, JP; Felson, DT. Glucosamine and chondroitin for treatment of osteoarthritis, a systematic quality assessment and meta-analysis. *JAMA.*, 2000 Mar 15; 283(11), 1469-1475.

[15] Clegg, DO; Reda, DJ; Harris, CL; Klein, MA; O'Dell, JR; Hooper, MM; et al. Glucosamine, chondroitin sulfate, and the two in combination for painful knee osteoarthritis. *N Engl J Med.*, 2006 Feb 23; 354(8), 795-808.

[16] Reginster, JY; Deroisy, R; Rovati, LC; Lee, RL; Lejeune, E; Bruyere, O; et al. Long-term effects of glucosamine sulphate on osteoarthritis progression, a randomised, placebo-controlled clinical trial. *Lancet.*, 2001 Jan 27; 357(9252), 251-256.

[17] Pavelka, K; Gatterova, J; Olejarova, M; Machacek, S; Giacovelli, G; Rovati, LC. Glucosamine sulfate use and delay of progression of knee osteoarthritis, a 3-year, randomized, placebo-controlled, double-blind study. *Arch Intern Med.*, 2002 Oct 14; 162(18), 2113-2123.

[18] Towheed, TE; Maxwell, L; Anastassiades, TP; Shea, B; Houpt, J; Robinson, V; et al. Glucosamine therapy for treating osteoarthritis. *Cochrane Database Syst Rev.*, 2005(2), CD002946.

[19] Leeb, BF; Schweitzer, H; Montag, K; Smolen, JS. A metaanalysis of chondroitin sulfate in the treatment of osteoarthritis. *J Rheumatol.*, 2000 Jan; 27(1), 205-211.

[20] Reichenbach, S; Sterchi, R; Scherer, M; Trelle, S; Burgi, E; Burgi, U; et al. Meta-analysis, chondroitin for osteoarthritis of the knee or hip. *Ann Intern Med.*, 2007 Apr 17; 146(8), 580-590.

[21] Schwartz, NB; Dorfman, A. Stimulation of chondroitin sulfate proteoglycan production by chondrocytes in monolayer. *Connect Tissue Res.*, 1975; 3(2), 115-122.

[22] Campo, GM; Avenoso, A; Campo, S; D'Ascola, A; Traina, P; Samà, D; et al. Glycosaminoglycans modulate inflammation and apoptosis in LPS-treated chondrocytes. *J Cell Biochem.*, 2009 Jan; 106(1), 83-92.

[23] Legendre, F; Baugé, C; Roche, R; Saurel, AS; Pujol, JP. Chondroitin sulfate modulation of matrix and inflammatory gene expression in IL-1beta-stimulated

chondrocytes--study in hypoxic alginate bead cultures. *Osteoarthritis Cartilage.*, 2008 Jan; 16(1), 105-114.

[24] Chan, PS; Caron, JP; Rosa, GJ; Orth, MW. Glucosamine and chondroitin sulfate regulate gene expression and synthesis of nitric oxide and prostaglandin E(2) in articular cartilage explants. *Osteoarthritis Cartilage.*, 2005 May; 13(5), 387-394.

[25] Uebelhart, D; Thonar, EJ; Zhang, J; Williams, JM. Protective effect of exogenous chondroitin 4, 6-sulfate in the acute degradation of articular cartilage in the rabbit. *Osteoarthritis Cartilage.* 1998 May; 6 Suppl A, 6-13.

[26] Jomphe, C; Gabriac, M; Hale, TM; Heroux, L; Trudeau, LE; Deblois, D; et al. Chondroitin sulfate inhibits the nuclear translocation of nuclear factor-kappaB in interleukin-1beta-stimulated chondrocytes. *Basic Clin Pharmacol Toxicol.*, 2008 Jan; 102(1), 59-65.

[27] Chan, PS; Caron, JP; Orth, MW. Effect of glucosamine and chondroitin sulfate on regulation of gene expression of proteolytic enzymes and their inhibitors in interleukin-1-challenged bovine articular cartilage explants. *Am J Vet Res.*, 2005 Nov; 66(11), 1870-1876.

[28] Tat, SK; Pelletier, JP; Vergés, J; Lajeunesse, D; Montell, E; Fahmi, H; et al. Chondroitin and glucosamine sulfate in combination decrease the pro-resorptive properties of human osteoarthritis subchondral bone osteoblasts, a basic science study. *Arthritis Res Ther.*, 2007; 9(6), R117.

[29] Campo, GM; Avenoso, A; Campo, S; Ferlazzo, AM; Calatroni, A. Antioxidant activity of chondroitin sulfate. *Adv Pharmacol.*, 2006; 53, 417-431.

[30] Egea, J; García, AG; Verges, J; Montell, E; López, MG. Antioxidant, antiinflammatory and neuroprotective actions of chondroitin sulfate and proteoglycans. *Osteoarthritis Cartilage.*, 2010 Jun; 18 Suppl 1, S24-27.

[31] Calamia, V; Lourido, L; Fernández-Puente, P; Mateos, J; Rocha, B; Montell, E; et al. Secretome analysis of chondroitin sulfate-treated chondrocytes reveals anti-angiogenic, anti-inflammatory and anti-catabolic properties. *Arthritis Res Ther.*, 2012 Oct; 14(5), R202.

[32] Lambert, C; Mathy-Hartert, M; Dubuc, JE; Montell, E; Vergés, J; Munaut, C; et al. Characterization of synovial angiogenesis in osteoarthritis patients and its modulation by chondroitin sulfate. *Arthritis Res Ther.*, 2012; 14(2), R58.

[33] Zhang, W; Moskowitz, RW; Nuki, G; Abramson, S; Altman, RD; Arden, N; et al. OARSI recommendations for the management of hip and knee osteoarthritis, Part II, OARSI evidence-based, expert consensus guidelines. *Osteoarthritis Cartilage.*, 2008 Feb; 16(2), 137-162.

[34] Zhang, W; Nuki, G; Moskowitz, RW; Abramson, S; Altman, RD; Arden, NK; et al. OARSI recommendations for the management of hip and knee osteoarthritis, part III, Changes in evidence following systematic cumulative update of research published through January 2009. *Osteoarthritis Cartilage.*, 2010 Apr; 18(4), 476-499.

[35] Zhang, W; Doherty, M; Arden, N; Bannwarth, B; Bijlsma, J; Gunther, KP; et al. EULAR evidence based recommendations for the management of hip osteoarthritis, report of a task force of the EULAR Standing Committee for International Clinical Studies Including Therapeutics (ESCISIT). *Ann Rheum Dis.*, 2005 May; 64(5), 669-681.

[36] Jordan, KM; Arden, NK; Doherty, M; Bannwarth, B; Bijlsma, JW; Dieppe, P; et al. EULAR Recommendations 2003, an evidence based approach to the management of knee osteoarthritis, Report of a Task Force of the Standing Committee for International Clinical Studies Including Therapeutic Trials (ESCISIT). *Ann Rheum Dis.*, 2003 Dec; 62(12), 1145-1155.

[37] Bali, JP; Cousse, H; Neuzil, E. Biochemical basis of the pharmacologic action of chondroitin sulfates on the osteoarticular system. *Semin Arthritis Rheum.*, 2001 Aug; 31(1), 58-68.

[38] Volpi, N. The pathobiology of osteoarthritis and the rationale for using the chondroitin sulfate for its treatment. *Curr Drug Targets Immune Endocr Metabol Disord.*, 2004 Jun; 4(2), 119-127.

[39] Campo, GM; Avenoso, A; Campo, S; D'Ascola, A; Traina, P; Calatroni, A. Chondroitin-4-sulphate inhibits NF-kB translocation and caspase activation in collagen-induced arthritis in mice. *Osteoarthritis Cartilage.*, 2008 Dec; 16(12), 1474-1483.

[40] Drynda, A; Quax, PH; Neumann, M; van der Laan, WH; Pap, G; Drynda, S; et al. Gene transfer of tissue inhibitor of metalloproteinases-3 reverses the inhibitory effects of TNF-alpha on Fas-induced apoptosis in rheumatoid arthritis synovial fibroblasts. *J Immunol.*, 2005 May; 174(10), 6524-6531.

[41] Omata, T; Itokazu, Y; Inoue, N; Segawa, Y. Effects of chondroitin sulfate-C on articular cartilage destruction in murine collagen-induced arthritis. *Arzneimittelforschung.*, 2000 Feb; 50(2), 148-153.

[42] Omata, T; Segawa, Y; Itokazu, Y; Inoue, N; Tanaka, Y. Effects of chondroitin sulfate-C on bradykinin-induced proteoglycan depletion in rats. *Arzneimittelforschung.*, 1999 Jul; 49(7), 577-581.

[43] Bayliss, MT; Osborne, D; Woodhouse, S; Davidson, C. Sulfation of chondroitin sulfate in human articular cartilage. The effect of age, topographical position, and zone of cartilage on tissue composition. *J Biol Chem.*, 1999 May; 274(22), 15892-15900.

[44] Lewis, S; Crossman, M; Flannelly, J; Belcher, C; Doherty, M; Bayliss, MT; et al. Chondroitin sulphation patterns in synovial fluid in osteoarthritis subsets. *Ann Rheum Dis.*, 1999 Jul; 58(7), 441-445.

[45] Shinmei, M; Miyauchi, S; Machida, A; Miyazaki, K. Quantitation of chondroitin 4-sulfate and chondroitin 6-sulfate in pathologic joint fluid. *Arthritis Rheum.* 1992 Nov; 35(11), 1304-1308.

[46] Volpi, N. Analytical aspects of pharmaceutical grade chondroitin sulfates. *J Pharm Sci.*, 2007 Dec; 96(12), 3168-3180.

[47] Volpi, N. Quality of different chondroitin sulfate preparations in relation to their therapeutic activity. *J Pharm Pharmacol.*, 2009 Oct; 61(10), 1271-1280.

[48] Volpi, N. Oral bioavailability of chondroitin sulfate (Condrosulf) and its constituents in healthy male volunteers. *Osteoarthritis Cartilage.*, 2002 Oct; 10(10), 768-777.

[49] Volpi, N. Oral absorption and bioavailability of ichthyic origin chondroitin sulfate in healthy male volunteers. *Osteoarthritis Cartilage.*, 2003 Jun; 11(6), 433-441.

[50] Ronca, F; Palmieri, L; Panicucci, P; Ronca, G. Anti-inflammatory activity of chondroitin sulfate. *Osteoarthritis Cartilage.* 1998 May; 6 Suppl A, 14-21.

[51] Rainsford, KD. Importance of pharmaceutical composition and evidence from clinical trials and pharmacological studies in determining effectiveness of chondroitin sulphate

and other glycosaminoglycans, a critique. *J Pharm Pharmacol.*, 2009 Oct; 61(10), 1263-1270.

[52] Reginster, JY; Gillot, V; Bruyere, O; Henrotin, Y. Evidence of nutriceutical effectiveness in the treatment of osteoarthritis. *Curr Rheumatol Rep.*, 2000 Dec; 2(6), 472-477.

[53] Curtis, CL; Harwood, JL; Dent, CM; Caterson, B. Biological basis for the benefit of nutraceutical supplementation in arthritis. *Drug Discov Today.*, 2004 Feb; 9(4), 165-172.

[54] Reginster, JY; Heraud, F; Zegels, B; Bruyere, O. Symptom and structure modifying properties of chondroitin sulfate in osteoarthritis. *Mini Rev Med Chem.*, 2007 Oct; 7(10), 1051-1061.

[55] Calamia, V; Ruiz-Romero, C; Rocha, B; Fernandez-Puente, P; Mateos, J; Montell, E; et al. Pharmacoproteomic study of the effects of chondroitin and glucosamine sulfate on human articular chondrocytes. *Arthritis Res Ther.* England; 2010, R138.

[56] Cillero-Pastor, B; Ruiz-Romero, C; Carames, B; Lopez-Armada, MJ; Blanco, FJ. Proteomic analysis by two-dimensional electrophoresis to identify the normal human chondrocyte proteome stimulated by tumor necrosis factor alpha and interleukin-1beta. *Arthritis Rheum.*, 2010 Mar; 62(3), 802-814.

[57] Fernández-Costa, C; Calamia, V; Fernández-Puente, P; Capelo-Martínez, JL; Ruiz-Romero, C; Blanco, FJ. Sequential depletion of human serum for the search of osteoarthritis biomarkers. *Proteome Sci.*, 2012; 10(1), 55.

[58] Ruiz-Romero, C; López-Armada, MJ; Blanco, FJ. Proteomic characterization of human normal articular chondrocytes, a novel tool for the study of osteoarthritis and other rheumatic diseases. *Proteomics.*, 2005 Aug; 5(12), 3048-3059.

[59] Ruiz-Romero, C; Lopez-Armada, MJ; Blanco, FJ. Mitochondrial proteomic characterization of human normal articular chondrocytes. *Osteoarthritis Cartilage.*, 2006 Jun; 14(6), 507-518.

[60] Ruiz-Romero, C; Carreira, V; Rego, I; Remeseiro, S; López-Armada, MJ; Blanco, FJ. Proteomic analysis of human osteoarthritic chondrocytes reveals protein changes in stress and glycolysis. *Proteomics.*, 2008 Feb; 8(3), 495-507.

[61] Ruiz-Romero, C; Calamia, V; Mateos, J; Carreira, V; Martínez-Gomariz, M; Fernández, M; et al. Mitochondrial dysregulation of osteoarthritic human articular chondrocytes analyzed by proteomics, a decrease in mitochondrial superoxide dismutase points to a redox imbalance. *Mol Cell Proteomics.*, 2009 Jan; 8(1), 172-189.

[62] Calamia, V; Rocha, B; Mateos, J; Fernández-Puente, P; Ruiz-Romero, C; Blanco, FJ. Metabolic labeling of chondrocytes for the quantitative analysis of the interleukin-1-beta-mediated modulation of their intracellular and extracellular proteomes. *J Proteome Res.*, 2011 Jun.

[63] Fernández-Puente, P; Mateos, J; Fernández-Costa, C; Oreiro, N; Fernández-López, C; Ruiz-Romero, C; et al. Identification of a panel of novel serum osteoarthritis biomarkers. *J Proteome Res.*, 2011 Nov; 10(11), 5095-5101.

[64] Mateos, J; Lourido, L; Fernández-Puente, P; Calamia, V; Fernández-López, C; Oreiro, N; et al. Differential protein profiling of synovial fluid from rheumatoid arthritis and osteoarthritis patients using LC-MALDI TOF/TOF. *J Proteomics.*, 2012 Jan.

[65] Rocha, B; Calamia, V; Mateos, J; Fernández-Puente, P; Blanco, FJ; Ruiz-Romero, C. Metabolic labeling of human bone marrow mesenchymal stem cells for the quantitative

analysis of their chondrogenic differentiation. *J Proteome Res.*, 2012 Nov; 11(11), 5350-5361.

[66] Archer, CW; Francis-West, P. The chondrocyte. *Int J Biochem Cell Biol.*, 2003 Apr; 35(4), 401-404.

[67] Behonick, DJ; Werb, Z. A bit of give and take, the relationship between the extracellular matrix and the developing chondrocyte. *Mech Dev.*, 2003 Nov; 120(11), 1327-1336.

[68] Lambrecht, S; Verbruggen, G; Verdonk, PC; Elewaut, D; Deforce, D. Differential proteome analysis of normal and osteoarthritic chondrocytes reveals distortion of vimentin network in osteoarthritis. *Osteoarthritis Cartilage.*, 2008 Feb; 16(2), 163-173.

[69] d'Abusco, AS; Calamia, V; Cicione, C; Grigolo, B; Politi, L; Scandurra, R. Glucosamine affects intracellular signalling through inhibition of mitogen-activated protein kinase phosphorylation in human chondrocytes. *Arthritis Res Ther.*, 2007; 9(5), R104.

[70] Chan, PS; Caron, JP; Orth, MW. Effects of glucosamine and chondroitin sulfate on bovine cartilage explants under long-term culture conditions. *Am J Vet Res.*, 2007 Jul; 68(7), 709-715.

[71] Piperno, M; Reboul, P; Hellio Le Graverand, MP; Peschard, MJ; Annefeld, M; Richard, M; et al. Glucosamine sulfate modulates dysregulated activities of human osteoarthritic chondrocytes in vitro. *Osteoarthritis Cartilage.*, 2000 May; 8(3), 207-212.

[72] Chan, PS; Caron, JP; Orth, MW. Short-term gene expression changes in cartilage explants stimulated with interleukin beta plus glucosamine and chondroitin sulfate. *J Rheumatol.*, 2006 Jul; 33(7), 1329-1340.

[73] Orth, MW; Peters, TL; Hawkins, JN. Inhibition of articular cartilage degradation by glucosamine-HCl and chondroitin sulphate. *Equine Vet J Suppl.*, 2002 Sep(34), 224-229.

[74] Chou, MM; Vergnolle, N; McDougall, JJ; Wallace, JL; Marty, S; Teskey, V; et al. Effects of chondroitin and glucosamine sulfate in a dietary bar formulation on inflammation, interleukin-1beta, matrix metalloprotease-9, and cartilage damage in arthritis. *Exp Biol Med* (Maywood)., 2005 Apr; 230(4), 255-262.

[75] Campo, GM; Avenoso, A; Campo, S; Ferlazzo, AM; Altavilla, D; Calatroni, A. Efficacy of treatment with glycosaminoglycans on experimental collagen-induced arthritis in rats. *Arthritis Res Ther.*, 2003; 5(3), R122-131.

[76] Fernandes, JC; Martel-Pelletier, J; Pelletier, JP. The role of cytokines in osteoarthritis pathophysiology. *Biorheology.*, 2002; 39(1-2), 237-246.

[77] White, IR; Pickford, R; Wood, J; Skehel, JM; Gangadharan, B; Cutler, P. A statistical comparison of silver and SYPRO Ruby staining for proteomic analysis. *Electrophoresis.*, 2004 Sep; 25(17), 3048-3054.

[78] Aebersold, R; Mann, M. Mass spectrometry-based proteomics. *Nature.*, 2003 Mar; 422(6928), 198-207.

[79] Afonso, V; Champy, R; Mitrovic, D; Collin, P; Lomri, A. Reactive oxygen species and superoxide dismutases, role in joint diseases. *Joint Bone Spine.*, 2007 Jul; 74(4), 324-329.

[80] Tat, SK; Pelletier, JP; Mineau, F; Duval, N; Martel-Pelletier, J. Variable effects of 3 different chondroitin sulfate compounds on human osteoarthritic cartilage/

chondrocytes, relevance of purity and production process. *J Rheumatol.*, 2010 Mar; 37(3), 656-664.

[81] Unlü, M; Morgan, ME; Minden, JS. Difference gel electrophoresis, a single gel method for detecting changes in protein extracts. *Electrophoresis.* 1997 Oct; 18(11), 2071-2077.

[82] Lilley, KS; Friedman, DB. All about DIGE, quantification technology for differential-display 2D-gel proteomics. *Expert Rev Proteomics.*, 2004 Dec; 1(4), 401-409.

[83] Marouga, R; David, S; Hawkins, E. The development of the DIGE system, 2D fluorescence difference gel analysis technology. *Anal Bioanal Chem.*, 2005 Jun; 382(3), 669-678.

[84] Calamia V, Fernández-Puente P, Mateos J, Lourido L, Rocha B, Montell E, et al. Pharmacoproteomic study of three different chondroitin sulfate compounds on intracellular and extracellular human chondrocyte proteomes. Mol Cell Proteomics. 2012 Jun; 11(6):M111.013417.

[85] Marshall, KW; Zhang, H; Yager, TD; Nossova, N; Dempsey, A; Zheng, R; et al. Blood-based biomarkers for detecting mild osteoarthritis in the human knee. *Osteoarthritis Cartilage.*, 2005 Oct; 13(10), 861-871.

[86] Lambrecht, S; Verbruggen, G; Verdonk, PC; Elewaut, D; Deforce, D. Differential proteome analysis of normal and osteoarthritic chondrocytes reveals distortion of vimentin network in osteoarthritis. *Osteoarthritis Cartilage.*, 2008 Feb; 16(2), 163-173.

[87] Catterall, JB; Rowan, AD; Sarsfield, S; Saklatvala, J; Wait, R; Cawston, TE. Development of a novel 2D proteomics approach for the identification of proteins secreted by primary chondrocytes after stimulation by IL-1 and oncostatin M. *Rheumatology* (Oxford)., 2006 Sep; 45(9), 1101-1109.

[88] Polacek, M; Bruun, JA; Johansen, O; Martinez, I. Differences in the secretome of cartilage explants and cultured chondrocytes unveiled by SILAC technology. *J Orthop Res.*, 2010 Aug; 28(8), 1040-1049.

[89] Haglund, L; Bernier, SM; Onnerfjord, P; Recklies, AD. Proteomic analysis of the LPS-induced stress response in rat chondrocytes reveals induction of innate immune response components in articular cartilage. *Matrix Biol.*, 2008 Mar; 27(2), 107-118.

[90] Mann, M. Functional and quantitative proteomics using SILAC. *Nat Rev Mol Cell Biol.*, England; 2006, 952-958.

[91] Eagle, H. Amino acid metabolism in mammalian cell cultures. *Science.*, 1959 Aug 21; 130(3373), 432-437.

[92] Silvestre, JS; Théry, C; Hamard, G; Boddaert, J; Aguilar, B; Delcayre, A; et al. Lactadherin promotes VEGF-dependent neovascularization. *Nat Med.*, 2005 May; 11(5), 499-506.

[93] Lambert, C; Mathy-Hartert, M; Dubuc, JE; Montell, E; Vergés, J; Munaut, C; et al. Characterization of synovial angiogenesis in osteoarthritis patients and its modulation by chondroitin sulfate. *Arthritis Res Ther.*, 2012 Mar; 14(2), R58.

[94] Hathout, Y. Approaches to the study of the cell secretome. *Expert Rev Proteomics.*, 2007 Apr; 4(2), 239-248.

[95] Kanaan, RA; Aldwaik, M; Al-Hanbali, OA. The role of connective tissue growth factor in skeletal growth and development. *Med Sci Monit.*, 2006 Dec; 12(12), RA277-281.

In: Chondroitin Sulfate
Editor: Vitor H. Pomin

ISBN: 978-1-62808-490-0
© 2013 Nova Science Publishers, Inc.

Chapter 7

Chondroitin Sulfate Regulates Growth Factor Signaling in Tissue Homeostasis and Disease

Dragana Nikitovic[1], Kallirroi Voudouri[1], Nikos Karamanos[2] and George Tzanakakis[1,*]
[1]Department of Histology--Embryology, Medical School, University of Crete, Heraklion, Greece
[2]Laboratory of Biochemistry, Department of Chemistry, University of Patras, Greece

Growth factors (GFs) are a group of biologically active polypeptides produced by the body that can stimulate cellular division, growth, and differentiation. Through the regulation of these key biological functions GFs participate in the development and homeostasis of tissues throughout life and are implicated in numerous pathological processes. Chondroitin sulfate (CS) is a glycosaminoglycan composed of repeating disaccharides of N-acetylgalactosamine and d-glucuronic acid or l-iduronic acid in the case of dermatansulfate (DS/CS-B), with various sulfation patterns. CS chains, covalently bound into proteoglycan (PGs) core proteins, are located to the extracellular space, at the cell membrane and also intracellularly. Through elegant feedback mechanisms CS can influence cellular processes by regulating the presentation and availability of growth factors to cells, matricinesignaling. This chapter focuses on the role of CS/DS in the regulation of growth factor signaling pathways crucial to development and tissue homeostasis as well as to disease conditions.

Introduction

Chondroitin sulfate (CS), is a glycosaminoglycan (GAG) composed of repeating disaccharide units of N-acetyl-galactosamine and of uronic acids (d-glucuronic acid or l-

---
[*]Corresponding author: Prof. George N Tzanakakis, Department of Histology-Embryology, Medical School, University of Crete, 711 10 Heraklion, Greece; Fax +30-2810-394786; Email: tzanakak@med.uoc.gr.

iduronic acid) being sulfated at various positions. CS is covalently bound into protein cores to form proteoglycans (PGs) and can be located to the interstitial matrix, basal membrane and cell surface (Iozzo & San Antonio, 2001). Growth factors (GFs) are a group of biologically active polypeptides that can stimulate cellular division, growth, and differentiation. *Via* modulation of these important biological functions GFs participate in the morphogenesis and homeostasis of tissues throughout life (Goldring et al., 2006; Bobick et al., 2009) and are involved in different disease states (Hayes & Ralphs, 2011). This review focuses on the regulation of GF-function by CS.

Glycosaminoglycans Are Ubiquitously Distributed to the Extracellular Matrices (ECMs) and Cells

GAGs comprise a class of linear, negatively charged polysaccharides composed of repeating disaccharide units of acetylated hexosamines (N-acetyl-galactosamine or N-acetyl-glucosamine) and mainly of uronic acids (d-glucuronic acid or l-iduronic acid) being sulfated at various positions. Based on the epimeric form of uronic acid and the type of hexosamine in their repeating disaccharide units, GAGs are classified into four major types; hyaluronan (HA), chondroitin sulfate (CS), heparin and heparan sulfate (HS) as well as keratan sulfate (KS). HA is synthesized in the absence of a protein core at the inner face of the plasma membrane and consequently found in the form of free chains whereas, other GAG types are covalently bound into protein cores to form PGs. With the exception of HA all GAG types are variably sulfated which contributes to the intricate complexity of their structures. Both free GAGs and those bound into PGs are essential components of the extracellular matrices (ECMs) and decorate the surface of most cells (Iozzo & San Antonio, 2001). The ECMs can be organised as a thin network of highly crosslinked glycoproteins, a basement membrane, or as a loose array of fibril-like macromolecules constituting the interstitial matrix. In addition highly specialized ECM structures, with characteristics of both the basement membrane and the interstitial matrix, form the reticular fibre network of secondary lymphoid organs (Sixt et al., 2005). ECM provides much more than just mechanical and structural support, but the signals originating therein are critically important for cell growth, survival, differentiation and key to various disease processes including inflammation and cancer (Hynes, 2009; Sorokin, 2010; Afratis et al., 2012; Nikitovic et al., 2012). Therefore, we can conclude that the ECM specific components, such as GAGs, impart spatial context for signaling events by various active molecules including GF and their respective cell surface growth factor receptors (GFR) (reviewed by: Rozario & DeSimone, 2010; Barkan et al., 2010).

CS Chains Typical Structure

The synthetic pathways involved in CS/DS biosynthesis include proteins, activated carbohydrate units (most of them as uridinediphosphate [UPD] derivatives), glycosyltransferases, and sulfotransferases (Paulsson & Heinegard, 1984; Pavão et al., 2006). CS are catabolized within the matrix by the action of lysosomal enzymes secreted by cells of the connective tissue such as glycosidases and chondroitinases that destroy the glucosidic bond between N-acetylglucosamine and glucuronic acid (Caterson et al., 1999).

The complex CS biosynthetic machinery creates CS chains typically consisting of repeating disaccharide units of -4GlcAβ1-3GalNAcβ1 which can be variously sulfated on GlcA and/or GalNAc residues. Highly represented are the monosulfated-4GlcAβ1-3GalNAc(4S) and -4GlcAβ1-3GalNAcβ(6S) designated as the A and C unit respectively. Oversulfated CS chains contain disulfated disaccharide units designated as D, E, H and K whereas iduronic acid -containing disaccharide units are known as CS-B or dermatan sulfate (DS) differing at C-5 of hexuronic acid moieties (Malavaki et al., 2008; Lamari & Karamanos, 2006). In addition to the sulfation pattern the number, configuration, arrangement and charge density of disaccharide units varies; resulting in highly variable and finely modulated structure of CS chains (Malavaki et al., 2008; Lamari & Karamanos, 2006).

CS Fine Structure Affects GF Binding and Biological Activities

The complex structures of CS chains allow specific interactions with discrete GF/GFR to regulate their biological activities. This was originally demonstrated for the heparin-binding GFs. Thus, it was shown that the activity of the heparin-binding GF midkine on neuronal cell adhesion was specifically inhibited by oversulfated CS-E with the other CS isoforms being inactive (Ueoka et al., 2000). Indeed, the majority of heparin-binding growth factors including the midkine, FGF and EGF families bind in a highly specific manner to CS-E (Deepa et al., 2002; Lander, 1998). Another heparin binding growth factor pleiotrophin was found to bind with high affinity to CS-D (Maeda et al., 2003). In a chronically injured spinal cord model CSPGs were targeted by chondroitinase ABC previous to transplantation of neural stem/ progenitor cells (NPCs) and transient infusion of heparin-binding EGF, bFGF and PDGF-AA. This combined strategy demonstrated that action of chondroitinase ABC facilitates combined GF action on NPC transplantation in chronic SCI (Karimi-Abdolrezeaee et al., 2010). In a later study, the same research team demonstrated that chondroitinase and GFs collectively enhance the activation and oligodendrocyte differentiation of endogenous neural precursor cells after SCI (Karimi-Abdolrezaee et al., 2012). These studies suggest that *in vivo* binding of GF to CS affects their actions. Moreover, since highly sulfated CS may cooperate with heparan sulfate (HS) chains to regulate GF activity the versatility in in the control of specific GF activities control is highly increased (Deepa et al., 2004; Nikitovic et al., 2008). Therefore, in conclusion the interactions among CS and GF/GFRs have recently become a target of many studies.

Signaling Pathways

The interplay between GFs and CS modulates cues transferred from the extracellular space to the cell nucleus through a complex system of signaling pathways, as depicted in Figure 1. The starting points of this system are the GFRs.GFRs are characterized as transmembrane proteins composed of three functional domains: an extracellular ligand binding domain bestowed with high binding specificity, a transmembrane section and an intracellular catalytic domain capable of activation through autophosphorylation, usually at multiple serine and threonine or tyrosine residues (Malarkey et al., 1995; Jiang & Hunter, 1999). In many cases the extracellular presence of corresponding ligand stabilizes a homo- or hetero-polymerization of more than one isoforms or receptor types required for the intracellular activation to occur (Heldin & Westermark, 1999; Klint & Claesson-Welsh, 1999; Reigstad et al., 2005; Moustakas & Heldin, 2009). The activation of GFRs, *i.e.* the phosphorylation of their intracellular domains triggers a cascade of successive phosphorylations/activations of intracellular signaling substrates targeting at the translation of the extracellular signal to the cell nucleus, and the consecutive modulation of gene expression. The key intracellular signaling pathways, at least regarding GF and CS action includethe highly conserved mitogen-activated protein kinase (MAPK) family, which in mammals is subdivided in at least four distinctly regulated sub-families: *i.e.* extracellular signal-regulated kinases 1 and 2 (ERK1/2), c-Jun-N-terminal kinases (JNKs), p38, and ERK5 (Chang & Karin, 2001). Indeed, the Rsa-Raf-ERK1/2 is the archetypal signal transduction pathway of many growth factors, such as PDGF, EGF and bFGF (App et al., 1991; Friesel & Maciag, 1995; Heldin & Westermark, 1999). One of the major downstream targets of MAPKs is the transcription factor activator protein-1 (AP-1), a heterodimeric protein complex assembled of different Jun (c-Jun, JunB, and JunD) and Fos (c-Fos, Fra-1, Fra-2, and FosB) subunits after phosphorylation by MAPKs (Whitmarsh & Davis, 1996), which in turn regulates the transcription of many targets genes including MMPs (Kajanne et al., 2007).

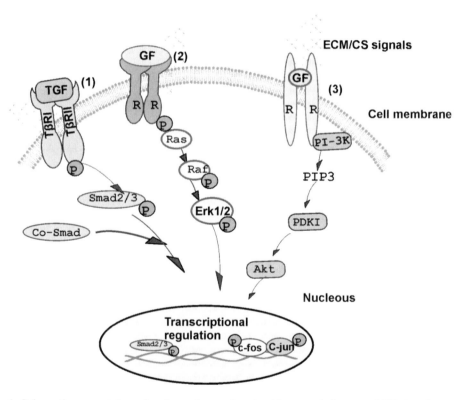

Figure 1. Schematic presentation of major pathways involved in growth factor and CS signal transduction from the cell membrane to the nucleus (see text).

The phosphoinositide 3-kinase (PI-3K) family comprises enzymes capable of phosphorylating phosphatidylinositol lipids at the D-3 position of their inositol ring after triggering by GFRs (Cantley, 2002). Upon generation of phosphatidylinositol (3,4,5)-trisphosphates, protein kinase-B, also called Akt (PKB/Akt) is recruited at the cell membrane, where it undergoes phosphorylation at serine and threonine residues by various kinases (Duronio et al., 1998). Consequently, PKB/Akt activates downstream signaling cascades to modulate various biological functions ranging from cell proliferation and apoptosis to cell migration (Brazil & Hemmings, 2001). Furthermore, various degrees of cooperation between these signaling pathways exist as illustrated in an oligodendrocyte model where activation of the PI3K pathway is required for PDGFR-a -induced migration of these cells, whereas activation of both PI3K and phospholipase Cgamma (PLCgamma) are required for their PDGFR-a-induced proliferation (McKinnon et al., 2005).

The Smads are a family of proteins, with inherent capability for nucleocytoplasmic shuttling, allowing them to directly transfer signals from transmembrane receptors to DNA-binding transcriptional complexes (Massague et al., 2005). Smads are the main transducers of the signals originating from the TGF-β superfamily (Attisano & Lee-Hoeflich, 2001). Smad proteins are subdivided into three groups in a manner dependent on their function: receptor-activated (R) Smads 2 and 3 directly phosphorylated after the binding of TGF-β (or activin) to GFR; Smad1, Smad5, and Smad8 activated upon binding of BMPs to respective GFR; and the inhibitory Smads (Smad6 and Smad7). The receptor activated Smads subsequently associate with the common-mediator, Smad4 to form a heterotrimer, which is transferred to the nucleus to modulate gene expression, while the inhibitory Smads negatively regulate signal strength and duration (Moustakas & Heldin, 2009).

Conclusion

CS Regulates Transforming Growth Factor-Beta (TGFβ) Actions

The transforming growth factor beta (TGFβ) is the prominent member of a superfamily of secreted dimeric cytokines that consists of TGFβs, activins, bone morphogenetic proteins (BMPs), and growth and differentiation factors (GDFs) (Wharton &Derynck, 2009; Moustakas & Heldin, 2009). Importantly, TGFβ which emerged during the evolution of multi-cellular organisms, gained an essential role in the development of the body plan during embryogenesis (Wu & Hill, 2009) and in the process of tissue homeostasis (Heldin et al., 2009). In mammals, three alternative TGFβisoforms exist, duly nominated TGFβ1, TGFβ2 and TGFβ3 (Roberts et al., 1991). TGFβ is synthesized and secreted by many cell types, as an integral part of a large molecule, the precursor-TGFβ containing the latency-associated proteins (LAPs) (ten Dijke & Arthur, 2007; Pohlers et al., 2009). The precursor TGFβ duly undergoes intracellular cleavage, subsequent secretion and binding to specific ECM components (Ruiz-Ortega et al., 2007; Bernabeu et al., 2009; Rozario & DeSimone, 2010). Release of mature TGFβ from this complex can be achieved by the action of various proteases (Leask & Abraham, 2004; Siegel & Massague, 2003). The released mature TGFβ perpetrates signaling through multiple cell surface receptors possessing intrinsic serine/threonine kinase activity (Massague et al., 2005; Wharton & Derynck, 2009). TGFβ cell surface receptors also contain a cytoplasmic kinase domain with a weaker tyrosine kinase activity, classifying the receptors thus, as dual specificity kinases (Heldin et al., 1997). The Smads are the main intracellular transducers of the signals originating from the TGF-β superfamily (Attisano & Lee-Hoeflich, 2001).

The TGFβ signaling pathway regulates key biological functions including proliferation, differentiation, apoptosis, adhesion, invasion as well as the constitution of the cellular microenvironment (Evanko et al., 1998; Padua & Massague 2009). Additionally, it plays a critical, dual role in the progression of human cancer (Meulmeester &Dijke, 2011). Thus, during the early phase, TGFβ acts as a tumor suppressor, but during the subsequent stages it promotes processes that support tumor progression (Meulmeester & Dijke, 2011).

The binding of TGFβ to ECM components is the main conduit for the regulation of TGFβ activity, the small leucine-rich repeat proteoglycans (SLRPs) being the key perpetrators (Schaefer & Iozzo, 2008). Namely, CS-containing SLRP members like decorin, biglycan and fibromodulin bind and regulate TGFβ by sequestering this GF within the ECM. The binding of TGFβ, perpetrated by the SLRPs respective protein cores, appears to be modulated negatively by their glycosylation status (Hildebrand et al., 1994). Namely, in an early study, Hildebrand et al., (1994) determined that tissue derived biglycan and decorin were less effective competitors for TGFβ1 binding than non-glycosylated fusion proteins. Indeed, removal of CS-A and –B sulfate chains of decorin and biglycan increased their binding affinity to TGFβ, suggesting that the GAG chains may hinder the interaction of the core proteins with TGFβ. However, the binding affinity of free CS/CS-B to TGFβ appears to be modulated by their sulfation patterns (Hintze et al., 2012). Thus, these authors constructed CS derivatives with different degree of sulfation and determined that non-physiological highly sulfated CS exhibited stronger interaction with TGFβ1. Also, it was observed that native, low-sulfated CS showed weak or no binding affinity. Independent studies provide further proof of modulatory effects of CS/CS-B on TGFβ1 activity *in vitro*. Namely, TGFβ1-induced signaling events in human articular chondrocytes concurrent with p38 and ERK1/2 activation levels, were influenced by exogenous CS (Holzmann et al., 2006) whereas, TGFβ-dependent osteoblast proliferation is affected by the addition of an osteoblast-derived GAG mixture (Manton et al., 2007). When combined with TGFβ1, cell-surface-derived CS appeared to potentiate the growth inhibitory effects of TGFβ1 at higher concentrations in osteoblast cell culture (Manton et al., 2007). These data on the potential CS regulation of TGFβ action could be highly relevant for tissues heavily dependent on TGFβ signaling including bone, cartilage and tendon.

TGFβ1 is one of the most abundant cytokines in the bone matrix. It coordinates bone formation by inducing migration of bone mesenchymal stem cells (MSC) as well as recruitment and proliferation of osteoblasts (Tang et al., 2009). In the bone ECM the concentration of free TGFβ1 is mostly regulated by its interaction with the SLRPs biglycan and decorin (Bi et al., 2005). Thus, TGFβ family members and CS are importantly suggested to play essential roles in the control of skeletogenesis (Alliston, 2010). TGFβ-activated phospho-Smad2 was increased with more prominent nuclear localization in chondroitin sulfate 4 transferase (C4ST)-deficient mice relative to wild-type controls. This illustrates that C4ST deficiency, resulting in lower CS expression, hyperactivates TGFβ signaling, perhaps at the expense of BMP function. Conclusively, C4ST-deficient mice reveal that CS maintains the balanced activity of two critical growth plate morphogens, TGFβ and BMP (Kluppel et al., 2005). The impact of CS on TGFβ signaling is corroborated by data obtained from studies of Mucopolysaccharidosis type VI (MPS VI). MPS VI, also called Maroteaux-Lamy syndrome is an autosomal recessive lysosomal storage disorder caused by deficiency of acetylgalactosamine-4-sulfatase (4S) enzyme, required for CS catabolism (Haskins et al., 2002). The partially degraded CS concentrated to ECM, in this syndrome, could conceivably interfere with the normal interactions between CS-containing PGs and TGFβ, modifying TGFβ signaling that is essential for skeletal development and function (Alliston, 2010). Indeed TGFβ was found to bind to immobilized C4S, but in a manner not optimal for cellular uptake (Hempel et al., 2012). Therefore, it can be concluded that CS regulates TGFβ function related to morphogenesis.

It is well established that the tumor stroma and tumor fibrotic tissues (Ioachim, 1976) contain abnormally high concentrations of CSPGs (Theocharis & Theocharis, 2002; Nikitovic et al., 2012). The enrichment of the tumorstroma with CS/DS chains is accompanied by structural modifications as to their type and sulfation pattern (Wegrowski & Maquart, 2004). The altered CS content could affect tumor related TGFβ signaling and be part of the dual phase role annotated to TGFβ during tumorigenesis. The role of CS/DS on TGFβ signaling in disease remains to be determined.

CS/DS has also been implicated in BMP signaling. Thus, it has been demonstrated thatoversulfated CS, which possesses 4,6-disulfates in N-acetyl-galactosamine, binds to BMP-4 and promotes osteoblast differentiation and subsequent mineralization (Miyazaki et al., 2008). Interestingly, the sulfation pattern appears to be of key importance as CS-E and CP-S had strong affinity for BMP-4, whereas CS-D and monosulfated CS (CS-B or CS-C) did not. Separate treatment with chondroitinase and heparitinase to deplete endogenous CS-A and -B did not effect human mesenchymal stem cells (hMSC) proliferation but rather increased their BMP bioactivity through SMAD1/5/8 intracellular signaling as well as enhancing canonical Wntsignaling through LEF1 activation. Increased BMP activity stimulated bone nodule formation, calcium accumulation, and the expression of such osteoblast markers as alkaline phosphatase, RUNX2, and osteocalcin (Manton et al., 2007). In conclusion, CS-conveyed cues are essential for the signaling of the TGFβ super family members in both physiological and transformed cells and represent potential therapeutic targets in the management of disease. The postulated effects of CS on GF signaling are schematically presented in Figure 2.

CS-Modulator of PDGF Activity

Platelet-derived growth factor (PDGF) is the major polypeptide mitogen for cells of mesenchymal origin (Zafiropoulos & Tzanakakis, 2008). The PDGF family consists of 4 variants e.g. PDGF-A, PDGF-B, PDGF-C and PDGF-D (Reigstad et al., 2005). The late inclusion of PDGF-C and -D to the PDGF family was based on the identification of a cDNA sequencing showing similarities to other members of the PDGF/VEGF growth factors PDGF-C (Li et al. 2000) and PDGF-D (Bergsten et al. 2001). The active form of PDGF is a homo- or hetero-dimer of polypeptide chains A, B, C or D (e.g. PDGF-AA, PDGF-AB, PDGF-BB, PDF-CC, PDGF-DD) with the monomers being inactive, as reviewed by Reigstad et al., (2005). Specifically, PDGF-AA, PDGF-BB and PDGF-AB are formed by heterodimerization or homodimerization of two distinct but highly homologous polypeptides, A and B (Kelly et al., 1985; Lustig et al., 1999). Interestingly, both A and B chains can be produced as long and short isoforms through the alternative splicing of exon 6 (Pollock & Richardson, 1992). The short isoforms are the most prevalent in the ECM and were shown to be more stable and active as compared to the long isoforms which are usually secreted in small quantities (Pollock & Richardson, 1992; Andersson et al. 1994). The long isoforms are immobilized on the cell surface through a stretch of positively charged amino acids called the retention motif and are destined to serve autocrine purposes (Pollock & Richardson, 1992; Andersson et al. 1994). The retention motif can interact with negatively charged molecules such as GAGs. This motif can be removed by proteolytic processing that occurs in the extracellular space and leads to the generation of the short PDGFs version (Andersson et al. 1994). The existence of short and long isoforms allows additional fine-tuning of the PDGF-dependent downstream pathways.

PDGF signaling is directly mediated *via* the specific binding to the respective high affinity receptors α and β, which possess tyrosine kinase properties (PDGFRs) (Garcia-Olivas et al., 2003). PDGFRα can bind PDGF-A, PDGF-B and PDFG-C whereas PDGFRβ can bind PDGF-B and PDGF-D (Li et al., 2003). The phosphorylation of PDGF receptor triggers downstream activation of a number of signaling proteins including Scr, phosphatidylinositol 3 kinase (PI-3 K), phospholipase Cγ (PLCγ) and MAPK/Ras (Tallquist & Kazlauskas, 2004).

The PDGF-responsive signaling pathways play important roles in embryogenesis and adult tissue maintenance (Lustig et al., 1999). Indeed, the action of these GFs is of special importance in the context of wound repair, fibrosis and angiogenesis (Garcia-Olivas et al., 2003). Moreover, several PDGFs have been suggested to participate in the pathogenesis of various diseases such as fibrosis (Heldin et al., 1992) and in malignant processes including autocrine transformation and human oncogenesis (Kelly et al., 1985; Heldin et al., 1992). The newest members of PDGFs were both found to be involved in progressive renal diseases, glioblastomas, medulloblastomas and fibrosis of a variety of tissues. PDGF-C appears to play an important role in Ewing family sarcomas while PDGF-D is linked to lung, prostate and ovarian cancers (Reigstad et al., 2005).

Importantly, the availability of PDGFs and the quality of their binding to respective PDGFRs was shown to be modulated by the interactions with free GAGs and PGs. Indeed, PDGF is suggested to interact with PGs mainly through their GAG chains (Zafiropoulos et al., 2008). This interaction is mediated by the electrostatic interaction of the negatively charged GAGs with the positively charged peptides in the PDGF sequence as well as with the retention motif of the long PDGF isoform (Fager et al., 1995). Both the long and the short isoforms can bind GAGs, the first with 10-100 fold greater affinity (Lustig et al., 1999). Importantly, PDGF isoforms have different binding patters and discrete affinities as regarding specific CS subtypes. Thus, Garcia-Olivas et al., (2003) showed in a CHO cell model that CS, uniquely among the naturally occurring GAGs, binds the long but not the short PDGF isoforms. Furthermore, these authors demonstrate that CS is an effective inhibitor of the PDGF-AA (long isoform) binding to low molecular weight heparin and to the cell surface GAGs. In addition, CS-A/CS-B are suggested to bind short PDGF-BB variant (Kozma et al., 2009). These authors conclude that the interaction is unaffected by the type of hexuronate isomer located at the binding site as judged from similar effectiveness of chondroitinase B and chondroitinase AC-I resistant chain fragments to inhibit short PDGF-BB binding to native decorin derived CS-B. Moreover, it was demonstrated that CS-A/CS-B binding to the short PDGF-BB involves 4-0 sulfated disaccharides and especially di-2,4-0-sulfated ones. Therefore, it appears that the suitable localization or local accumulation of the latter disaccharides would influence the binding capabilities of CS-A and -B and not their total content. Conclusively PDGF variants may recognize and bind distinct GAG sequences. The distinct GAG binding properties may result from the fact that they demonstrate different configurations of polypeptide chain motifs potentially involved in the interaction (Kozma et al., 2009).

This interplay of PDGFs with matrix GAGs can regulate their biological functions. Specifically, it has been shown that exogenous CS-B (Fager et al., 1995) prevents the proliferation of human smooth muscle cells (SMCs) induced by PDGF, while CS-A does not. Similarly, CS-B was found to inhibit the proliferation of normal fibroblasts (Ferrao & Mason, 1993; Westergrem-Thorsson et al., 1991). On the other hand a significant co-stimulatory activity of exogenous CSA in combination with PDGF-BB on the growth of HT1080 and B6FS human fibrosarcoma cells was demonstrated (Fthenou et al., 2006). Moreover, the removal of endogenous cell surface CS in both HT1080 and B6FS cells had minor effects on short PDGF-BB function (Fthenou et al., 2006), which is corroborated by an earlier study showing that chondroitinase ABC treatment did not reduce the binding of short PDGF-BB on CHO cells' membrane (Garcia-Olivas et al., 2003). Indeed, it is suggested that the co-stimulatory effect of exogenous CSA was not due to transcriptional up-regulation of PDGF receptors but rather due to enhanced signaling of tyrosine kinases. Indeed, it is suggested that cell surface GAGs are not essential for receptor-mediated activity of PDGF and may contribute basically to the retention and accumulation of long PDGF isoforms (Garcia-Olivas et al., 2007). Therefore, the activities of CS chains appear to be discrete both as regarding their subtype and PDGF variants form (Figure 2).

In human lung fibrobrasts (DLF), it was determined that PDGF-BB receptor signaling and mitogenic responses can be significantly affected both by exogenous and endogenous CS chains (Fthenou et al., 2006). CS chains were found to downregulate the proliferative responses of DLF cells by reducing the phosphorylation of PDGF-Rβ (Fthenou et al., 2006; Zafiropoulos et al., 2008). Indeed, the CS- bearing decorin in smooth muscle cells (SMCs) (Nili et al., 2003) and β-D-xyloside (which is known to induce CS/DS synthesis) in human lung fibroblasts (Fthenou et al., 2008) can significantly reduce PDGF-Rβ phosphorylation. CS-A and B produced by arterial smooth muscle cells may bind PDGF competitively in atherogenesis but only CS-B inhibits cellular DNA synthesis. It is therefore, suggested that PDGF deposition may occur by binding to GAGs derived from smooth muscle cells within atherosclerotic lesions (Fager et al., 1995).

PDGF-BB has been shown to promote cell motility and to function as chemotactic signal for cells of mesenchymal origin (Schneller et al., 1997; Woodard et al., 1998). Indeed, it was demonstrated that both these functions were affected by the presence of free CS chains indicating that CS causes a generalized blockade of the PDGF-BB signaling pathway (Fthenou et al., 2008). On the other hand CS-chains bound into Neuropilin-1, which is a co-receptor for VEGFR, have been positively correlated to PDGF-regulated cell migration. In a recent report neuropilin-1 in a manner dependent on its CS chains was found to enhance PDGF-induced VSMC migration, possibly by acting as a co-receptor for PDGFRα and via selective mobilization of a novel p130Cas tyrosine phosphorylation pathway (Pellet-Many et al., 2011). Conclusively, the above data support the notion that the interaction between CS subtypes and PDGF may regulate the bioavailabity of PDGF through storage and/or controlled release (Fthenou et al., 2008).

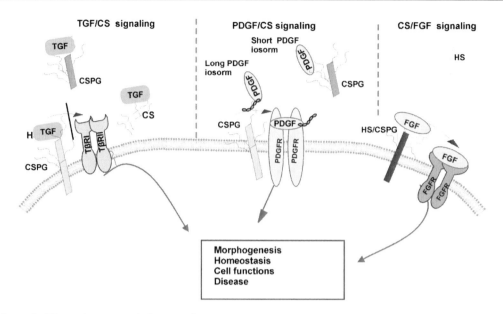

Figure 2. CS regulates growth factor action.

CS, Likely in Cooperation with HS Modulates FGF Signaling

Fibroblast Growth Factors (FGFs) comprise a structurally related family of 22 polypeptide growth factors that are found in organisms ranging from nematodes to humans (Ornitz & Itoh, 2001; Zhang et al., 2006). The members of the FGF family range in molecular mass from 11 to 34 kDa and share 17-71% amino acid identity (Ornitz&Itoh, 2001). FGFs can be grouped into seven subfamilies based on their sequence similarities and functional properties (Itoh & Ornitz, 2004; Popovici et al., 2005).

These GFs are expressed by various cell types and are involved in regulating growth, differentiation and gene expression at the cellular level, thereby regulating development, homeostasis and metabolism at the organ level (Asada et al., 2009). FGFs possess a large range of activities in embryonic development and physiological functions in the adult (Zhang et al., 2006). Thus, in the embryo, FGFs often signal across mesenchymal - epithelial boundaries, thereby regulating organogenesis and pattern formation (Boilly et al., 2000; Ornitz, 2005). Moreover, in the adult, FGFs play important roles in regulating homeostasis; wound healing and tissue repair (Finch & Rubin, 2004). Thus it was demonstrated that, FGF-2 promotes the recruitment of inflammatory cells to the wound site during the inflammatory phase of wound healing (Kibe et al., 2000), Furthermore, this GF, stimulates cellular proliferation and has been suggested to play a role in endothelial cell migration. The expression of FGF-10 increases considerably during wound repair (Radek et al., 2009). FGF-7 (keratinocyte growth factor) was initially identified as a highly specific paracrine growth factor for epithelial cells (Finch et al., 1989; Rubin et al., 1989). These GFs are implicated in tumorigenesis, not only due to their mitogenic and angiogenic effects, but also due to their migratory effects on tumor and endothelial cells (Boilly et al., 2000).

The activities of FGFs are mainly exerted through their high affinity binding to the respective FGF receptor tyrosine kinases (FGFR1-4) on the cell surface (Basilico &

Moscatelli, 1992; Ornitz, 2000). Each FGF receptor contains an extracellular ligand binding domain, a single transmembrane domain and an intracellular tyrosine kinase domain (Ornitz, 2000). FGF binding to the cell surface receptors induces FGFR dimerisation, subsequent activation of receptor tyrosine kinases and autophosphorylation of the cytoplasmic domains of receptors (Klint & Claesson-Welsh, 1999). Target enzymes such as PLCγ and Src bind to the tyrosine autophosphorylation sites and in turn themselves become phosphorylated. The autophosphorylation sites also serve as binding sites for adaptor proteins such as Grb2 and Shc. Grb2 bind to the Ras- guanine nucleotide-releasing factor Sos. The formation of Grb2-Sos complex results in recruitment of the oncogene Ras, and its further activation. Indeed, it is well established that the Ras signaling pathway is crucial for the FGF-induced proliferation of many cell types (Boilly et al., 2000). Thus, activated Ras leads to activation of a signaling cascade involving the Ser/Thr kinase Raf, the dual specificity MAP kinase (MEK), and MAP kinase (ERK1/2) (Lewis et al., 1998). Interestingly, the role and downstream signaling of PKC, Src or PI-3 kinase seem to depend on cell type, even though the final effect of the FGF-2 induced signal is to promote cellular proliferation (Boilly et al., 2000). Activation of FGF receptors by their ligands may elicit a diverse set of cellular responses, including proliferation, migration and differentiation (Boilly et al., 2000).

FGFR activation is modulated by heparin, HS or other GAG chains (Rapraeger et al., 1991). Indeed, heparin, modulates the specificity of the receptor-ligand binding having an active role in the establishing an active FGF-FGFR complex. Therefore, heparin and its structural analogue HS have been characterized as cofactors (Zhang et al., 2006). Some FGFs were found to interact with CS (Asada et al., 2009). Furthermore, it is postulated that variations in the structure of CS and their spatiotemporal expression may modulate the biological activity of these FGFs (Asada et al., 2009). Specifically it was show that even though the majority of FGFs have little or no affinity for CS-E, members FGF-3, -6, -8, -16, -18 and -22 bind effectively to CS-E. FGF-5 showed moderate affinity for CS-D, but no FGF exhibited any affinity for CS-B. Interestingly, the primary structures of involved FGFs as well as the positioning of their basic amino acids are not very similar making mechanistic aspects of the binding not well understood (Asada et al., 2009). In an earlier study on FGFs' binding, Deepa et al., (2002) revealed that particular FGF-16 and FGF-18 bind to CS-E. These authors report that FGF-2 and FGF-19 bind to CS-E with lower affinity as compared to heparin whereas FGF-1 exhibits almost no affinity to CS-E. Furthermore, CSA/CSB hybrid chains isolated from embryonic pig brain exhibited strong binding affinity towards FGF2, -10 and 18 and not CS isolated from adult pig brain (Deepa et al., 2004). There is also evidence that in some cases GAGs have the capacity to protect FGF from proteolytic cleavage. According to Coltrini et al., (1993) this capacity decreases in the following order: heparin > HS > CS > DS >hyaluronan. Thus, the different protective capacities of various GAGs seem to be at least partly related to differences in their degree of sulfation.

A rising amount of evidence has implicated that CSPGs also participate in FGF-2 signaling (Bao et al., 2004; Molteni et al., 1999; Smith et al., 2007). CSPGs were shown to modulate the binding of FGF-2 to FGFRs, either autonomously in the role of low affinity binding sites (Smith et al., 2007) or in cooperation with the HS chains (Deepa et al., 2004). Moreover, it was demonstrated that, in addition to HS chains, CS/DS modulated both basal and FGF-2-induced growth of WM9 and M5 human metastatic melanoma cells (Nikitovic et al., 2008). Upon utilization of sodium chlorate, a competent inhibitor of GAG sulfation (Fannon & Nugent, 1996), a significant inhibition in WM9 and M5 cell growth was observed which was not duly restored by the addition of FGF-2. Therefore, Nikitovic et al., (2008) suggest that CSPGs, likely in cooperation with HS, participate in metastatic melanoma cell FGF-2-induced mitogenic response, which is postulated to represent a novel finding establishing the central role of sulfated GAGs on melanoma growth. This is in accordance with earlier studies reporting that sulfation of GAGs are critical for the mitogenic effect of FGF-2 (Ashikari-Hada et al., 2004; Taylor et al., 2005). CS is suggested to exert its effect by modulating the FGF-2 - FGFRs interactions. Thus, it was shown that the removal of DS (CS-B) inhibited the proliferative response of human fibroblasts to FGF-2 (Denholm et al., 2000). These results corroborate to the suggestion that the removal of CS-B from the cell surface might interfere with the binding of this GF to its receptors (Denholm et al., 2000). In a recent study it was reported that CS are essential for proliferation, self-renewal and maintenance of FGF-2 responsive Neural Stem / Progenitor Cells (NSPCs) (Sirko et al., 2010). Furthermore, these authors show that the removal of CS chains by chondroitinase ABC reduced FGF-2 mediated MAP kinase activation, resulting in the reduction of the FGF-induced neural stem cell/progenitor proliferation. Therefore, it is postulated that CSPGs act as essential cofactors for FGF-2 mediated MAP kinase signaling and proliferation of primary NSPCs (Sirko et al., 2010).

FGF-7 (keratinocyte growth factor), is expressed in dermal tissue (Rubin et al., 1995) and is suggested to be involved in wound healing (Werner et al., 1998). The expression of this GF is activated upon injury and induces the proliferation of keratinocytes (Trowbridge et al., 2002). It was shown that CS-B (DS), abundantly expressed in dermal tissues (Tajima et al., 1982), enhances the FGF-7-induced keratinocyte proliferation in a manner selective for FGF-7 (Trowbridge et al., 2002). In addition, in this study it was demonstrated that the size and the sulfation level of CS-B affect both proliferation and FGF-7 receptor binding. In contrast, Asada et al., (2009) show only a weak interaction between FGF-7 and CS-B and attribute this discrepancy to the fact that the earlier investigators did not take into account the direct interactions among the proteins within the signaling complex (*i.e.* CS-B, FGF-7 and FGFR). Further structural analysis will be needed to shed light on this issue.

In a keratinocyte cell model it was demonstrated that the function of FGF-10 during injury is dependent upon the expression of specific cutaneous GAGs produced (Radek et al., 2009). Thus, it is postulated that DS (CS-B) released from the dermis acts as a cofactor for FGF-10 and promotes FGF-10 and FGF-7 dependent keratinocyte proliferation and migration. Moreover, it is suggested that cleavage of wound derived-DS, generating small, more bioactive DS fragments specifically promotes FGF-10 activity. Interestingly, the sulfation pattern of DS appears to be important on the ability of this GAG to promote cell proliferation through FGF-7 and FGF-10 (Radek et al., 2009). In a separate study it was reported that human FGF-19, an endocrine metabolic regulator that controls bile acid synthesis in the liver, requires hepatic sulfated GAGs, such as heparin, HS and CS, for its signaling *via* FGFR4 (Nakamura et al., 2011).

Syndecans are the major cell surface PGs expressed by virtually all epithelial cells (Bernfield at al., 1992). The majority of GAG chains bound into the syndecan core proteins are of the HS type, although syndecan-1 (Rapraeger et al., 1985) and syndecan-4 (Shworak et al., 1994) are additionally modified by CS chains. CS chains of syndecan-1 and syndecan-4 were found to have a higher degree of sulfation than their HS counterparts (Deepa et al., 2004). Indeed, the HS chains of syndecan-1 and syndecan-4 were structurally and functionally similar but, the CS chains were distinct in both respects and appear to have regulatory roles in modulating GF functions through the cooperation with the HS chains (Deepa et al., 2004). The removal of HS chains resulted in a complete loss of FGF-2 binding whereas the removal of the CS chains from both syndecans in this study accelerated the association and dissociation of FGF-2 from their HS counterparts (Deepa et al., 2004). These results prompted the authors to postulate the formation a ternary or quaternary complex involving syndecan CS chains, HS chains and FGF and possibly involving the syndecan core protein depending on the nature of the growth factor. This complex is suggested to efficiently transfer the FGF to its corresponding cell surface receptor (Deepa et al., 2004).

Take Home Message

CS is an emerging essential cellular effector that integrates and responds to the environmental stimuli through the regulation of GF signaling pathways. Correct integration of the GF-CS signaling regulates key biological functions that participate in the development and homeostasis of tissues throughout life whereas, abnormalities in these interactions are implicated in some pathological processes. Until now, the application of CS/DS and their derivatives has been limited due to fact that in most cases the precisely sulfated distinct structures of CS/DS, which specifically bind to functional proteins, have not been elucidated. Therefore, structural elucidation of the functional domains of CS/DS is desired to fully characterise the roles and possible utilisation of these versatile molecules.

References

Afratis, N., Gialeli, C., Nikitovic, D., Tsegenidis, T., Karousou, E., Theocharis, A. D., Pavao, M. S., Tzanakakis, G. N. &Karamanos, N. K. (2012). Glycosaminoglycans: key players in cancer cell biology and treatment. *Febs J*, *279*, 1177-1197.

Alliston, T. (2010). Chondroitin sulfate and growth factor signaling in the skeleton: Possible links to MPS VI. *J PediatrRehabil Med.*,*3*, 129-138.

Andersson, M., Ostman, A., Westermark, B. &Heldin, C. H. (1994). Characterization of the retention motif in the C-terminal part of the long splice form of platelet-derived growth factor A-chain. *J BiolChem*, 269, 926-930.

App, H., Hazan, R., Zilberstein, A., Ullrich, A., Schlessinger, J. & Rapp, U. (1991). Epidermal growth factor (EGF) stimulates association and kinase activity of Raf-1 with the EGF receptor. *Mol Cell Biol*, *11*, 913-919.

Asada, M., Shinomiya, M., Suzuki, M., Honda, E., Sugimoto, R., Ikekita, M. & Imamura, T. (2009). Glycosaminoglycan affinity of the complete fibroblast growth factor family. *BiochimBiophysActa*, *1790*, 40-48.

Ashikari-Hada, S., Habuchi, H., Kariya, Y., Itoh, N., Reddi, A. H. &Kimata, K. (2004). Characterization of growth factor-binding structures in heparin/heparan sulfate using an octasaccharide library. *J BiolChem*, *279*, 12346-12354.

Attisano, L. & Lee-Hoeflich, S. T. (2001). The Smads. *Genome Biol*, 2, REVIEWS3010.

Bao, X., Nishimura, S., Mikami, T., Yamada, S., Itoh, N. &Sugahara, K. (2004). Chondroitin sulfate/dermatan sulfate hybrid chains from embryonic pig brain, which contain a higher proportion of L-iduronic acid than those from adult pig brain, exhibit neuritogenic and growth factor binding activities. *J Biol Chem, 279,* 9765-9776.

Barkan, D., Green, J. E. & Chambers, A. F. (2010). Extracellular matrix: a gatekeeper in the transition from dormancy to metastatic growth. *Eur J Cancer, 46,* 1181-1188.

Basilico, C. &Moscatelli, D. (1992). The FGF family of growth factors and oncogenes. *Adv Cancer Res, 59,* 115-165.

Bergsten, E., Uutela, M., Li, X., Pietras, K., Ostman, A., Heldin, C. H., Alitalo, K. & Eriksson, U. (2001). PDGF-D is a specific, protease-activated ligand for the PDGF beta-receptor. *Nat Cell Biol, 3,* 512-516.

Bernabeu, C., Lopez-Novoa, J. M. & Quintanilla, M. (2009). The emerging role of TGF-beta superfamily coreceptors in cancer. *Biochim Biophys Acta, 1792,* 954-973.

Bernfield, M., Kokenyesi, R., Kato, M., Hinkes, M. T., Spring, J., Gallo, R. L. & Lose, E. J. (1992). Biology of the syndecans: a family of transmembraneheparan sulfate proteoglycans. *Annu Rev Cell Biol, 8,* 365-393.

Bi, Y., Stuelten, C. H., Kilts, T., Wadhwa, S., Iozzo, R. V., Robey, P. G., Chen, X. D. & Young, M. F. (2005). Extracellular matrix proteoglycans control the fate of bone marrow stromal cells. *J Biol Chem, 280,* 30481–30489.

Bobick, B. E., Chen, F. H., Le, A. M. & Tuan, R. S. (2009). Regulation of the chondrogenic phenotype in culture. *Birth Defects Res C Embryo Today, 87,* 351-371.

Boilly, B., Vercoutter-Edouart, A. S., Hondermarck, H., Nurcombe, V. & Le Bourhis, X. (2000). FGF signals for cell proliferation and migration through different pathways. *Cytokine Growth Factor Rev, 11,* 295-302.

Brazil, D. P. &Hemmings, B. A. (2001). Ten years of protein kinase B signalling: a hard Akt to follow. *Trends Biochem Sci, 26,* 657-664.

Cantley, L. C. (2002). The phosphoinositide 3-kinase pathway. *Science, 296,* 1655-1657.

Caterson, B., Flanerry, C. R., Hughes,C. E. & Little, C. B. (1999). Mechanisms of proteoglycan metabolism that lead to cartilage destruction in the pathogenesis of arthritis. *Drugs Today, 35,* 397-402.

Chang, L. & Karin, M. (2001). Mammalian MAP kinase signalling cascades. *Nature, 410,* 37-40.

Coltrini, D., Rusnati, M., Zoppetti, G., Oreste, P., Isacchi, A., Caccia, P., Bergonzoni, L. &Presta, M. (1993). Biochemical bases of the interaction of human basic fibroblast growth factor with glycosaminoglycans. New insights from trypsin digestion studies. *Eur J Biochem, 214,* 51-58.

Deepa, S. S., Umehara, Y., Higashiyama, S., Itoh, N. &Sugahara, K. (2002). Specific molecular interactions of oversulfated chondroitin sulfate E with various heparin-binding growth factors. Implications as a physiological binding partner in the brain and other tissues. *J Biol Chem, 277,* 43707-43716.

Deepa, S. S., Yamada, S., Zako, M., Goldberger, O. &Sugahara, K. (2004). Chondroitin sulfate chains on syndecan-1 and syndecan-4 from normal murine mammary gland epithelial cells are structurally and functionally distinct and cooperate with heparan sulfate chains to bind growth factors. A novel function to control binding of midkine, pleiotrophin, and basic fibroblast growth factor. *J Biol Chem, 279,* 37368-37376.

Denholm, E. M., Cauchon, E., Poulin, C. & Silver, P. J. (2000). Inhibition of human dermal fibroblast proliferation by removal of dermatan sulfate. *Eur J Pharmacol, 400,* 145-153.

Duronio, V., Scheid, M. P. &Ettinger, S. (1998). Downstream signalling events regulated by phosphatidylinositol 3-kinase activity. *Cell Signal, 10*, 233-239.

Evanko, S. P., Raines, E. W., Ross, R., Gold, L. I. & Wight, T. N. (1998). Proteoglycan distribution in lesions of atherosclerosis depends on lesion severity, structural characteristics, and the proximity of platelet-derived growth factor and transforming growth factor-beta. *Am J Pathol, 152*, 533-546.

Fager, G., Camejo, G., Olsson, U., Ostergren-Lunden, G., Lustig, F. &Bondjers, G. (1995). Binding of platelet-derived growth factor and low density lipoproteins to glycosaminoglycan species produced by human arterial smooth muscle cells. *J Cell Physiol, 163*, 380-392.

Fannon, M. & Nugent, M. A. (1996). Basic fibroblast growth factor binds its receptors, is internalized, and stimulates DNA synthesis in Balb/c3T3 cells in the absence of heparan sulfate. *J Biol Chem, 271*, 17949-17956.

Ferrao, A. V. & Mason, R. M. (1993). The effect of heparin on cell proliferation and type-I collagen synthesis by adult human dermal fibroblasts. *Biochim Biophys Acta, 1180*, 225-230.

Finch, P. W. & Rubin, J. S. (2004). Keratinocyte growth factor/fibroblast growth factor 7, a homeostatic factor with therapeutic potential for epithelial protection and repair. *Adv Cancer Res, 91*, 69-136.

Finch, P. W., Rubin, J. S., Miki, T., Ron, D. &Aaronson, S. A. (1989). Human KGF is FGF-related with properties of a paracrine effector of epithelial cell growth. *Science, 245*, 752-755.

Friesel, R. E. &Maciag, T. (1995). Molecular mechanisms of angiogenesis: fibroblast growth factor signal transduction. *Faseb J, 9*, 919-925.

Fthenou, E., Zafiropoulos, A., Katonis, P., Tsatsakis, A., Karamanos, N. K. &Tzanakakis, G. N. (2008). Chondroitin sulfate prevents platelet derived growth factor-mediated phosphorylation of PDGF-R beta in normal human fibroblasts severely impairing mitogenic responses. *J Cell Biochem, 103*, 1866-1876.

Fthenou, E., Zafiropoulos, A., Tsatsakis, A., Stathopoulos, A., Karamanos, N. K. &Tzanakakis, G. N. (2006). Chondroitin sulfate A chains enhance platelet derived growth factor-mediated signalling in fibrosarcoma cells. *Int J Biochem Cell Biol, 38*, 2141-2150.

Garcia-Olivas, R., Hoebeke, J., Castel, S., Reina, M., Fager, G., Lustig, F. &Vilaro, S. (2003). Differential binding of platelet-derived growth factor isoforms to glycosaminoglycans. *Histochem Cell Biol, 120*, 371-382.

García-Olivas, R., Vilaro, S., Reina, M. & Castel, S. (2007). PDGF-stimulated cell proliferation and migration of human arterial smooth muscle cells. Colocalization of PDGF isoforms with glycosaminoglycans. *Int J Biochem Cell Biol., 39*, 1915-1929.

Goldring, M. B., Tsuchimochi, K. &Ijiri, K. (2006). The control of chondrogenesis. *J Cell Biochem, 97*, 33-44.

Haskins, M., Casal, M., Ellinwood, N. M., Melniczek, J., Mazrier, H. &Giger, U. (2002). Animal models for mucopolysaccharidosis and their clinical relevance. *Acta Paediatr Suppl, 91*, 88–97.

Hayes, A. J. & Ralphs, J. R. (2011). The response of fetal annulus fibrosus cells to growth factors: modulation of matrix synthesis by TGF-beta1 and IGF-1. *Histochem Cell Biol, 136*, 163-175.

Heldin, C. H. (1992). Structural and functional studies on platelet-derived growth factor. *Embo J*, *11*, 4251-4259.

Heldin, C. H., Landstrom, M. &Moustakas, A. (2009). Mechanism of TGF-beta signaling to growth arrest, apoptosis, and epithelial-mesenchymal transition. *Curr Opin Cell Biol*, *21*, 166-176.

Heldin, C. H., Miyazono, K. & ten Dijke, P. (1997). TGF-beta signaling from cell membrane to nucleus through SMAD proteins. *Nature*, *390*, 465-471.

Heldin, C. H. &Westermark, B. (1999). Mechanism of action and in vivo role of platelet-derived growth factor. *Physiol Rev*, *79*, 1283-1316.

Hempel, U., Hintze, V., Möller, S., Schnabelrauch, M., Scharnweber, D. & Dieter, P. (2012). Artificial extracellular matrices composed of collagen I and sulfated hyaluronan with adsorbed transforming growth factor β1 promote collagen synthesis of human mesenchymal stromal cells. *Acta Biomater*, *8*, 659-666.

Hildebrand, A. (1994). Interaction of the small interstitial proteoglycans biglycan, decorin and fibromodulin with transforming growth factor beta, *Biochem J*, *302*, 527–534.

Hintze, V., Miron, A., Moeller, S., Schnabelrauch, M., Wiesmann, H. P., Worch, H. &Scharnweber, D. (2012). Sulfated hyaluronan and chondroitin sulfate derivatives interact differently with human transforming growth factor-beta1 (TGF-beta1). *Acta Biomater*, *8*, 2144-2152.

Holzmann, J., Brandl, N., Zemann, A., Schabus, R., Marlovits, S., Cowburn, R. &Huettinger, M. (2006). Assorted effects of TGF beta and chondroitin sulfate on p38 and ERK1/2 activation levels in human articular chondrocytes stimulated with LPS. *Osteoarthritis Cartilage*, *14*, 519–525.

Hynes, R. O. (2009). The extracellular matrix: not just pretty fibrils. *Science*, *326*, 1216-1219.

Ioachim, H. L. (1976). The stromal reaction of tumors: an expression of immune surveillance. *J Natl Cancer Inst*, *57*, 465-475.

Iozzo, R. V. & San Antonio, J. D. (2001). Heparan sulfate proteoglycans: heavy hitters in the angiogenesis arena. *J Clin Invest*, *108*, 349-355.

Itoh, N. &Ornitz, D. M. (2004). Evolution of the Fgf and Fgfr gene families. *Trends Genet*, *20*, 563-569.

Jiang, G. & Hunter, T. (1999). Receptor signaling: when dimerization is not enough. *Curr Biol*, *9*, R568-571.

Kajanne, R., Miettinen, P., Mehlem, A., Leivonen, S. K., Birrer, M., Foschi, M., Kahari, V. M. &Leppa, S. (2007). EGF-R regulates MMP function in fibroblasts through MAPK and AP-1 pathways. *J Cell Physiol*, *212*, 489-497.

Karimi-Abdolrezaee, S., Eftekharpour, E., Wang, J., Schut, D. &Fehlings, M. G. (2010). Synergistic effects of transplanted adult neural stem/progenitor cells, chondroitinase, and growth factors promote functional repair and plasticity of the chronically injured spinal cord. *J Neurosci*, *30*, 1657-1676.

Karimi-Abdolrezaee, S., Schut, D., Wang, J. &Fehlings, M. G. (2012). Chondroitinase and growth factors enhance activation and oligodendrocyte differentiation of endogenous neural precursor cells after spinal cord injury. *PLoS One*, *7*, e37589.

Kelly, J. D., Raines, E. W., Ross, R. & Murray, M. J. (1985). The B chain of PDGF alone is sufficient for mitogenesis. *Embo J*, *4*, 3399-3405.

Kibe, Y., Takenaka, H. &Kishimoto, S. (2000). Spatial and temporal expression of basic fibroblast growth factor protein during wound healing of rat skin. *Br J Dermatol, 143*, 720-727.

Klint, P. &Claesson-Welsh, L. (1999). Signal transduction by fibroblast growth factor receptors. *Front Biosci, 4*, D165-177.

Kluppel, M., Wight, T. N., Chan, C., Hinek, A. &Wrana, J. L. (2005). Maintenance of chondroitin sulfation balance by chondroitin-4-sulfotransferase 1 is required for chondrocyte development and growth factor signaling during cartilage morphogenesis, *Development, 132*, 3989–4003.

Kozma, E. M., Wisowski, G. &Olczyk, K. (2009). Platelet derived growth factor BB is a ligand for dermatan sulfate chain(s) of small matrix proteoglycans from normal and fibrosis affected fascia. *Biochimie, 91*, 1394-1404.

Lamari, F. N. &Karamanos, N. K. (2006). Structure of chondroitin sulfate. *Adv Pharmacol, 53*, 33-48.

Lander, A. D. (1998). Proteoglycans: master regulators of molecular encounter? *Matrix Biol, 17*, 465-472.

Leask, A. & Abraham, D. J. (2004). TGF-beta signaling and the fibrotic response. *Faseb J, 18*, 816-827.

Lewis, T. S., Shapiro, P. S. &Ahn, N. G. (1998). Signal transduction through MAP kinase cascades. *Adv Cancer Res, 74*, 49-139.

Li, X. & Eriksson, U. (2003). Novel PDGF family members: PDGF-C and PDGF-D. *Cytokine Growth Factor Rev, 14*, 91-98.

Li, X., Ponten, A., Aase, K., Karlsson, L., Abramsson, A., Uutela, M., Backstrom, G., Hellstrom, M., Bostrom, H., Li, H., Soriano, P., Betsholz, C., Heldin, C. H., Alitalo, K., Ostman, A. & Eriksson, U.(2000). PDGF-C is a new protease-activated ligand for the PDGF alpha-receptor. *Nat Cell Biol, 2*, 302-309.

Lustig, F., Hoebeke, J., Simonson, C., Ostergren-Lunden, G., Bondjers, G., Ruetchi, U. &Fager, G. (1999). Processing of PDGF gene products determines interactions with glycosaminoglycans. *J MolRecognit, 12*, 112-120.

Maeda, N., He, J., Yajima, Y., Mikami, T., Sugahara, K. & Yabe, T. (2003). Heterogeneity of the chondroitin sulfate portion of phosphacan/6B4 proteoglycan regulates its binding affinity for pleiotrophin/heparin binding growth-associated molecule. *J BiolChem, 278*, 35805-35811.

Malarkey, K., Belham, C. M., Paul, A., Graham, A., McLees, A., Scott, P. H. &Plevin, R. (1995). The regulation of tyrosine kinase signaling pathways by growth factor and G-protein-coupled receptors. *Biochem J, 309*, 361-375.

Malavaki, C., Mizumoto, S., Karamanos, N. &Sugahara, K. (2008). Recent advances in the structural study of functional chondroitin sulfate and dermatan sulfate in health and disease. *Connect Tissue Res, 49*, 133-139.

Manton, K. J., Leong, D. F., Cool, S. M. &Nurcombe, V. (2007). Disruption of heparan and chondroitin sulfate signaling enhances mesenchymal stem cell-derived osteogenic differentiation via bone morphogenetic protein signaling pathways. *Stem Cells, 25*, 2845-2854.

Manton, K. J., Haupt, L. M., Vengadasalam, K., Nurcombe, V. & Cool, S. M. (2007). Glycosaminoglycan and growth factor mediated murine calvarial cell proliferation. *J Mol Histol,38*, 415–424.

Massague, J., Seoane, J. & Wotton, D. (2005). Smad transcription factors. *Genes Dev, 19*, 2783-2810.

McKinnon, R. D., Wardon, S. & Kiel, M. E.(2005). PDGF alpha-receptor signal strength controls an RTK rheostat that integrates phosphoinositol 3'-kinase and phospholipase Cgamma pathways during oligodendrocyte maturation. *J Neurosci., 25*, 3499-3508.

Meulmeester, E. & Ten Dijke, P. (2011). The dynamic roles of TGF-beta in cancer. *J Pathol, 223*, 205-218.

Miyazaki, T., Miyauchi, S., Tawada, A., Anada, T., Matsuzaka, S. & Suzuki, O. (2008). Oversulfated chondroitin sulfate-E binds to BMP-4 and enhances osteoblast differentiation. *J Cell Physiol., 217*, 769-777.

Molteni, A., Modrowski, D., Hott, M. & Marie, P. J. (1999). Alterations of matrix- and cell-associated proteoglycans inhibit osteogenesis and growth response to fibroblast growth factor-2 in cultured rat mandibular condyle and calvaria. *Cell Tissue Res, 295*, 523-536.

Moustakas, A. &Heldin, C. H. (2009). The regulation of TGFbeta signal transduction. *Development, 136*, 3699-3714.

Nakamura, M., Uehara, Y., Asada, M., Honda, E., Nagai, N., Kimata, K., Suzuki, M. & Imamura, T. (2011). Sulfated glycosaminoglycans are required for specific and sensitive fibroblast growth factor (FGF) 19 signaling via FGF receptor 4 and betaKlotho. *J Biol Chem, 286*, 26418-26423.

Nikitovic, D., Assouti, M., Sifaki, M., Katonis, P., Krasagakis, K., Karamanos, N. K. &Tzanakakis, G. N. (2008). Chondroitin sulfate and heparan sulfate-containing proteoglycans are both partners and targets of basic fibroblast growth factor-mediated proliferation in human metastatic melanoma cell lines. *Int J Biochem Cell Biol, 40*, 72-83.

Nikitovic, D., Chatzinikolaou, G., Tsiaoussis, J., Tsatsakis, A., Karamanos, N. K. &Tzanakakis, G. N. (2012). Insights into targeting colon cancer cell fate at the level of proteoglycans / glycosaminoglycans. *Curr Med Chem, 19*, 4247-4258.

Nili, N., Cheema, A. N., Giordano, F. J., Barolet, A. W., Babaei, S., Hickey, R., Eskandarian, M. R., Smeets, M., Butany, J., Pasterkamp, G. & Strauss, B. H.(2003). Decorin inhibition of PDGF-stimulated vascular smooth muscle cell function: potential mechanism for inhibition of intimal hyperplasia after balloon angioplasty. *Am J Pathol, 163*, 869-878.

Ornitz, D. M. (2005). FGF signaling in the developing endochondral skeleton. *Cytokine Growth Factor Rev, 16*, 205-213.

Ornitz, D. M. (2000). FGFs, heparan sulfate and FGFRs: complex interactions essential for development. *Bioessays, 22*, 108-112.

Ornitz, D. M. &Itoh, N. (2001). Fibroblast growth factors. *Genome Biol, 2*, REVIEWS3005.

Padua, D. &Massague, J. (2009). Roles of TGFbeta in metastasis. *Cell Res, 19*, 89-102.

Paulsson, M. & Heinegard, D. (1984). Noncollagenous cartilage proteins current status of an emerging research field. *Coll Relat Res, 4*, 219-229.

Pavao, M. S., Vilela-Silva, A. C. &Mourao, P. A. (2006). Biosynthesis of chondroitin sulfate: from the early, precursor discoveries to nowadays, genetics approaches. *AdvPharmacol, 53*, 117-140.

Pellet-Many, C., Franklel, P., Evans, I. M., Herzog, B., Jünemann-Ramírez, M. & Zachary, I. C. (2011). Neuropilin-1 mediates PDGF stimulation of vascular smooth muscle cell migration and signalling via p130Cas. *Biochem J.,435*, 609-618.

Pohlers, D., Brenmoehl, J., Loffler, I., Muller, C. K., Leipner, C., Schultze-Mosgau, S., Stallmach, A., Kinne, R. W. & Wolf, G. (2009). TGF-beta and fibrosis in different organs - molecular pathway imprints. *BiochimBiophysActa*, *1792*, 746-756.

Pollock, R. A. & Richardson, W. D. (1992). The alternative-splice isoforms of the PDGF A-chain differ in their ability to associate with the extracellular matrix and to bind heparin in vitro. *Growth Factors*, *7*, 267-277.

Popovici, C., Roubin, R., Coulier, F. & Birnbaum, D. (2005). An evolutionary history of the FGF superfamily. *Bioessays*, *27*, 849-857.

Radek, K. A., Taylor, K. R. & Gallo, R. L. (2009). FGF-10 and specific structural elements of dermatan sulfate size and sulfation promote maximal keratinocyte migration and cellular proliferation. *Wound Repair Regen*, *17*, 118-126.

Rapraeger, A. &Bernfield, M. (1985). Cell surface proteoglycan of mammary epithelial cells. Protease releases a heparan sulfate-rich ectodomain from a putative membrane-anchored domain. *J Biol Chem*, *260*, 4103-4109.

Rapraeger, A. C., Krufka, A. &Olwin, B. B. (1991). Requirement of heparan sulfate for bFGF-mediated fibroblast growth and myoblast differentiation. *Science*, *252*, 1705-1708.

Reigstad, L. J., Varhaug, J. E. &Lillehaug, J. R. (2005). Structural and functional specificities of PDGF-C and PDGF-D, the novel members of the platelet-derived growth factors family. *Febs J*, *272*, 5723-5741.

Roberts, A. B., Kim, S. J., Noma, T., Glick, A. B., Lafyatis, R., Lechleider, R., Jakowlew, S. B., Geiser, A., O'Reilly, M. A., Danielpour, D. et al. (1991). Multiple forms of TGF-beta: distinct promoters and differential expression. *Ciba Found Symp.*, *157*, 7-15.

Rozario, T. &DeSimone, D. W. (2010). The extracellular matrix in development and morphogenesis: a dynamic view. *Dev Biol*, *341*, 126-140.

Rubin, J. S., Bottaro, D. P., Chedid, M., Miki, T., Ron, D., Cheon, G., Taylor, W. G., Fortney, E., Sakata, H., Finch, P. W. et al. (1995). Keratinocyte growth factor. *Cell Bio lInt*, *19*, 399-411.

Ruiz-Ortega, M., Rodriguez-Vita, J., Sanchez-Lopez, E., Carvajal, G. &Egido, J. (2007). TGF-beta signaling in vascular fibrosis. *Cardiovasc Res*, *74*, 196-206.

Schaefer, L. &Iozzo, R. V. (2008). Biological functions of the small leucine-rich proteoglycans: from genetics to signal transduction. *J BiolChem*, *283*, 21305-21309.

Schneller, M., Vuori, K. &Ruoslahti, E. (1997). Alphavbeta3 integrin associates with activated insulin and PDGFbeta receptors and potentiates the biological activity of PDGF. *Embo J*, *16*, 5600-5607.

Shworak, N. W., Shirakawa, M., Mulligan, R. C. & Rosenberg, R. D. (1994). Characterization of ryudocan glycosaminoglycan acceptor sites. *J Biol Chem*, *269*, 21204-21214.

Siegel, P. M. &Massague, J. (2003). Cytostatic and apoptotic actions of TGF-beta in homeostasis and cancer. *Nat Rev Cancer, 3*, 807-821.

Sirko, S., von Holst, A., Weber, A., Wizenmann, A., Theocharidis, U., Gotz, M. &Faissner, A. (2010). Chondroitin sulfates are required for fibroblast growth factor-2-dependent proliferation and maintenance in neural stem cells and for epidermal growth factor-dependent migration of their progeny. *Stem Cells*, *28*, 775-787.

Sixt, M., Kanazawa, N., Selg, M., Samson, T., Roos, G., Reinhardt, D. P., Pabst, R. Lutz, M. B. & Sorokin, L. (2005). The conduit system transports soluble antigens from the afferent lymph to resident dendritic cells in the T cell area of the lymph node. *Immunity*, *22*, 19-29.

Smith, S. M., West, L. A., Govindraj, P., Zhang, X., Ornitz, D. M. &Hassell, J. R. (2007). Heparan and chondroitin sulfate on growth plate perlecan mediate binding and delivery of FGF-2 to FGF receptors. *Matrix Biol*, *26*, 175-184.

Sorokin, L. (2010). The impact of the extracellular matrix on inflammation. *Nat Rev Immunol*, *10*, 712-723.

Tajima, S., Nishikawa, T., Hatano, H. & Nagai, Y. (1982). Distribution of macromolecular components in human dermal connective tissue. *Arch Dermatol Res*, *273*, 115-120.

Tallquist, M. &Kazlauskas, A. (2004). PDGF signaling in cells and mice. *Cytokine Growth Factor Rev*, *15*, 205-213.

Tang, Y., Wu, X., Lei, W., Pang, L., Wan, C., Shi, Z., Zhao, L., Nagy, T.R., Peng, X., Hu, J., Feng, X., Van Hul, W., Wan, M. & Cao X. (2009). TGF-beta1-induced migration of bone mesenchymal stem cells couples bone resorption with formation. *Nat Med*, *15*, 757–765.

Taylor, K. R., Rudisill, J. A. & Gallo, R. L. (2005). Structural and sequence motifs in dermatan sulfate for promoting fibroblast growth factor-2 (FGF-2) and FGF-7 activity. *J BiolChem*, *280*, 5300-5306.

ten Dijke, P. & Arthur, H. M. (2007). Extracellular control of TGFbetasignalling in vascular development and disease. *Nat Rev Mol Cell Biol*, *8*, 857-869.

Theocharis, A. D. &Theocharis, D. A. (2002). High-performance capillary electrophoretic analysis of hyaluronan and galactosaminoglycan-disaccharides in gastrointestinal carcinomas. Differential disaccharide composition as a possible tool-indicator for malignancies. *Biomed Chromatogr*, *16*, 157-161.

Trowbridge, J. M., Rudisill, J. A., Ron, D. & Gallo, R. L. (2002). Dermatan sulfate binds and potentiates activity of keratinocyte growth factor (FGF-7). *J Biol Chem*, *277*, 42815-42820.

Ueoka, C., Kaneda, N., Okazaki, I., Nadanaka, S., Muramatsu, T. &Sugahara, K. (2000). Neuronal cell adhesion, mediated by the heparin-binding neuroregulatory factor midkine, is specifically inhibited by chondroitin sulfate E. Structural and functional implications of the over-sulfated chondroitin sulfate. *J Biol Chem*, *275*, 37407-37413.

Wegrowski, Y. &Maquart, F. X. (2004). Involvement of stromal proteoglycans in tumour progression. *Crit Rev Oncol Hematol*, *49*, 259-268.

Westergren-Thorsson, G., Onnervik, P. O., Fransson, L. A. &Malmstrom, A. (1991). Proliferation of cultured fibroblasts is inhibited by L-iduronate-containing glycosaminoglycans. *J Cell Physiol*, *147*, 523-530.

Wharton, K. &Derynck, R. (2009). TGFbeta family signaling: novel insights in development and disease. *Development*, *136*, 3691-3697.

Whitmarsh, A. J. & Davis, R. J. (1996). Transcription factor AP-1 regulation by mitogen-activated protein kinase signal transduction pathways. *J Mol Med* (Berl), *74*, 589-607.

Woodard, A. S., Garcia-Cardena, G., Leong, M., Madri, J. A., Sessa, W. C. &Languino, L. R. (1998). The synergistic activity of alphavbeta3 integrin and PDGF receptor increases cell migration. *J Cell Sci*, *111*, 469-478.

Wu, M.Y. & Hill, C.S. (2009). Tgf-beta superfamily signaling in embryonic development and homeostasis. *Dev Cell*, *16*, 329-343.

Zafiropoulos, A., Fthenou, E., Chatzinikolaou, G. &Tzanakakis, G. N. (2008). Glycosaminoglycans and PDGF signaling in mesenchymal cells. *Connect Tissue Res, 49*, 153-156.

Zhang, X., Ibrahimi, O. A., Olsen, S. K., Umemori, H., Mohammadi, M. &Ornitz, D. M. (2006). Receptor specificity of the fibroblast growth factor family. The complete mammalian FGF family. *J Biol Chem, 281*, 15694-15700.

In: Chondroitin Sulfate
Editor: Vitor H. Pomin

ISBN: 978-1-62808-490-0
© 2013 Nova Science Publishers, Inc.

Chapter 8

Fucosylated Chondroitin Sulfate: A Serpin-Independent Anticoagulant Polysaccharide

Vitor H. Pomin[*]

Program of Glycobiology, Institute of Medical Biochemistry, University Hospital
Clementino Fraga Filho, Federal University of Rio de Janeiro, Rio de Janeiro, Brazil

Abstract

Marine organisms are a rich source of sulfated polysaccharides with unique structures. Fucosylated chondroitin sulfate (FucCS) from the sea cucumber *Ludwigothuria grisea* is one of these unusual molecules since it shows a saccharide backbone similar to the regular chondroitin sulfate from mammals, however, with uneven branches of sulfated fucosyl units. Besides the uncommon structures of marine polysaccharides, they also may exhibit important therapeutic properties when assayed in clinical systems that resemble parts of the human physiology. The mostly studied and highly desirable therapeutic action of FucCS is its anticoagulant and antithrombotic activity. The capacity for these activities is mainly attributed to the presence of the branching fucosyl unit since the regular chondroitin sulfate composed only of the alternating galactosamine and glucuronic acid backbone is devoid of these biological actions. Earlier, it was considered that the anticoagulant activities of FucCS was driven mainly by a catalytic serpin-dependent mechanism likewise the mammalian heparins. Its serpin-dependent anticoagulant action relies on promoting thrombin and/or factor Xa inhibition by their specific natural inhibitors (the serpins antithrombin and heparin cofactor II). However, unlikely heparins, the FucCS proved still capable in promoting coagulation inhibition when using serpin-free plasmas. This puzzle observation was further investigated and clearly demonstrated that the echinoderm FucCS has an unusual serpin-independent anticoagulant effect by inhibiting the formation of factor Xa and/or thrombin through the pro-coagulant tenase and prothrombinase complexes, respectively. The marine FucCS with unusual anticoagulant mechanism opens clearly new

---

[*] Corresponding author: E-mail: pominvh@bioqmed.ufrj.br.

perspectives for the development of new antithrombotic drugs, especially in clinical cases of related serpins-compromised patients.

Keywords: Anticoagulant; antithrombotic; fucosylated chondroitin sulfate; marine organisms; marine drugs

1. Introduction

1.1. Fucosylated Chondroitin Sulfate from Sea Cucumber

1.1.1. Structure and Anticoagulant Properties

Fucosylated chondroitin sulfate (FucCS) is a marine sulfated polysaccharide (MSP) obtained from the body wall of the sea cucumber *Ludwigothurea grisea*. The backbone of this polysaccharide is made up of repeating disaccharide units of alternating 4-linked β-D-glucuronic acid (GlcA) units and 3-linked N-acetyl-β-D-galactosamine (GalNAc) (Figure 1A), the same structure of mammalian CS backbone. In the sea cucumber polysaccharide however the β-D-GlcA residues bear sulfated Fuc*p* branches bound at 3-position and the GalNAc units from the central core with also a complex sulfation pattern (see Figure 2G of Chapter 8). Approximately, 12% are 4,6-di-sulfated, 53% are 6-mono-sulfated, 4% are 4-mono-sulfated and 31% are non-sulfated GalNAcs [1-3].

The physiological role of this SP in the sea cucumber is not completely understood but it is speculated that it plays a structural role in assembling the body wall of the invertebrate. FucCS is present on the connective tissue and perhaps with its high negatively charge density and consequent capacity to retain water in the extracellular-matrix it might produce a "space" among muscle fibers allowing the tissue to change its length rapidly and reversibly by more than 200% [4].

L. grisea FucCS exhibits potential pharmacological actions in mammalian system such as anti-metastatic and anti-inflammatory activities [5, 6]. However this FucCS has been better explored as an anticoagulant and antithrombotic candidate [7]. Unlike mammalian CSs which do not show anticoagulant behavior, FucCS is an effective anticoagulant and antithrombotic molecule when administrated orally or by intravascular routes in rats [7, 8]. Because of its potency as an anticoagulant agent, FucCS could be an alternative drug candidate for the treatments of thrombosis, with many advantages over heparin, the most exploited anticoagulant glycosaminoglycan (GAG). Like heparin, FucCS has a serine-protease inhibitor (serpin)-dependent anticoagulant activity due to its capacity to increase thrombin (IIa)-inhibition more by heparin cofactor II (HCII) than by antithrombin (AT). However unlike heparin, FucCS also shows a serpin-independent anticoagulant activity by inhibiting tenase and prothrombinase procoagulant complexes [9] as explained below. In this chapter we give some basis and details about these uncommon inhibiting mechanisms.

Anticoagulant and antithrombotic activities of FucCS are dependent on its molecular weight and can be attributable to some of its structural features. The native FucCS has an average molecular weight (MW) of ~ 40 kDa and a very low polydispersity when compared with mammalian CSs [1]. Reduction on the MW diminishes its antithrombotic and anticoagulant efficacy [8]. Sulfated Fuc*p* units play a crucial role for the anticoagulant activity of FucCS. Removal of these branches by mild acid hydrolysis (Figure 1b), as well as desulfation reaction, reduces considerably its anticoagulant and antithrombotic activities to the same low levels of mammalian CS [1, 8, 9]. Moreover, sulfated Fuc*p* branches in FucCS molecules prevent its rapid digestion by enzymes, especially hialuronidase that normally degrade GAGs in the gastrointestinal tract of vertebrates [2, 3]. Due to this fact FucCS was proved to be effective when administrated by oral routes, differently from heparin treatments [7].

Previous studies using MSPs from invertebrates have shown that the occurrence of 2,4-di-sulfated Fuc*p* units amplifies the effect of the AT-mediated anticoagulant activity of 3-linked α-L-fucans [10-12] (see also Chapter 8 for details). Surprisingly, these 2,4-di-sulfated Fuc*p* units when occurred as branches, they did not favor interaction with AT in a similar way. Clearly, the anticoagulant effect of FucCS is mostly via potentiating HCII, as proved in the work of [11].

The reduction of the carboxyl groups of the GlcA residues to glucose (Figure 1c, in gray ellipse) does not affect its anticoagulant activity [1, 8, 9], meaning no such big influence of the negatively charged carboxyl groups for interaction. In contrast, carboxyl-reduced FucCS (cr-FucCS) are still able to retain the anticoagulant activity but with no traces of bleeding adverse effects as native FucCS and heparin have, indicating therefore an even more favorable antithrombotic action than the native unmodified molecule [8].

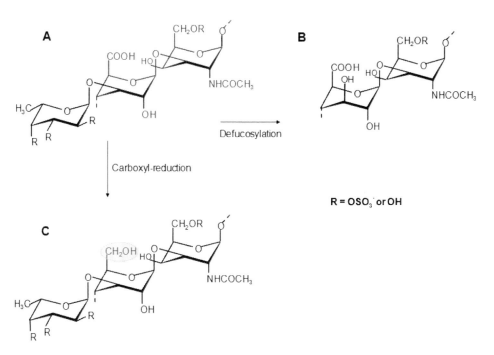

Figure 1. Structure of the sea cucumber fucosylated chondroitin sulfate (FucCS) (a), its defucosylated (b), and carboxyl-reduced (cr-FucCS) (c) derivatives. The backbone of this polysaccharide (highlighted in blue) is made up of repeating disaccharide units of alternating 4-linked â-D-glucuronic acid (GlcA) and 3-linked N-acetyl-â-D-galactosamine (GalNAc), the same structure as mammalian chondroitin sulfate (CS). But, in the sea cucumber polysaccharide, the â-D-glucuronic acid residues bear sulfated fucose branches at the 3-position. These branches are removed by mild acid hydrolysis while the hexuronic acid carboxyl groups can be reduced by 1-ethyl-3-(3-dimethylaminopropyl) carbodiimide/NaBH4 [1, 9]. Dashed line represents glycosidic bonds.

cr-FucCS also has differences regarding its interaction with some plasma proteases. It possesses anticoagulant activity by potentiating inhibition of IIa through its natural inhibitor HCII while FucCS increases IIa inhibition by activating the HCII and, in a lesser extent, through AT as well [9]. Furthermore, in contrast with the native compound, cr-FucCS is proved to not activate factor XII from the contact system of coagulation [7]. The importance of this activation has been highlighted by the observation that chemically oversulfated CS (OSCS), found as the main contaminant of pharmaceutical heparin preparations, activates factor XII and induces severe hypotension in patients associated with kallikrein release, when administered by intravenous injection [13]. Like OSCS, FucCS has also usually more sulfate groups than the mammalian CS. However, these two highly sulfated CSs differ significantly in their effects on coagulation and thrombosis [14].

These findings illustrates that the structural requirement for the interaction of these SPs with coagulation factors are very stereospecific and not only a mere consequence of sulfate content and increased charge density. Above all, while some non-specific electrostatic interactions of SPs exist for binding to basic proteins, evidence continues to push the idea that many of the effects of SPs involve specific structural moieties [15]. Taking the anticoagulant action of heparin as an example, approximately two-thirds of native heparin is unable to form a stable complex with AT. This is essentially due to the presence of specific binding sequence (discussed more in details below) in only few specific regions of the heparin chain [16]. Obviously, the identification of specific structural requirements in the invertebrate SP necessary for its interaction with coagulation cofactors is an essential step for more rational development of anticoagulant drugs.

1.1.2. Methods of Extraction

The body wall of sea cucumbers must be carefully separated from other tissues, immediately immersed in acetone and kept at low temperature for transportation or storage before handle for extraction. Acidic glycans can be extracted from the dry tissue by papain as previously described [2, 3]. About 20 mg of the crude acidic glycans from the body wall of L. grisea can be recovered and further dissolved in 1.5 ml of 0.3 M pyridinelacetate buffer (pH 6.0) for subjection into a gel-permeation chromatography on a Sepharose CL-4B column (115 x 1.5 cm), consequently eluted with the same buffer plus 4.0 M guanidine hydrochloride in 0.3 M pyridinelacetate buffer (pH 6.0). Columns can be successfully eluted at a flow rate of 6 ml/h and aliquots of approximately 1.0 ml might be collected. The presence of sulfated glycans in each fraction can be easily detected by the DuBois reaction and/or by metachromatic property [2, 3]. Columns might be calibrated using blue dextran (2 thousands kDa) as a marker to V0 and cresol red (~ 0.35 kDa) as a marker to Vt. After chromatography on Sepharose CL-4B column, the obtained crude polysaccharide must be further applied to a DEAE-cellulose column (3.5 x 2 cm) equilibrated with 0.1 M sodium acetate buffer (pH 6.0) and washed with 100 ml of the same buffer. The column is then developed by a linear gradient prepared by mixing 35 ml of 0.1 M sodium acetate buffer (pH 6.0) with 35 ml of 1.0 M NaCl and 35 ml of 2.0 M NaCl in the same buffer. The flow rate of the column could be set to 10 ml/h, and fractions of 2.5 ml might be collected. The resultant fractions can be checked by the DuBois reaction, ultraviolet absorption and conductivity. Fractions must be finally pooled, and dialyzed against distilled water and lyophilized for future assays.

2. MSPs and Anticoagulation

2.1. The Heart- and Blood-Related Diseases

Cardiovascular diseases (CVD) are the leading cause of death and illness throughout the world. It has been estimated that cardiovascular diseases are responsible for more than one million deaths annually in the United States [17, 18]. After myocardial infarction and stroke, venous thromboembolism is the third major cause of cardiovascular-associated death [19]. Venous thromboembolism (VTE) consists of deep vein thrombosis, which typically involves deep veins of the leg or pelvis, and its complication, pulmonary embolism (PE). VTE contributes to more than 250 thousands hospital admissions per year. Thirty percent die within 30 days, one fifth suffer from sudden death due to PE and 30% developed episodic recurrence of VTE within 10 years in the United States [17, 18]. It is estimated that 12% of the annual deaths occurring in the European Union are associated with VTE [20]. In the United States, PE causes about 300 thousands deaths per year [21].

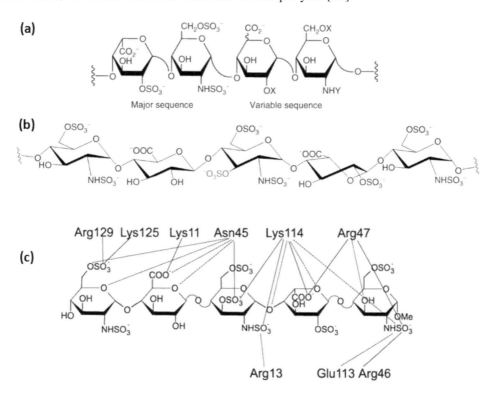

Figure 2. Structure of heparin and the pentasaccharide motif with high affinity for AT. (a) Structure of heparin major and minor variable sequences (X = SO_3^- or H, Y = SO_3^-, $COCH_3$, or H). (b) Heparin pentasaccharide antithrombin (AT) binding sequence. The red highlighted sulfonate group at the C-3 position of the center glucosamine (GlcN) residue is critical for the interaction with AT (Kemp and Linhardt 2009). (c) The AT residues (mostly cationic ones) that interact specifically with the Heparin-pentasaccharide are highlighted. The intermolecular interactions involved are also indicated (solid lines are ionic and dashed are hydrogen bonds).

Arterial thromboembolism is also an important contributor to the growing burden of cardiovascular disease [18]. Atherosclerosis is a progressive disease characterized by accumulation of lipids and fibrous elements in the large arteries that can grow sufficiently to block blood flow. The most important clinical complication is an acute occlusion due to formation of a thrombus resulting in myocardial infarction or stroke [22].

Anticoagulant drugs are highly effective for prevention of arterial and venous thromboembolism [23]. The conventional management of thrombotic and cardiovascular disorders is based on the use of heparin and its derivatives of low molecular weight (LMWH) [24]. Heparin has been used in the clinic as an anticoagulant for more than 50 years [25]. Anticoagulation treatment with heparin is necessary to prevent thrombus growth and reduce the risk of thromboembolism. Furthermore, any condition that predicts an increased risk of thrombosis requires the preventive use of anticoagulants. Heparin is also required for extracorporeal circulation during cardiovascular surgeries and renal dialysis [13].

Heparin is a mixture of heterogeneous SPs chains varying from ~ 3 to ~ 30 kDa [24]. It consists of a disaccharide repeating unit composed of an uronic acid (iduronic, IdoA, or glucuronic acid, GlcA) and a glucosamine (GlcN), with the majority of disaccharides units containing IdoA and di-sulfated GlcA (Figure 2a) [26]. Heparin acts as an anticoagulant by activating the physiological inhibitors of blood coagulation proteases serpins: AT and HCII. Serpins inhibits blood coagulation proteases, including IIa, the final protease generated in the blood coagulation cascade, responsible for the cleavage of fibrinogen to form fibrin clot [27]. In the presence of heparin, the rates of IIa-inhibition by AT is increased ~ 2 thousands-fold [28]. This interaction is specific via a pentasaccharide with high affinity for AT (Figure 2b) and the hydrogen-bonds involved in such interaction of the heparin pentasaccharide with the positively charged amino acid residues have been characterized [29]. Figure 3c shows the hydrogen bond network involved in such molecular interaction.

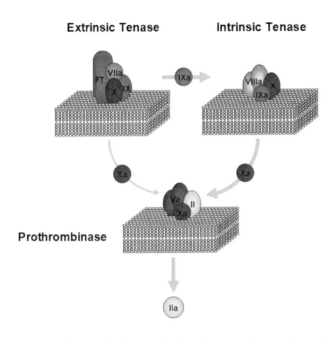

Figure 3. Schematic representation of the vitamin K-dependent complexes of coagulation. Each serine protease is shown in association with the appropriate cofactor on the membrane surface.

A number of limitations associated with pharmacokinetic and biophysical properties of heparin have complicated its use. Heparin has a narrow therapeutic window and a highly variable dose-response relationship, necessitating frequent coagulation monitoring. The main side effects of this drug are bleedings, thrombocytopenia and osteoporosis. Moreover, the heparin source is limited. It is obtained from pig intestine or bovine lung, and contamination of samples with pathogens is a serious concern in the extraction procedure [30]. The situation was further complicated recently due to contamination of heparin preparations with OSCS [31]. As mentioned before, this contaminant induces hypotension associated with kallikrein release when administered by intravenous injection [32].

The incidence of CVD remains high (WHO estimates that by 2030 the number of annual deaths caused by CVD will rise from 17 to 23 millions) and as a consequence, the use of heparin will increase strikingly. Hence, there is a current need for new anticoagulant drugs or alternative sources of heparin in anticoagulation. Fortunately, heparin is not the only SP capable of inhibiting blood coagulation proteases. Marine organisms are an abundant source of SPs with anticoagulant and antithrombotic activities as well [10, 13, 17, 30]. In this chapter we present in detail the MSP from the sea cucumber *L. grisea* FucCS with an unusual and promising serpin-independent anticoagulant action which is not observed in the mechanism of action of Heparin.

2.2. Biochemical Mechanisms of Blood Coagulation and Thrombus Formation

Efficient functioning of the coagulation system is vital to human health. The maintenance of normal blood flow depends completely on the haemostatic system. Hemostasis must be tightly regulated and coordinated to prevent consequent diseases. Failure of its regulation and coordination leads to hemorrhagic disorders and thromboembolic events. The hemostasis system involves activation, regulation, and coordination of numerous proteases. Three catalytic complexes are involved in hemostasis and culminate in the generation of IIa, a key enzyme responsible for the cleavage of fibrinogen to ultimately form the fibrin-clot. Each complex involves a vitamin K-dependent serine protease and a cofactor protein assembled on a phospholipid membrane surface provided by an activated or damaged cell, platelets and endothelial cells (Figure 3) [33].

In normal physiologic conditions hemostasis is naturally initiated, controlled, and terminated. The response of the coagulation process is generally limited to the site of injury and is proportional to the extent of vascular damage. Coagulation response occurs somehow in a localized, amplified, and modulated manner. However, genetic or physiologic perturbations can lead to severe dysfunctions on one or more of these systems.

The physiologic response to vascular damage culminates in the rapid generation of precise and balanced amounts of thrombin at the site of injury. The blood coagulation cascade is triggered when sub-endothelial tissue-factor (TF) is exposed to the blood flow as a consequence of a lesion of the vessel wall or activation of endothelium by chemicals, cytokines, or inflammatory and metastatic processes [34-36]. The contact of TF exposed with already circulating factor VIIa [37], in the presence of phospholipids and calcium ions, leads to the formation of extrinsic tenase complex which can activate factor X, responsible to convert small amounts of prothrombin (II) to thrombin (IIa) (Figures 5 and 6) [38]. Albeit rather inefficiently, this initial thrombin formation is necessary to accelerate coagulation process by activating platelets, factor V and factor VIII [39, 40]. The extrinsic tenase complex can also activate factor IX. Factor IXa and cofactor VIIIa combine to form the intrinsic tenase complex assembled on a membrane surface, which activate large amount of factor X to supply the prothrombinase complex (Figures 3 and 4) [38]. The intrinsic tenase complex is the major activator of factor X. Fifty times more factor X is activated by intrinsic tenase complex than extrinsic tenase complex [41]. The factor IXa-factor VIIIa complex is 10^5-fold more active than factor IXa alone as a factor X activator [42]. In the absence of factor VIIIa or factor IXa, the intrinsic tenase complex cannot be assembled; thus, no amplification of the factor Xa generation occurs. This is the principal defect observed in hemophilia A and B types [43]. Factor Xa generated and cofactor Va assemble on a membrane surface to form the prothrombinase complex, which converts II to IIa (Figures 3 and 4). Prothrombinase is 300 thousand-fold more active than factor Xa alone in catalyzing II activation [44]. Finally, IIa cleaves fibrinogen and factor XIII to form the insoluble cross linked fibrin clot [45].

Alternatively, coagulation may be initiated through the "intrinsic pathway" when factor XII is activated on a negatively charged surface by a process called contact activation [46, 47]. Activation of factor XII is followed sequentially by activation of factor XI and factor IX. The intrinsic and extrinsic pathways (Factor VIIa-tissue factor) converge at the level of factor X activation (formation of Xa) to converts consequently fibrinogen to fibrin [48-51]. Typically, the intrinsic pathway is illustrated as a sequence of proteolytic reactions culminating in factor IXa (Figures 4 and 5). However, the hemorrhagic profiles of patients deficient in components of the intrinsic pathway suggest more complex interactions. The deficiency of factor IX or its cofactor (factor VIII), cause hemophilia B and hemophilia A respectively, associated with severe hemorrhage into joints and muscles, and soft tissue bleeding that can be life threatening [52]. In contrast, factor XI deficiency is associated with a milder disorder characterized by trauma or soft tissue-related hemorrhage [53]. While, factor XII-deficient patients do not exhibit an abnormal bleeding tendency, even with surgery, despite having markedly prolonged clotting times on the activated partial thromboplastin time (aPPT) in assays used currently for clinical evaluation [54, 55]. These observations suggest that these proteases are not exclusively activated in a linear sequential way.

Although the relative participation of these two mechanisms for factor IX activation are not clear, the activation by factor VIIa-TF is reported as the major physiological contributor mechanism. Factor XI may be activated by proteases other than factor XIIa, providing an explanation for the absence of a bleeding tendency in factor XII deficiency. Thrombin can convert factor XI to the active protease factor XIa [56, 57] and it is postulated that the early thrombin generated in clot formation activates factor XI, creating a feedback loop that sustains coagulation (Figure 5) [58]. In animal models of hemostasis using deficient factor XII mouse, factor XII was not required for fibrin formation [59-61].

As deficiency of some coagulation factors causes hemorrhagic phenotypes, upper regulated production of these proteases can also predicts thrombotic diseases. Increased levels of factor VIII, IX, for example, are correlated with bigger incidence of venous thromboembolism [62, 63]. Moreover, there are some indications that the deficiency of factor VIII and IX provides some protection from arterial thrombosis events [64, 65]. These findings are supported by the observation that venous thrombosis is rare in hemophiliacs. Because of the rarity of factor XI disorders and the lack of available data about factor XII deficiency is not clear whether these disorders contributes positively or negatively to thrombotic diseases.

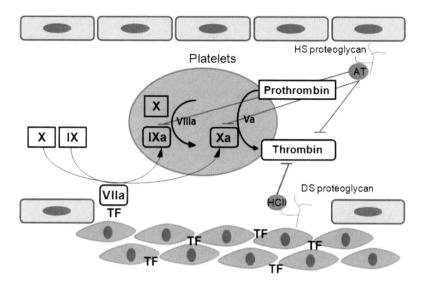

Figure 4. Phospholipid-bound reactions that are involved in the activation of coagulation and the potentiation of antithrombin (AT) and heparin cofactor II (HCII) by glycosaminoglycans (GAGs) *in vivo*. Tissue-factor (TF) is exposed on extravascular cells after vascular injury and binds circulating factor VIIa. The extrinsic tenase complex (FT-VIIa) accelerates factor X and factor IX activation. Factors IXa and Xa assemble with their protein cofactors (VIIIa and Va, respectively) on the surface of aggregated platelets form the intrinsic tenase and prothrombinase complexes. This leads to local generation of large amounts of Xa and thrombin (IIa), followed by conversion of fibrinogen to fibrin. IIa is originated by a catalytic modification on prothrombin (II). AT inhibits coagulation factors IXa, Xa, and IIa when bound to heparan sulfate (HS) proteoglycans associated with vascular endothelial cells. After disruption of the endothelium, HCII is activated by dermatan sulfate (DS) proteoglycans in the vessel wall and inhibits IIa.

Consequently, tight regulation of thrombin generation and/or thrombin activity is essential to prevent excessive thrombosis [44]. Different anticoagulant principles are utilized such as proteolytic degradation of the enzyme cofactors factor Va and VIIIa and enzyme inhibition. The protein C anticoagulant system inhibits the procoagulant functions of factor VIIIa and Va, the cofactors in the tenase and prothrombinase complexes respectively. Activated protein C (APC) cleaves a few peptide bonds in each of the phospholipid membrane-bound cofactors Va and VIIIa (Figure 5). The tissue factor pathway inhibitor (TFPI) regulates the initial steps of blood coagulation involving factor VIIa and TF (Figure 5). For further explanations see references [66, 67].

However, the most important regulators are the serine proteases inhibitors (serpins): antithrombin (AT) and heparin cofactor II (HCII) that inhibits procoagulant enzymes such as factor Xa and thrombin (IIa).

2.3. The Classical Inhibiting Mechanism via Serpins

The principal procoagulant components of blood coagulation are serine proteases. Inasmuch, serpins are the predominant modulator of this system and controls inappropriate, excessive or mislocalized clotting in the blood flow. Two major serpins are involved in hemostasis: AT that inhibits several coagulation proteases, mostly important factor Xa and IIa; and HCII that inhibits exclusively IIa (Figure 5). Circulating AT and HCII are relatively inefficient inhibitors. GAGs such as heparin, heparan sulfate (HS) and DS have been found to significantly accelerate the interactions between serpins and coagulation proteases, providing maximal inhibitory activity (Figure 6) [27].

AT is the most important serpin in hemostasis. Its importance is demonstrated by the high association of AT deficiency with venous thrombosis [68], by the embryonic lethal phenotype in the mouse knockout model [69], and by the success of heparin therapy [16]. The concentration of AT in plasma (2-3 μM) greatly exceeds that of any of the target proteases generated during coagulation [70]. AT is a single chain, 58 kDa glycoprotein and inhibits several of the proteases involved in blood coagulation, including thrombin, factor Xa, IXa, XIa and XIIa. Based on rates of inhibition, its primary targets are factor Xa and IIa (Figure 5) [71].

The physiological role of AT is to protect the circulation from liberated enzymes and to limit the coagulation process to sites of vascular injury. This is consistent with the observation that the free enzymes are readily inhibited by AT while clot bound IIa and factor Xa are protective from inactivation by AT [72, 73].

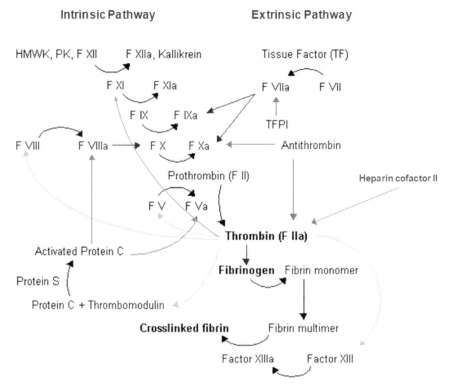

Figure 5. The intrinsic and extrinsic coagulation pathway. The beginning of the coagulation cascade occurs after a vascular injury and exposure of tissue factor to the blood. This fact triggers the extrinsic pathway of coagulation (right side). The intrinsic pathway (left side) can be triggered *in vitro* when factor XII, prekallikrein, and high-molecular weight kininogen (HMWK) bind to kaolin, glass, or another artificial surface. Once bound, reciprocal activation of XII and prekallikrein occurs. Factor XIIa triggers clotting via the sequential activation of factors XI, IX and X. The two pathways converge in the formation of thrombin (IIa).

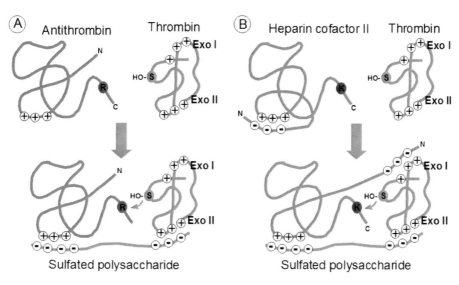

Figure 6. Molecular schematic representation of (A) antithrombin and (B) heparin cofactor II activation by glycosaminoglycans. The thrombin (IIa, in blue) can be inhibited by serpins such as antithrombin (AT, in green) or heparin cofactor II (HCII, in orange). In both cases, the glycosaminoglycans (GAGs) or other sulfated polysaccharides (SPs, gray line) bring together the serpins and the protease (IIa) mainly through electrostatic interactions of their opposite charges. In the thrombin, this charged cluster is the EXO II. Next, the hydroxyl groups of a serine (S) residue from thrombin will bind to the C-terminus of the serpins, actually to an arginine (R) residue of the AT, or to a lysine (K) residue in the case of the HCII. In the bind-states, a conformational change will occur in both serpins, although this change is more predominant and necessary at the HCII case. Note that the N-terminus of the HCII will interact also with the EXO I of IIa through also electrostatic contacts. With the examples described throughout the text, it's clear that the template mechanism between SPs, serpins (AT, HCII) and protease (IIa) has differential stabilities or formation kinetics directly related to the structural features of the SPs.

AT, as other serpins, inhibits serine proteases by forming a tight equimolar complex (Figure 6). The inhibition occurs through the cleavage of a peptide bond, present in an exposed loop of AT. The enzyme attacks the bond and remains attached to the inhibitor through a covalent bond. The cleavage causes a conformational change in AT, which irreversibly binds the protease to AT [74-78]. This interaction can be enhanced by heparin. The anticoagulant effect of commercially available heparin and its LMW derivatives is mediated predominantly through the activation of AT [16]. Heparin can bind AT and provide the conformational change necessary in the inhibitor resulting in accelerated interaction with IIa or other proteases and as consequence AT inhibition rate [79, 80]. This binding occurs through a "heparin binding site" on AT that interacts with a unique pentasaccharide sequence found in one third of the heparin chains (Figure 2c). The 3-O-sulfonated GlcN unit present in the middle of the pentasaccharide, is essential for this affinity with AT [81, 82] (Figure 4b, in red). Following complex formation with thrombin, AT loses its high affinity for heparin, which will be released and ready to activate another AT molecule [83].

The conformational change of the AT molecule is an important contributor to the rate enhancement, but a minimum chain length of ~18 saccharides is required to enhance the rates of thrombin inhibition [84]. These findings are better explained by an additional mechanism, which predicted that heparin was acting as a surface or bridge of both proteins to the same heparin chain. So, heparin accelerates IIa inhibition rate through activation of AT by an allosteric modification of the structure of AT and by providing a template on which inhibitor and protease can interact (via exosite II on the protease) (Figure 6). The template mechanism accelerates the interaction of AT with IIa, one thousand-fold and with fXa 10 thounsand-fold [85, 86].

Although both factor Xa and IIa are capable of forming a ternary complex with AT and heparin, the inhibition of factor Xa by AT can be accelerated only by the pentasaccharide sequence (Figures 2b and c). The pentasaccharide alone accelerates the inhibition of factor Xa by 300-fold and of IIa by only 2-fold [77]. Heparin enhancement of FXa inhibition is said to be through an "allosteric mechanism", whereas the enhancement of thrombin inhibition requires "template mechanism".

Recently, the crystal structure of heparin-catalyzed AT-templated within IIa has been shown. The bridging role of heparin is clear on the structure (Figure 7). The observation that the pentasaccharide sequence alone does not catalyze AT-mediated IIa-inhibition was confirmed. The pentasaccharide binding only facilitates the interaction of AT with IIa by increasing the flexibility of exposed loop.

Heparin is not the real physiological activator of AT. Presumably, heparin-like molecules, such as HS anchored to the surface of endothelial cells by its proteoglycan core, are responsible for the activation of AT and contribute to the non thrombogenic properties of blood vessels *in vivo* (Figure 6) [80]. The pentasaccharide sequence (Figure 2b) is also present on HS chains [87], although at much lower concentration than found in heparin chains. Nowadays, there is an intense debate whether HS is actually antithrombotic or not, since generated mice deficient in 3-*O*-sulfotransferase-1 failed to show accelerated thrombosis in injured arteries compared with wild type mice [87, 88].

HCII that occurs in plasma at μM concentration is a single-chain 66 kDa glycoprotein [89] that also inactivates thrombin by formation of a stable complex (Figure 6). HCII has more restricted protease specificity than AT. HCII does not react with factor Xa and other coagulation proteases (Figure 5) [90]. In the absence of a GAG, the inhibition of IIa is very slow. In this case, DS is the more important activator of HCII. Heparin also stimulates HCII, but does not require the specific pentasaccharide structure shown in Figure 4b for stimulation by heparin [91, 92]. However, the affinity of HCII for DS is higher than for heparin and a ten-fold higher concentration of heparin is required to accelerate IIa inhibition by HCII [90]. Its relatively low affinity for heparin explains why the antithrombotic effect of therapeutic heparin is mediated mainly through activation of AT.

Like heparan sulfate, DS is a component of proteoglycans on the cell surface and in the extracellular matrix. DS is a repeating polymer of D-GlcA/L-IdoA and GalNAc units [93]. *O*-sulfonation at IdoA residues in the C2 position and at GalNAc residues in the C4 and C6 positions occurs to a variable extent, yielding heterogeneous structures within the polymer. The high affinity binding site for HCII in DS consists of three repeated 2-sulfated IdoA and 4-sulfated GalNAc disaccharide subunits. The 4-*O*-sulfonation of GalN is essential for activity with HCII [94, 95]. The high affinity hexasaccharide increases the rate of inhibition of thrombin by HCII about 50-times [92], although DS chains containing up to 14 monosaccharide units are required for maximal stimulation [96].

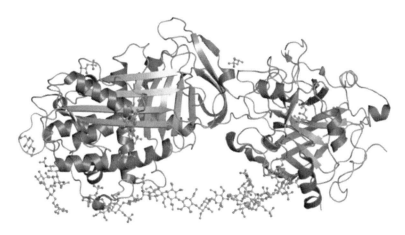

Figure 7. Crystal structure of ternary Hep-AT-IIa complex reveals antithrombotic template-mechanism for Heparin. Left-hand side ribbon-model structure is AT, right-hand side is IIa, and ball-and-stick model structure in green and red represent the Heparin chain.

The stimulatory effect of heparin and DS appears to be allosteric and uses conformational activation of the serpin. The activation of HCII depends on the presence of an acidic polypeptide domain near the N-terminus of HCII [97]. Heparin and DS displaces the N-terminal acidic domain to interact with exosite I of thrombin [98-100]. Thrombin binds to the acidic domain of HCII and facilitates inhibition by bringing the active site of thrombin into approximation with the reactive site of HCII (Figure 5).

The function of HCII *in vivo* remains obscure. Individuals with inherited partial deficiency of HCII (~ 50 percent of normal) have been reported in association with histories of thrombotic disease [101]. The AT deficiency is not compensated by HCII [102]. Some reports suggest that *in vivo* HCII assumes special relevance after vascular endothelial injury. DS is the predominant antithrombotic GAG in the vessel walls and is synthesized by cells from the sub-endothelial cells (Figure 3) [103].

HCII and AT could be activated by several MSPs. While HS and DS are physiological activators of AT and HCII, heparin and many different polyanions, including MSPs are able to accelerate the serpin inhibition of some coagulation proteases [9, 22, 30, 104]. SFs isolated from the brown algae as *Fucus vesiculosus* and *Ecklonia kurome* possesses anticoagulant activity due to activation of HCII [105, 106]. In contrast, the anticoagulant effect of the SF from *Ascophylum nodosum* is mediated mainly via AT [107].

2.4. The Uncommon Serpin-Independent Anticoagulant Mechanism

Besides the common serpin-dependent anticoagulant activity above-described for the sea cucumber FucCS, this glycan can also exhibit a serpin-independent complementary mechanism that contributes to their anticoagulant action. This MSP is able to inhibit the procoagulant tenase and prothrombinase complexes. Initially, its anticoagulant action was attributed only by its capacity of potentiate factor Xa and IIa inhibition by AT and HCII. Currently, FucCS is known to inhibit the generation of factor Xa and IIa by these complexes. Factor Xa is activated mainly by the intrinsic tenase complex and IIa is converted from II by the prothrombinase complex (Figure 3). FucCS inhibits Xa and IIa activation by these complexes [9]. These are critical steps for the amplification of coagulation process. Protease activation by these complexes can be inhibiting through direct inactivation of the enzyme and/or the cofactor or by impairing assembling of all components of the complex on the phospholipid surface.

The contribution of serpins to the anticoagulant activity of FucCS was determined in a plasmatic system using an aPTT test. Basically, aPTT tests are used to evaluate the anticoagulant effect of the SPs. In this assay, the anticoagulant effect of this MSP was evaluated by the measure of the time necessary to plasma clotting. Normal plasma and depleted plasma (free of serpins) were used in these tests. FucCS prolonged the clotting time potentially, even when the serpins are not present (Table 1). This result suggested an anticoagulant activity that persist independent of the inhibitory action based on serpins activity. More importantly, addition of FucCS to either normal or serpin-free plasmas increased the clotting time with similar potency, demonstrating that the serpin-independent anticoagulant effect predominates over the serpin-dependent action. The result was unexpected because heparin and other GAGs with anticoagulant and antithrombotic effect are usually known to catalyze inhibition of factor Xa and thrombin by AT and HCII [16, 89]. According to the literature, heparin has no effect on AT depleted plasma [108, 109].

Further evidence was demonstrated by a factor Xa and IIa generation tests where the generation of these proteases was quantified. In these assays, normal or serpin-free plasma was incubated with the SPs, and then activated to induce the coagulation. The assay is characterized by an initial lag-phase, followed by an explosive generation of factor Xa or IIa until a plateau is reached. When the SPs were added to plasma a delay in the generation of the proteases and a decrease in the maximum amounts formed was observed (panels A-D of Figure 8). Again, when similar assays were performed with AT+HCII-free plasma, the effect of heparin was totally abolished. In contrast, FucCS stills retain the activities. Overall, these experiments clearly confirmed that FucCS has an additional uncommon serpin-independent anticoagulant activity.

FucCS interferes with the activation of factor X and II by the intrinsic tenase and prothrombinase complexes, respectively. In these assays, all the purified proteases of the complexes, calcium and phospholipids are used. This glycan inhibits the generation of factor Xa and IIa by the complexes. The effect of FucCS on IIa generation was even demonstrated by monitoring II activation by SDS-PAGE assay (Figure 8E-G). As shown at panels E-G of Figure 8, the conversion of II into IIa was almost complete after II incubation with the prothrombinase compounds. Heparin did not impair the conversion while FucCS abolishes the activation process (Figure 8 F *vs* G) [9].

Additional experiments with FucCS demonstrated that the inactivation of the prothrombinase complex is not due to an interference with prothrombinase complex assembly on the phospholipid membrane. Probably, the invertebrate SP may complicate the assembly of factor Va on the complex. It is possible that the predominant target of FucCS in the prothrombinase complex is related to the interaction of factor Va and factor Xa (Figure 9).

Table 1. Concentrations of GAGs required for doubling APTT in normal, AT-and/or HCII-free plasmas

GAG	Plasma (values in µg/mL)			
	Normal	AT-free	HCII-free	AT + HCII-free
Heparin	0.60	NA	0.43	NA
Native FucCS	2.80	2.08	2.60	3.04
Carboxyl-reduced FucCS	7.31	3.06	4.62	3.60

NA, not achieved.

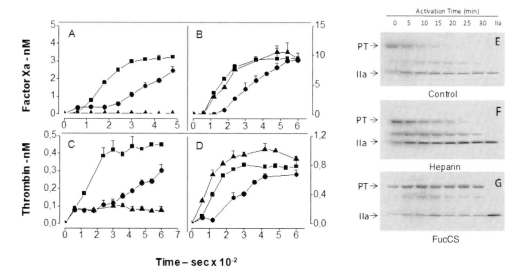

Figure 8. Factor Xa (A, and B) and thrombin (C and D) generation tests in normal (A and C) and serpin-free (B and D) plasmas. Defibrinated plasmas (50 µL) were incubated in the absence (■) or in the presence of 0.2 µg/mL of heparin (▲) or fucosylated chondroitin sulfate (FucCS) (●) with 50 µL of TS/PEG buffer and 10 µL of Cephalin reagent. After incubation for 2 min at room temperature, the protease generation reaction was started by addition of 100 µL 12.5 mM $CaCl_2$, and aliquots of 10 µL were removed each 15 sec into microplate wells containing 40 µL TS/PEG buffer + 50 mM EDTA. The amounts of factor Xa or thrombin generated were determined using the chromogenic substrates S-2765 or S-2238 respectively. Substrate hydrolysis was detected using a Thermomax Microplate Reader. Reactions were recorded continuously at 405 nm for 15 min at 37°C. The panels show mean±SD, n=3. Effect of sulfated polysaccharides on thrombin generation by the prothrombinase complex (E-G). The effect of sulfated polysaccharides on prothrombinase complex was analyzed on 12% SDS-PAGE. The incubation mixtures contain: 1 nM plasma-derived factor Xa, 3 nM factor Va, 20 µM phospholipids and 10 µg/mL sulfated polysaccharide in TS/PEG buffer containing 10 mM $CaCl_2$, final volume 500 µL. After incubation for 10 min at 37°C, the activation reaction was started by addition of 0.5 µM prothrombin. Aliquots from each reaction mixture were removed at the time point indicated in the panels and immediately quenched in SDS-PAGE loading buffer. The gel was stained with Coomassie blue and band intensities for prothrombin and thrombin were monitored by densitometric analysis. PT, prothrombin and IIa, thrombin. *$p < 0.05$ for □ vs. ●.

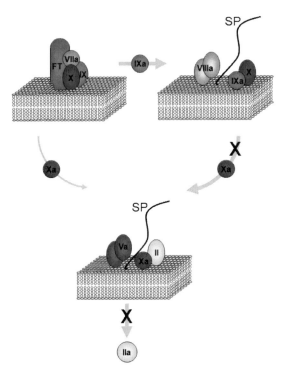

Figure 9. Proposed mechanism of inhibition of factor Xa, and thrombin activation by intrinsic tenase, and prothrombinase complexes. Sulfated polysaccharides (SPs) may difficult the assembly of the cofactors, VIIIa and Va, on the complexes. It is possible that the predominant target of SPs in procoagulant complexes are related to the interaction of the cofactors and the proteases, factor IXa, and factor Xa.

The main factor Xa residues responsible for its association with heparin were determined [110]. These same residues permit the binding of factor Xa with cofactor Va and/or the substrate in the prothrombinase complex [72]. These domains are conserved in vitamin K-dependent serine proteases, including factor IXa and participate in the binding of factor IXa to cofactor VIIIa in the intrinsic tenase complex [111-113]. Perhaps the site of action of FucCS is the same in both systems. Possibly, FucCS binds through this same region on factor IXa and factor Xa, since both proteases exhibit structural homology, thus hindering the binding of proteases to their cofactors in the formation of the complexes (Figure 9) [9].

The carboxyl-reduced derivative of FucCS (cr-FucCS) (Figure 3c) reveals an effect on these systems very similar to the native compound. The potent effect of FucCS on inhibit the tenase and prothrombinase complex is clearly associated with the presence of sulfated Fuc*p* branches and the pattern of sulfation of the molecule, since other GAGs such as DS and CS have no effect on these complexes [9, 114, 115].

Similar results were found for two other SPs. One of these polysaccharides is the pentosan polysulfate, obtained by chemical oversulfation of naturally occurring pentosan [116]. The other is also obtained by an invertebrate and is denominated "depolymerized FucCS" [108, 114]. Depolymerized FucCS also inhibits intrinsic tenase activity through interactions with the heparin binding exosite present on factor IXa [104]. However, the absence of a clear description of its structure makes it difficult to trace a comparison with

FucCS. Pentosan polysulfate has a critical limitation for its use as an antithrombotic drug due to a potent bleeding effect [117].

These findings demonstrates that FucCS has an unusual serpin independent anticoagulant activity in addition to its ability to potentiate the inhibitory action of AT and HCII. This effect is due to inhibition of factor Xa and IIa generation by the tenase and prothrombinase complexes, respectively.

3. Advantages of FucCS in Medicine

The amount of serine protease is amplified at each step in the coagulation system. Because of that, it is interesting that the selective inhibition of coagulation factors above IIa might be highly blocked as well. Furthermore, by not inhibiting all IIa activity directly, such anticoagulant agents might allow traces of IIa to escape neutralization thereby facilitating hemostasis and leading to a favorable profile with respect to bleeding. Thus, there is a suggestion that the removal of all AT-dependent actions of heparin could further reduce the bleeding risk and increase the therapeutic action [115]. Given the critical role of tenase and prothrombinase enzyme complexes in hemostasis, antithrombotic drugs that act on these complexes are promising candidates. These observations led several authors to look for SPs, prepared from either new natural sources or by chemical modification of standard heparin, with serpin-independent anticoagulant action and, perhaps, with additional antithrombotic effects.

Heparin is not able to inhibit procoagulant complexes. The approach to obtain a derivative with predominant action on the intrinsic tenase complex, like FucCS, involved periodate oxidation of LMWH, which reduces its affinity for AT followed by oversulfation of the saccharide chain. This chemically modified heparin became a potent inhibitor of the intrinsic tenase and prothrombinase complexes [109]. However, the serpin-independent anticoagulant effect of FucCS and SG do not require any additional chemical modification or laborious synthetic route. The structural requirement for its activity is clear, namely, sulfated Fuc$p$ branches linked to the polysaccharide core [9].

Even, serpin-dependent anticoagulant drugs used nowadays are synthesized or chemically modified. For example, LMWH are also commonly used in the treatment of thromboembolic and cardiovascular disorders. They are generally prepared by chemical or enzymatical depolymerization method of porcine unfractionated heparins (UFHs). In comparison to UFHs, LMWHs possess an antithrombotic property with fewer side effects [118]. Another strategy for the development of new antithrombotics was the synthetic heparin pentasaccharide (Figure 2b), called fondaparinux. This drug induces a conformational change in AT that increases the affinity of the serpin for factor Xa, potentiating the natural inhibitory effect of AT against factor Xa [119]. Recently, a chemoenzymatically pentasaccharide was reconstructed in milligrams quantities by following the heparin biosynthetic pathway [120]. However, these methods are complex, expensive, increase the treatment costs and are more time-consuming than compared to extraction-based procedures of natural sources.

In contrast with those observations, FucCS occurs at high concentrations in the sea cucumber. This marine organism is abundant in nature. There is now more interest in therapeutics prepared from non-mammalian sources which avoids the risk of contamination with pathogens agents. The yield obtained from each sea cucumber specimen is ~7% per dry weight and about 35 mg of purified polysaccharide. FucCS has clear advantages over heparin and other anticoagulant drugs that are currently used in the clinic of thrombosis. First of all, FucCS is absorbed after oral administration and the peak in plasma is achieved about 2 h after oral administration in parallel with the antithrombotic effect [7]. Its carboxyl-reduced derivative does not cause bleeding and retains the serpin-independent anticoagulant activity indicating an even more favorable antithrombotic effect than the native polysaccharide [8].

These results concerning the serpin-independent anticoagulant activity of MSPs may help to design new drugs with specific actions on coagulation and thrombosis. For example, these new MSPs may be active in patients with inherited AT deficiency due to a mutation in the heparin-binding site [121].

In conclusion, certain mechanisms have to be explored before defining FucCS as definitive antithrombotic drugs of practical use. Critical points are related to the bioavailability, half-life and safety of these compounds. In addition, the magnitude of serpin-independent effect for the antithrombotic activity of these MSPs should be more carefully evaluated.

References

[1]   Mourão, PAS; Pereira, MS; Pavão, MSG; Mulloy, B; Tollefsen, DM; Mowinckel, M-C; Abildgaard, U. Structure and Anticoagulant Activity of a Fucosylated Chondroitin Sulfate from Echinoderm. *Journal of Biological Chemistry*, 1996, 271, 23973-84.

[2]   Vieira, RP; Mourão, PA. Occurrence of a unique fucose-branched chondroitin sulfate in the body wall of a sea cucumber. *Journal of Biological Chemistry*, 1988, 263, 18176-83.

[3]   Vieira, RP; Mulloy, B; Mourão, PA. Structure of a fucose-branched chondroitin sulfate from sea cucumber. Evidence for the presence of 3-O-sulfo-beta-D-glucuronosyl residues. *Journal of Biological Chemistry*, 1991, 266, 13530-6.

[4]   Landeira-Fernandez, AM; Aiello, KRM; Aquino, RS; Silva, L-CF; Meis, Ld; Mourão, PAS. A sulfated polysaccharide from the sarcoplasmic reticulum of sea cucumber smooth muscle is an endogenous inhibitor of the Ca2+-ATPase. *Glycobiology*, 2000, 10, 773-9.

[5]   Melo-Filho, NM; Belmiro, CL; Gonçalves, RG; Takiya, CM; Leite, M; Pavão, MSG; Mourão, PAS. Fucosylated chondroitin sulfate attenuates renal fibrosis in animals submitted to unilateral ureteral obstruction: a P-selectin-mediated event? *American Journal of Physiology - Renal Physiology*, 2010, 299, F1299-F307.

[6]   Borsig, L; Wang, L; Cavalcante, MCM; Cardilo-Reis, L; Ferreira, PL; Mourão, PAS; Esko, JD; Pavão, MSG. Selectin Blocking Activity of a Fucosylated Chondroitin Sulfate Glycosaminoglycan from Sea Cucumber. *Journal of Biological Chemistry*, 2007, 282, 14984-91.

[7]   Fonseca, RJC; Mour; atilde; o, PAS. Fucosylated chondroitin sulfate as a new oral antithrombotic agent2006.

[8] Zancan, P; Mourão, PA. Venous and arterial thrombosis in rat models: dissociation of the antithrombotic effects of glycosaminoglycans. *Blood Coagulation & Fibrinolysis*, 2004, 15, 45-54.

[9] Glauser, BF; Pereira, MS; Monteiro, RQ; Mour; atilde; o, PAS. Serpin-independent anticoagulant activity of a fucosylated chondroitin sulfate2008.

[10] Pereira, MS; Melo, FR; Mourão, PAS. Is there a correlation between structure and anticoagulant action of sulfated galactans and sulfated fucans? *Glycobiology*, 2002, 12, 573-80.

[11] Fonseca, RJC; Santos, GRC; Mour; atilde; o, PAS. *Effects of polysaccharides enriched in 2,4-disulfated fucose units on coagulation, thrombosis and bleeding.* Practical and conceptual implications2009.

[12] Pereira, MS; Vilela-Silva, A-CES; Valente, A-P, Mourão, PAS. A 2-sulfated, 3-linked α-l-galactan is an anticoagulant polysaccharide. *Carbohydrate Research*, 2002, 337, 2231-8.

[13] Blossom, DB; Kallen, AJ; Patel, PR; Elward, A; Robinson, L; Gao, G; Langer, R; Perkins, KM; Jaeger, JL; Kurkjian, KM; Jones, M; Schillie, SF; Shehab, N; Ketterer, D; Venkataraman, G; Kishimoto, TK; Shriver, Z; McMahon, AW; Austen, KF; Kozlowski, S; Srinivasan, A; Turabelidze, G; Gould, CV; Arduino, MJ; Sasisekharan, R. Outbreak of Adverse Reactions Associated with Contaminated Heparin. *New England Journal of Medicine*, 2008, 359, 2674-84.

[14] Fonseca, RJC; Oliveira, S-NMCG; Pomin, VH; Mecawi, A; eacute; Araujo, IG; Mour; atilde; o, PAS. *Effects of oversulfated and fucosylated chondroitin sulfates on coagulation.* Challenges for the study of anticoagulant polysaccharides2010.

[15] Pomin, VH. Review: An overview about the structure–function relationship of marine sulfated homopolysaccharides with regular chemical structures. *Biopolymers*, 2009, 91, 601-9.

[16] Gray, E; Mulloy, B; Barrowcliffe, TW. Heparin and low-molecular-weight heparin. *Thrombosis and haemostasis*, 2008, 99, 807-18.

[17] WHO. The global burden of desease: 2004 update. Geneva: WHO; 2004, 160.

[18] AHA. Heart desease and stroke statistics: 2010 update at a glance.: AHA; 2010, 20.

[19] Cushman, M. Epidemiology and Risk Factors for Venous Thrombosis. *Seminars in hematology*, 2007, 44, 62-9.

[20] Cohen, AT; Agnelli, G; Anderson, FA; Arcelus, JI; Bergqvist, D; Brecht, JG; Greer, IA; Heit, JA; Hutchinson, JL; Kakkar, AK; Mottier, D; Oger, E; Samama, MM; Spannagl, M; Europe, VTEIAGi. Venous thromboembolism (VTE) in Europe. The number of VTE events and associated morbidity and mortality. *Thrombosis and haemostasis*, 2007, 98, 756-64.

[21] Heit, J; Cohen, A; Anderson, F; on Behalf of the VTEIAG. Estimated Annual Number of Incident and Recurrent, Non-Fatal and Fatal Venous Thromboembolism (VTE) Events in the US. *ASH Annual Meeting Abstracts*, 2005, 106, 910.

[22] Lusis, AJ. Atherosclerosis. *Nature*, 2000, 407, 233-41.

[23] Gresele, P; Agnelli, G. Novel approaches to the treatment of thrombosis. *Trends in Pharmacological Sciences*, 2002, 23, 25-32.

[24] Hirsh, J; Warkentin, TE; Shaughnessy, SG; Anand, SS; Halperin, JL; Raschke, R; Granger, C; Ohman, EM; Dalen, JE. Heparin and low-molecular-weight heparin:

mechanisms of action, pharmacokinetics, dosing, monitoring, efficacy, and safety. *Chest*, 2001, 119, 64S-94S.

[25] Spyropoulos, AC. Brave new world: the current and future use of novel anticoagulants. *Thrombosis research*, 2008, 123 Suppl 1, S29-35.

[26] Li, W; Johnson, DJD; Esmon, CT; Huntington, JA. Structure of the antithrombin-thrombin-heparin ternary complex reveals the antithrombotic mechanism of heparin. *Nat Struct Mol Biol*, 2004, 11, 857-62.

[27] Bourin, MC; Lindahl, U. Glycosaminoglycans and the regulation of blood coagulation. *The Biochemical journal*, 1993, 289 (Pt 2), 313-30.

[28] Ofosu, FA; Smith, LM; Anvari, N; Blajchman, MA. An approach to assigning in vitro potency to unfractionated and low molecular weight heparins based on the inhibition of prothrombin activation and catalysis of thrombin inhibition1988.

[29] Carter, WJ; Cama, E; Huntington, JA. Crystal structure of thrombin bound to heparin. *Journal of Biological Chemistry*, 2005, 280, 2745-9.

[30] Mourao, PA; Pereira, MS. Searching for alternatives to heparin: sulfated fucans from marine invertebrates. *Trends in cardiovascular medicine*, 1999, 9, 225-32.

[31] Guerrini, M; Beccati, D; Shriver, Z; Naggi, A; Viswanathan, K; Bisio, A; Capila, I; Lansing, JC; Guglieri, S; Fraser, B; Al-Hakim, A; Gunay, NS; Zhang, Z; Robinson, L; Buhse, L; Nasr, M; Woodcock, J; Langer, R; Venkataraman, G; Linhardt, RJ; Casu, B; Torri, G; Sasisekharan, R. Oversulfated chondroitin sulfate is a contaminant in heparin associated with adverse clinical events. *Nat Biotech*, 2008, 26, 669-75.

[32] Kishimoto, TK; Viswanathan, K; Ganguly, T; Elankumaran, S; Smith, S; Pelzer, K; Lansing, JC; Sriranganathan, N; Zhao, G; Galcheva-Gargova, Z; Al-Hakim, A; Bailey, GS; Fraser, B; Roy, S; Rogers-Cotrone, T; Buhse, L; Whary, M; Fox, J; Nasr, M; Dal Pan, GJ; Shriver, Z; Langer, RS; Venkataraman, G; Austen, KF; Woodcock, J; Sasisekharan, R. Contaminated Heparin Associated with Adverse Clinical Events and Activation of the Contact System. *New England Journal of Medicine*, 2008, 358, 2457-67.

[33] Mann, K; Nesheim, M; Church, W; Haley, P; Krishnaswamy, S. Surface-dependent reactions of the vitamin K-dependent enzyme complexes. *Blood*, 1990, 76, 1-16.

[34] Camera, M; Giesen, PLA; Fallon, J; Aufiero, BM; Taubman, M; Tremoli, E; Nemerson, Y. Cooperation Between VEGF and TNF-α Is Necessary for Exposure of Active Tissue Factor on the Surface of Human Endothelial Cells. *Arteriosclerosis, Thrombosis, and Vascular Biology*, 1999, 19, 531-7.

[35] Wilcox, JN; Smith, KM; Schwartz, SM; Gordon, D. Localization of tissue factor in the normal vessel wall and in the atherosclerotic plaque. *Proceedings of the National Academy of Sciences*, 1989, 86, 2839-43.

[36] Weiss, H; Turitto, V; Baumgartner, H; Nemerson, Y; Hoffmann, T. Evidence for the presence of tissue factor activity on subendothelium. *Blood*, 1989, 73, 968-75.

[37] Morrissey, J; Macik, B; Neuenschwander, P; Comp, P. Quantitation of activated factor VII levels in plasma using a tissue factor mutant selectively deficient in promoting factor VII activation. *Blood*, 1993, 81, 734-44.

[38] Lawson, JH; Mann, KG. Cooperative activation of human factor IX by the human extrinsic pathway of blood coagulation. *Journal of Biological Chemistry*, 1991, 266, 11317-27.

[39] Lawson, JH; Kalafatis, M; Stram, S; Mann, KG. A model for the tissue factor pathway to thrombin. I. An empirical study. *Journal of Biological Chemistry*, 1994, 269, 23357-66.

[40] Butenas, S; van 't Veer, C; Mann, KG. Evaluation of the Initiation Phase of Blood Coagulation Using Ultrasensitive Assays for Serine Proteases. *Journal of Biological Chemistry*, 1997, 272, 21527-33.

[41] Mann, KG; Krishnaswamy, S; Lawson, JH. Surface-dependent hemostasis. *Seminars in hematology*, 1992, 29, 213-26.

[42] Hockin, MF; Jones, KC; Everse, SJ; Mann, KG. A Model for the Stoichiometric Regulation of Blood Coagulation. *Journal of Biological Chemistry*, 2002, 277, 18322-33.

[43] Cawthern, KM; van 't Veer, C; Lock, JB; DiLorenzo, ME; Branda, RF; Mann, KG. Blood Coagulation in Hemophilia A and Hemophilia C. *Blood*, 1998, 91, 4581-92.

[44] Mann, KG; Butenas, S; Brummel, K. The Dynamics of Thrombin Formation. *Arteriosclerosis, Thrombosis, and Vascular Biology*, 2003, 23, 17-25.

[45] Brummel, KE; Butenas, S; Mann, KG. An Integrated Study of Fibrinogen during Blood Coagulation. *Journal of Biological Chemistry*, 1999, 274, 22862-70.

[46] Renné, T; Gailani, D. Role of Factor XII in hemostasis and thrombosis: clinical implications. *Expert Review of Cardiovascular Therapy*, 2007, 5, 733-41.

[47] Gailani, D; Renné, T. The intrinsic pathway of coagulation: a target for treating thromboembolic disease? *Journal of Thrombosis and Haemostasis*, 2007, 5, 1106-12.

[48] Mann, KG. Biochemistry and physiology of blood coagulation. *Thrombosis and haemostasis*, 1999, 82, 165-74.

[49] Davie, EW; Kulman, JD. An overview of the structure and function of thrombin. *Seminars in thrombosis and hemostasis*, 2006, 32 Suppl 1, 3-15.

[50] Furie, B; Furie, BC. Molecular and Cellular Biology of Blood Coagulation. *New England Journal of Medicine*, 1992, 326, 800-6.

[51] Dahlbäck, B. Blood coagulation. *The Lancet*, 2000, 355, 1627-32.

[52] Skinner, MW. Haemophilia: provision of factors and novel therapies: World Federation of Hemophilia goals and achievements. *British Journal of Haematology*, 2011, 154, 704-14.

[53] Salomon, O; Steinberg, DM; Seligshon, U. Variable bleeding manifestations characterize different types of surgery in patients with severe factor XI deficiency enabling parsimonious use of replacement therapy. *Haemophilia*, 2006, 12, 490-3.

[54] Kaplan, AP. Intrinsic coagulation, thrombosis, and bleeding1996.

[55] Lammle, B; Wuillemin, WA; Huber, I; Krauskopf, M; Zurcher, C; Pflugshaupt, R; Furlan, M. Thromboembolism and bleeding tendency in congenital factor XII deficiency--a study on 74 subjects from 14 Swiss families. *Thrombosis and haemostasis*, 1991, 65, 117-21.

[56] Gailani, D; Broze, G. Factor XI activation in a revised model of blood coagulation. *Science*, 1991, 253, 909-12.

[57] Naito, K; Fujikawa, K. Activation of human blood coagulation factor XI independent of factor XII. Factor XI is activated by thrombin and factor XIa in the presence of negatively charged surfaces. *Journal of Biological Chemistry*, 1991, 266, 7353-8.

[58] von dem Borne, P; Meijers, J; Bouma, B. Feedback activation of factor XI by thrombin in plasma results in additional formation of thrombin that protects fibrin clots from fibrinolysis. *Blood*, 1995, 86, 3035-42.

[59] Morrissey, JH. Tissue factor: a key molecule in hemostatic and nonhemostatic systems. *International journal of hematology*, 2004, 79, 103-8.

[60] Mackman, N. Role of Tissue Factor in Hemostasis, Thrombosis, and Vascular Development. *Arteriosclerosis, Thrombosis, and Vascular Biology*, 2004, 24, 1015-22.

[61] Rapaport, SI; Rao, LV. The tissue factor pathway: how it has become a "prima ballerina". *Thromb Haemost*, 1995, 74, 7-17.

[62] Meijers, JCM; Tekelenburg, WLH; Bouma, BN; Bertina, RM; Rosendaal, FR. High Levels of Coagulation Factor XI as a Risk Factor for Venous Thrombosis. *New England Journal of Medicine*, 2000, 342, 696-701.

[63] Vlieg, AvH; van der Linden, IK; Bertina, RM; Rosendaal, FR. High levels of factor IX increase the risk of venous thrombosis. *Blood*, 2000, 95, 3678-82.

[64] Triemstra, M; Rosendaal, FR; Smit, C; Van der Ploeg, HM; Briet, E. Mortality in Patients with Hemophilia: Changes in a Dutch Population from 1986 to 1992 and 1973 to 1986. *Annals of Internal Medicine*, 1995, 123, 823-7.

[65] Rosendaal, FR; Briét, E; Stibbe, J; Herpen, Gv; Leuven, JAG; Hofman, A; Vandenbroucke, JP. Haemophilia protects against ischaemic heart disease: a study of risk factors. *British Journal of Haematology*, 1990, 75, 525-30.

[66] Dahlbäck, B; Villoutreix, BO. The anticoagulant protein C pathway. *FEBS Letters*, 2005, 579, 3310-6.

[67] Broze, GJ. Tissue factor pathway inhibitor. *Thrombosis and haemostasis*, 1995, 74, 90-3.

[68] Hirsh, J. Blood tests for the diagnosis of venous and arterial thrombosis. *Blood*, 1981, 57, 1-8.

[69] Kojima, T. Targeted gene disruption of natural anticoagulant proteins in mice. *International journal of hematology*, 2002, 76 Suppl 2, 36-9.

[70] Conard, J; Brosstad, F; Lie Larsen, M; Samama, M; Abildgaard, U. Molar Antithrombin Concentration in Normal Human Plasma. *Pathophysiology of Haemostasis and Thrombosis*, 1983, 13, 363-8.

[71] Olson, ST; Bjork, I; Shore, JD. Kinetic characterization of heparin-catalyzed and uncatalyzed inhibition of blood coagulation proteinases by antithrombin. *Methods in enzymology*, 1993, 222, 525-59.

[72] Rezaie, AR. Prothrombin protects factor Xa in the prothrombinase complex from inhibition by the heparin-antithrombin complex. *Blood*, 2001, 97, 2308-13.

[73] Weitz, JI; Buller, HR. Direct Thrombin Inhibitors in Acute Coronary Syndromes. *Circulation*, 2002, 105, 1004-11.

[74] Ye, S; Cech, AL; Belmares, R; Bergstrom, RC; Tong, Y; Corey, DR; Kanost, MR; Goldsmith, EJ. The structure of a Michaelis serpin-protease complex. *Nat Struct Biol*, 2001, 8, 979-83.

[75] Kaslik, G; Kardos, J; Szabó, E; Szilágyi, L; Závodszky, P; Westler, WM; Markley, JL; Gráf, L. Effects of Serpin Binding on the Target Proteinase: Global Stabilization, Localized Increased Structural Flexibility, and Conserved Hydrogen Bonding at the Active Site†. *Biochemistry*, 1997, 36, 5455-64.

[76] Huntington, JA; Read, RJ; Carrell, RW. Structure of a serpin-protease complex shows inhibition by deformation. *Nature*, 2000, 407, 923-6.

[77] Olson, ST; Björk, I; Sheffer, R; Craig, PA; Shore, JD; Choay, J. Role of the antithrombin-binding pentasaccharide in heparin acceleration of antithrombin-proteinase reactions. Resolution of the antithrombin conformational change contribution to heparin rate enhancement. *Journal of Biological Chemistry*, 1992, 267, 12528-38.

[78] Björk, I; Ylinenjärvi, K; Olson, ST; Bock, PE. Conversion of antithrombin from an inhibitor of thrombin to a substrate with reduced heparin affinity and enhanced conformational stability by binding of a tetradecapeptide corresponding to the P1 to P14 region of the putative reactive bond loop of the inhibitor. *Journal of Biological Chemistry*, 1992, 267, 1976-82.

[79] Olson, ST; Björk, I. Predominant contribution of surface approximation to the mechanism of heparin acceleration of the antithrombin-thrombin reaction. Elucidation from salt concentration effects. *Journal of Biological Chemistry*, 1991, 266, 6353-64.

[80] Damus, PS; Hicks, M; Rosenberg, RD. Anticoagulant Action of Heparin. *Nature*, 1973, 246, 355-7.

[81] Choay, J; Petitou, M; Lormeau, JC; Sinay, P; Casu, B; Gatti, G. Structure-activity relationship in heparin: a synthetic pentasaccharide with high affinity for antithrombin III and eliciting high anti-factor Xa activity. *Biochemical and biophysical research communications*, 1983, 116, 492-9.

[82] Rosenberg, RD; Shworak, NW; Liu, J; Schwartz, JJ; Zhang, L. Heparan sulfate proteoglycans of the cardiovascular system. Specific structures emerge but how is synthesis regulated? *The Journal of Clinical Investigation*, 1997, 99, 2062-70.

[83] Olson, ST; Shore, JD. Transient kinetics of heparin-catalyzed protease inactivation by antithrombin III. The reaction step limiting heparin turnover in thrombin neutralization. *Journal of Biological Chemistry*, 1986, 261, 13151-9.

[84] Shore, JD; Olson, ST; Craig, PA; Choay, J; BjÖRk, I. Kinetics of Heparin Actiona. *Annals of the New York Academy of Sciences*, 1989, 556, 75-80.

[85] Danielsson, A; Raub, E; Lindahl, U; Björk, I. Role of ternary complexes, in which heparin binds both antithrombin and proteinase, in the acceleration of the reactions between antithrombin and thrombin or factor Xa. *Journal of Biological Chemistry*, 1986, 261, 15467-73.

[86] Griffith, MJ. The heparin-enhanced antithrombin III/thrombin reaction is saturable with respect to both thrombin and antithrombin III. *Journal of Biological Chemistry*, 1982, 257, 13899-302.

[87] Weitz, JI. Heparan sulfate: Antithrombotic or not? *The Journal of Clinical Investigation*, 2003, 111, 952-4.

[88] HajMohammadi, S; Enjyoji, K; Princivalle, M; Christi, P; Lech, M; Beeler, D; Rayburn, H; Schwartz, JJ; Barzegar, S; de Agostini, AI; Post, MJ; Rosenberg, RD; Shworak, NW. Normal levels of anticoagulant heparan sulfate are not essential for normal hemostasis. *The Journal of Clinical Investigation*, 2003, 111, 989-99.

[89] Tollefsen, DM; Pestka, CA; Monafo, WJ. Activation of heparin cofactor II by dermatan sulfate. *Journal of Biological Chemistry*, 1983, 258, 6713-6.

[90] Tollefsen, DM; Majerus, DW; Blank, MK. Heparin cofactor II. Purification and properties of a heparin-dependent inhibitor of thrombin in human plasma. *Journal of Biological Chemistry*, 1982, 257, 2162-9.

[91] Hurst, RE; Poon, MC; Griffith, MJ. Structure-activity relationships of heparin. Independence of heparin charge density and antithrombin-binding domains in thrombin inhibition by antithrombin and heparin cofactor II. *The Journal of Clinical Investigation*, 1983, 72, 1042-5.

[92] Maimone, MM; Tollefsen, DM. Activation of heparin cofactor II by heparin oligosaccharides. *Biochemical and biophysical research communications*, 1988, 152, 1056-61.

[93] Conrad, HE. Structure of Heparan Sulfate and Dermatan Sulfate. *Annals of the New York Academy of Sciences*, 1989, 556, 18-28.

[94] Halldórsdóttir, AM; Zhang, L; Tollefsen, DM. N-Acetylgalactosamine 4,6-O-sulfate residues mediate binding and activation of heparin cofactor II by porcine mucosal dermatan sulfate. *Glycobiology*, 2006, 16, 693-701.

[95] Pavao, MS; Mourao, PA; Mulloy, B; Tollefsen, DM. A unique dermatan sulfate-like glycosaminoglycan from ascidian. Its structure and the effect of its unusual sulfation pattern on anticoagulant activity. *The Journal of biological chemistry*, 1995, 270, 31027-36.

[96] Tollefsen, DM; Peacock, ME; Monafo, WJ. Molecular size of dermatan sulfate oligosaccharides required to bind and activate heparin cofactor II. *Journal of Biological Chemistry*, 1986, 261, 8854-8.

[97] Van Deerlin, VM; Tollefsen, DM. The N-terminal acidic domain of heparin cofactor II mediates the inhibition of alpha-thrombin in the presence of glycosaminoglycans. *Journal of Biological Chemistry*, 1991, 266, 20223-31.

[98] Ragg, H; Ulshöfer, T; Gerewitz, J. On the activation of human leuserpin-2, a thrombin inhibitor, by glycosaminoglycans. *Journal of Biological Chemistry*, 1990, 265, 5211-8.

[99] Myles, T; Church, FC; Whinna, HC; Monard, D; Stone, SR. Role of Thrombin Anion-binding Exosite-I in the Formation of Thrombin-Serpin Complexes. *Journal of Biological Chemistry*, 1998, 273, 31203-8.

[100] Liaw, PCY; Austin, RC; Fredenburgh, JC; Stafford, AR; Weitz, JI. Comparison of Heparin- and Dermatan Sulfate-mediated Catalysis of Thrombin Inactivation by Heparin Cofactor II. *Journal of Biological Chemistry*, 1999, 274, 27597-604.

[101] Tollefsen, DM. Heparin Cofactor II Deficiency. *Archives of Pathology & Laboratory Medicine*, 2002, 126, 1394-400.

[102] Griffith, M; Carraway, T; White, G; Dombrose, F. Heparin cofactor activities in a family with hereditary antithrombin III deficiency: evidence for a second heparin cofactor in human plasma. *Blood*, 1983, 61, 111-8.

[103] Tovar, AMF; de Mattos, DA; Stelling, MP; Sarcinelli-Luz, BSL; Nazareth, RA; Mourão, PAS. Dermatan sulfate is the predominant antithrombotic glycosaminoglycan in vessel walls: Implications for a possible physiological function of heparin cofactor II. *Biochimica et Biophysica Acta (BBA) - Molecular Basis of Disease*, 2005, 1740, 45-53.

[104] Sheehan, JP; Walke, EN. Depolymerized holothurian glycosaminoglycan and heparin inhibit the intrinsic tenase complex by a common antithrombin-independent mechanism. *Blood*, 2006, 107, 3876-82.

[105] Nishino, T; Aizu, Y; Nagumo, T. Antithrombin activity of a fucan sulfate from the brown seaweed Ecklonia kurome. *Thrombosis research*, 1991, 62, 765-73.

[106] Cumashi, A; Ushakova, NA; Preobrazhenskaya, ME; D'Incecco, A; Piccoli, A; Totani, L; Tinari, N; Morozevich, GE; Berman, AE; Bilan, MI; Usov, AI; Ustyuzhanina, NE; Grachev, AA; Sanderson, CJ; Kelly, M; Rabinovich, GA; Iacobelli, S; Nifantiev, NE. A comparative study of the anti-inflammatory, anticoagulant, antiangiogenic, and antiadhesive activities of nine different fucoidans from brown seaweeds. *Glycobiology*, 2007, 17, 541-52.

[107] Mauray, S; Sternberg, C; Theveniaux, J; Millet, J; Sinquin, C; Tapon-Bretaudiere, J; Fischer, AM. Venous antithrombotic and anticoagulant activities of a fucoidan fraction. *Thrombosis and haemostasis*, 1995, 74, 1280-5.

[108] Nagase, H; Enjyoji, K; Minamiguchi, K; Kitazato, K; Kitazato, K; Saito, H; Kato, H. Depolymerized holothurian glycosaminoglycan with novel anticoagulant actions: antithrombin III- and heparin cofactor II-independent inhibition of factor X activation by factor IXa-factor VIIIa complex and heparin cofactor II-dependent inhibition of thrombin. *Blood*, 1995, 85, 1527-34.

[109] Anderson, JAM; Fredenburgh, JC; Stafford, AR; Guo, YS; Hirsh, J; Ghazarossian, V; Weitz, JI. Hypersulfated Low Molecular Weight Heparin with Reduced Affinity for Antithrombin Acts as an Anticoagulant by Inhibiting Intrinsic Tenase and Prothrombinase. *Journal of Biological Chemistry*, 2001, 276, 9755-61.

[110] Rezaie, AR. Identification of Basic Residues in the Heparin-binding Exosite of Factor Xa Critical for Heparin and Factor Va Binding. *Journal of Biological Chemistry*, 2000, 275, 3320-7.

[111] Stenflo, J. Structure-function relationships of epidermal growth factor modules in vitamin K-dependent clotting factors. *Blood*, 1991, 78, 1637-51.

[112] Furie, B; Furie, BC. The molecular basis of blood coagulation. *Cell*, 1988, 53, 505-18.

[113] Mathur, A; Bajaj, SP. Protease and EGF1 Domains of Factor IXa Play Distinct Roles in Binding to Factor VIIIa. *Journal of Biological Chemistry*, 1999, 274, 18477-86.

[114] Nagase, H; Enjyoji, K-i, Shima, M; Kitazato, K; Yoshioka, A; Saito, H; Kato, H. Effect of Depolymerized Holothurian Glycosaminoglycan (DHG) on the Activation of Factor VIII and Factor V by Thrombin. *Journal of Biochemistry*, 1996, 119, 63-9.

[115] Barrow, RT; Parker, ET; Krishnaswamy, S; Lollar, P. Inhibition by heparin of the human blood coagulation intrinsic pathway factor X activator. *Journal of Biological Chemistry*, 1994, 269, 26796-800.

[116] Sie, P; Ofosu, F; Fernandez, F; Buchanan, MR; Petitou, M; Boneu, B. Respective role of antithrombin III and heparin cofactor II in the in vitro anticoagulant effect of heparin and of various sulphated polysaccharides. *British Journal of Haematology*, 1986, 64, 707-14.

[117] Buchanan, MR; Ofosu, FA; Fernandez, F; Van Ryn, J. Lack of relationship between enhanced bleeding induced by heparin and other sulfated polysaccharides and enhanced catalysis of thrombin inhibition. *Seminars in thrombosis and hemostasis*, 1986, 12, 324-7.

[118] Glauser, BF; Vairo, BC; Oliveira, CPM; Cinelli, LP; Pereira, MS; MourÃO, PAS. Generic versions of enoxaparin available for clinical use in Brazil are similar to the original drug. *Journal of Thrombosis and Haemostasis*, 2011, 9, 1419-22.

[119] Wienbergen, H; Zeymer, U. Management of acute coronary syndromes with fondaparinux. *Vascular health and risk management*, 2007, 3, 321-9.

[120] Xu, Y; Masuko, S; Takieddin, M; Xu, H; Liu, R; Jing, J; Mousa, SA; Linhardt, RJ; Liu, J. Chemoenzymatic Synthesis of Homogeneous Ultralow Molecular Weight Heparins. *Science*, 2011, 334, 498-501.

[121] Patnaik, MM; Moll, S. Inherited antithrombin deficiency: a review. *Haemophilia*, 2008, 14, 1229-39.

In: Chondroitin Sulfate   ISBN: 978-1-62808-490-0
Editor: Vitor H. Pomin   © 2013 Nova Science Publishers, Inc.

Chapter 9

Chondroitin Sulfate in Treatment of Tissue Degeneration

Michele Marcolongo[1] and Katsiaryna Prudnikova[2]
[1]Materials Science & Engineering, Drexel University
[2]Materials Science & Engineering, Drexel University, Philadelphia, PA, US

Abstract

Chondroitin sulfate (CS) is a negatively charged linear glycosaminoglycan (GAG) composed of individual sulfated monosaccharides. CS is an essential component of the extracellular matrix of soft and connective tissues and is a structural unit of large macromolecules, proteoglycans, such as aggrecan and versican, organized in a 3D bottle-brush architecture. Sulfation of CS allows water uptake providing tissue hydration and contributing to the osmotic pressure and compressive resistance. Elegant 3D organization of CS in proteoglycans provides an additional contribution to compressive stiffness of the tissue due to electro repulsive forces between CS molecules. With age and degeneration, GAG content in tissue is reduced due to low cell activity and increased enzymatic attacks, which results in a host of mechanical, hydration and nutritional deficits to tissue function. This, in turn, can manifest in pain, joint stiffness and loss of mobility. Most common examples of tissue degeneration associated with loss of GAG content are osteoarthritis and intervertebral disc degeneration. Conservative treatments of these diseases include physical exercise to reduce mechanical stress on joints and analgesics to reduce pain, or even surgical joint replacements or disc fusions in severe cases. However, these methods do not address underlying cause of the problem. Therefore, there have been increased efforts in developing alternative strategies, which aim to restore structural integrity of the degenerated tissue. Application of CS to restore reduced GAG content is one of the potential ways to treat degenerated tissue. Most well known approach, which has undergone clinical trials, involves an oral administration of CS, however it does not provide a local effect, and long-time hydration/restoration effects are limited due to diffusion of low-molecular weight CS out of the tissue. Other ongoing research efforts include studies on effect of chondroitin sulfate on cell synthetic activity in tissue; various chondroitin-hyaluronic acid-collagen scaffolds to mimic extracellular matrix; organization of CS in larger aggregates to mimic natural proteoglycans and their effect on biological and mechanical tissue function. An overview of these research initiatives will be provided in the current article.

Introduction

Chondroitin Sulfate Structure

Chondroitin sulfate (CS) is a negatively charged linear glycosaminoglycan (GAG) composed of individual sulfated monosaccharides (Glucuronic acid GlcUA and N-acetylgalactosamine GalNac). Each CS chain consists of 10-50 repeating disaccharide units of GlcUA and GalNAc and is approximately 20 kDa with a length of 40 nm [2]. Negative charge density is brought by sulfated groups in addition to carboxylic acid groups present on monosaccharide units. Two most common CS types have being identified with respect to position of the sulfated group on N-acetylgalactosamine. As shown in Figure 1, CS can be sulfated at either 4- or 6-position with resulting structures being labeled as Chondroitin-4-sulfate or Chondroitin-6-sulfate, respectively. Additionally, Chondroitin-2,6-sulfate and Chondroitin-4,6-sulfate have been identified [3].

Originally, CS molecules are not present in tissue individually, but constitute a structural unit of larger molecules, proteoglycans (PGs), where they are linked to the protein core of proteoglycans in a 3D architecture resembling a bottle brush. Aggrecan and versican are examples of such large proteoglycans.

Versican is present in a variety of soft tissues and has a molecular mass of more than 1,000 kDa. Versican consists of G1, GAG-binding and G3 domains with four isoforms being identified based on core molecular weight and a number of GAG-binding sites [4]. The largest versican isoform V0 consists of a large core (370 kDa) but only contains ~20 CS chains per GAG domain [5].

In the case of aggrecan, approximately 100 CS chains are covalently attached to the core protein in the CS region with a grafting density of approximately 0.25 to 0.5 nm^{-1} [6-8] (Figure 2). Protein core of aggrecan is approximately 250-300 kDa and 400 nm in contour length, and the molecular mass of aggrecan can reach ~2,200 kDa. It consists of several domains, which allow for the molecules flexibility (IGD) attachment to hyaluronic acid (G1 globular domain), attachment of chondroitin sulfate (CS1 and CS2 domains) and keratan sulfate (KS) (KS domain) and cell signaling (G3 globular domain). N- and O-linked oligosaccharides also decorate the aggrecan core protein throughout the CS and KS regions. The KS region of the aggrecan core protein is smaller with only ~30 KS chains (5-15 kDa) attached. Aggrecan is the most abundant proteoglycan in cartilage and nucleus pulposus region of the intervertebral disc and is essential for tissue integrity and functional behavior.

Functional Properties of Chondrotin Sulfate

Approximately 8,000-10,000 negatively charged groups are present on the aggrecan bottle brush via the charged sulfate and carboxylic acids of the attached CS and KS chains [8]. Charged groups of CS allow water uptake by the tissue, which, in part, provide tissue osmotic pressure [9]. Additional contribution to osmotic pressure comes from electrostatic repulsion between CS bristles due to the elegant 3D macromolecular bottle brush [10]. Together, they provide compressive resistance of soft and connective tissue. Interestingly, the hydrostatic pressure from the hydration of the molecule itself does not provide sufficient pressure in the absence of the macromolecular architecture. Electrostatic forces between CS chains on the aggrecan molecule account for 50% (290 kPa) of the equilibrium compressive elastic modulus as predicted by theoretical modeling [10]. Together with other constituents of the extracellular matrix (ECM), such as type I and type II collagen fibrils and hyaluronic acid (HA), aggrecan plays the main role in determining the mechanical properties of the tissue matrix.

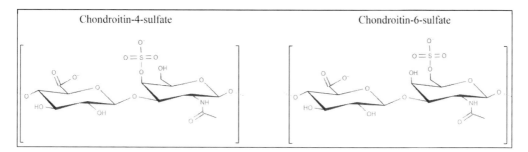

Figure 1. Chondroitin sulfate structures.

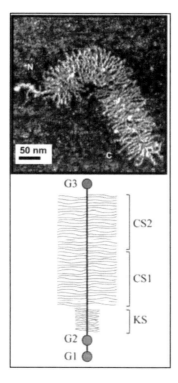

Figure 2. Aggrecan is a bottle brush molecule with a protein core and chondroitin and keratin sulfate bristles. AFM image reproduced from [1].

Aggrecan is assembled intracellularly through a complex series of enzymatic reactions [11]. Resulting sulfation sequence of CS is poorly understood, but it is believed to depend on tissue origin and function. After intracellular assembly, the aggrecan macromolecule is secreted to the extracellular space where it is able to assemble into larger aggregate structures with hyaluronic acid and link protein [11]. Although aggrecan is able to associate with HA and link protein extracellularly, large HA-aggrecan aggregates are only predominant in infancy. For example, by 6 months of age only approximately 30% of aggrecan in the nucleus pulposus region of the intervertebral disc is in the aggregate form and levels as low as 10% aggregation are seen in the adult NP [12, 13]. In addition to their contribution to the organization of the tissue, CS chains on aggrecan can also participate in a wide range of cellular events by regulating cell division and cytokinesis and providing binding sites for growth factors [3, 14, 15].

With age and degeneration, a loss of nutrient supply to the tissue results in a reduction of the synthesis of proteoglycans with a concordant increase in enzymatic attacks. Enzymatic cleavage of aggrecan is targeted to the core protein of the molecule and does not affect the CS region. However, this results in fragmentation of the PG molecule; aggrecan fragments vary in functional capacity, such as electrostatic repulsion and osmotic potential, as well as increased tendency to migrate out of the tissue over time. Matrix metalloproteinases (MMP) and aggrecanases (ADAMTS) are the main enzymes that contribute to the degradation of aggrecan [16-20]. In particular MMPs 1, 3, 7, 9 and 13 demonstrated increased activity with degeneration as well as aggrecanase 1, 4, 9, 5 and 15.

As a result, GAG content in tissue decreases, leading to loss of hydration, and results in a host of mechanical, hydration and nutritional deficits to tissue function, when tissue losses its ability to sustain and redistribute mechanical loads. This, in turn, can manifest in pain, joint stiffness and loss of mobility. Most common examples of tissue degeneration associated with loss of GAG content are osteoarthritis (cartilage degeneration) and intervertebral disc degeneration (nucleus pulposus tissue degeneration), which affect significant portion of U.S. population. Thus, lower back pain resulting from intervertebral disc degeneration is one of the leading musculoskeletal disorders confronting our health system with 15%-20% of the population experiencing lower back pain annually [7, 21]. Osteoarthritis (OA), in turn, is the most common form of arthritis and one of the leading causes of disabilities in the elderly population, affecting more than 20 million people in the U.S. [22, 23].

Most conservative treatments of tissue degeneration diseases involve gentle physical exercises to reduce mechanical stress on joints, chiropractic and osteopathic treatments, anti-inflammatory medications, and analgesics to reduce pain. The most common surgical approaches treat the end-stage of degeneration and include joint replacement (for OA) or fusion and total disc replacement (for IVD degeneration), with over 441,000 fusions performed in the U.S. in 2007 [24]. However, both non-surgical and surgical treatments of OA aim at reducing symptoms of the disease but do not address the potential underlying cause of reduced GAG content within tissue. Clinical and research efforts have focused on CS application as an individual therapeutic agent as well as a part of a more complex scaffold applied to degenerated tissue to restore its integrity, improve hydration and mechanical stability.

Chondroitin Sulfate in Treatment of Tissue Degeneration

Oral Administration of CS

Most well-known approach, which has undergone clinical trials, involves oral administration of CS, which is sold as a dietary supplement in the United States (regulated by the Food and Drug Administration) and is a prescription drug in Europe (symptomatic slow-acting drug). CS has been recommended by the Osteoarthritis Research Society International (OARSI) for treatment of knee OA and by the European League Against Rheumatism (EULAR) for treatment of hip and knee OA [25-27]. An average dose of CS ranges between 800 – 1200 mg/day, and CS is often being used in combination with glucosamine.

While the exact mechanism of CS therapeutic action in this treatment is under debate, the effect of CS administration could be a combination of anti-inflammatory activity, up-regulation of proteoglycan synthesis and inhibition of the synthesis of proteolytic enzymes which attack and degrade existing PGs [28]. For example, several *in vitro* studies have shown that CS can stimulate the proteoglycan synthesis of chondrocytes [29-31] and also decrease expression of matrix metalloproteinase and aggrecanase [31-33]. Anti-inflammatory ability of CS may be attributed to the reported reduction in cyclooxygenase and prostaglandin expressions [34, 35].

There have been a number of clinical trials that showed mixed results. Uebelhart et al. conducted a 1-year pilot study that included 42 patients with symptomatic knee OA. The patients were treated orally with CS and placebo was used as a control. They reported that CS significantly reduced pain in patients and improved joint mobility [36]. In recent study by Wildi et al., CS treatment was shown to reduce cartilage volume loss (as compared to placebo) in 6 months in a group of 69 patients and was associated with reduced number of subchondral bone marrow lesions [37]. Hochnberg conducted a meta-analysis of three 2-year long placebo-controlled clinical trials and concluded that a prolonged intake of CS can be effective for reducing the rate of joint space narrowing in patients with knee OA [38].

Despite positive reviews, efficacy of CS supplements has been questioned in a review of 7 clinical trials by Leeb et al., who noted that in some cases CS administration was accompanied by intake of additional drugs such as analgesics or non-steroidal anti-inflammatory drugs making it a poorly controlled treatment [39].

Reichenbach et al. reported a systematic review of 20 clinical trials (3846 patients) and concluded that CS treatment resulted in zero or minimal effects thus discouraging further application of CS in human trials [40]. Recent Glucosamine/Chondroitin Sulfate Arthritis Intervention Trial (GAIT) (6-month long, multicenter, 662 patients with knee OA) funded by NIH has demonstrated that CS had no statistically significant effect on OA symptoms in overall patient population, but combination of CS and glucosamine had some efficacy in reducing pain for a group of patients with mild to severe tissue degeneration [41, 42].

While most trials are focusing on application of CS for treatment of osteoarthritis, little information is available on efficacy of CS administration for lower back pain. In a study conducted by Blitterswijk et al., a 56-year old man with recurrent lower back pain was administered CS in combination with glucosamine and manganese ascorbate over a 2 year period [43]. T2-weighted MRI was used to monitor the state of L3-4 (mild degeneration) and L4-5 (severe degeneration) intervertebral discs. In 2 years, the condition of severely degraded disc L4-5 didn't change, however restoration of disc height and reduction in disc protrusion was observed for the L3-4 disc. Despite some positive outcome reported, this study is clearly not conclusive due to only one patient participating. In a trial by Leffler et al., CS/glucosamine/manganese ascorbate was used in a 16-week randomized, double-blind, placebo-controlled trial with 34 males suffering from degenerative joint disease of knee or lower back. While the treatment was shown to have an effect for knee osteoarthritis, the results on lower back pain remained largely inconclusive, and as authors suggested, the therapy needs to be re-evaluated in a larger trial [44].

Further studies are definitely needed to deduce the effects of CS administration and determine the actual mechanism of the therapeutic action, but results evaluation and comparison may be complicated due to the variety of forms of CS and differences in precise composition of each dietary supplement. Most currently available CS is extracted from different animal sources (cow, pig, shark tissues) with varied sulfation pattern and molecular weight, and is regulated in compliance with food processing standards but not the pharmaceutical ones.

Up to date, clinical studies have not yet identified any significant side effects of CS intake and absence of drug-drug interactions was demonstrated for CS, making it a safe therapeutic agent. However more efficient ways of CS delivery may be needed to improve treatment efficacy. For example, while increased CS concentration in plasma levels were detected as early as 2 hours after an intake [45], and presence of labeled CS in joint tissues was confirmed after oral administration [46], it was noticed that only 10% of CS reached the blood compartment in its original molecular weight state, while remaining 90% were depolymerized [47]. This can result in non-systematic delivery of CS to degenerated tissue what will further complicate interpretation of the treatment efficacy.

Injections of CS

To target local sites of tissue degeneration, CS can be potentially administered through injections with an idea to increase local hydration and osmotic pressure thus helping tissue to resist compressive loading and stabilize the affected joint. CS may also induce proteoglycan secretion and down regulate synthesis of enzymes, thus helping damaged matrix to restore its PG concentration within natural levels [29-33]. As a current treatment for OA, hyaluronic acid is being injected into knee joints where it contributes to the synovial fluid lubricating properties [48]. It helps to ease pain and stiffness resulting from excessive joint friction associated with degenerative state of adjacent cartilage. HA is, however, known for its short life-time period in tissue [49].

While local injections of CS can potentially increase hydration and affect cellular activity, long-term effects of this treatment might be limited due to diffusion of low-molecular weight CS out of the tissue, as it happens with fragments of enzymatically digested proteoglycans.

Nevertheless, in a study conducted by Uebelhart et al., the effect of the intramuscular injection of the commercially available chondroitin-4,6-sulfate (Chondrosulf®) was studied in a rabbit model [50]. Cartilage degeneration in a rabbit knee was modeled with an injection of chemopapain, which causes loss of articular cartilage PGs. Chondrosulf® was administered orally and via an intramuscular injection for 21 days (starting 11 days prior chemopapain treatment), leading to a reduction in weight-bearing articular cartilage PG loss in both cases. While this study didn't show any significant differences in outcomes between oral intake of CS and intramuscular injections, both treatments produced results that were significantly different from untreated samples (oral intake $P=0.0036$, intramuscular injection $P=0.0457$).

Recently, Hui et al. evaluated the effect of the intra-articular delivery of CS to joint defects in a rabbit model [51]. Instead of direct injections of CS, injectable hydrogels progressively releasing CS were implanted into the knee joints near sites of chondral defects created with punches. CS treatment resulted in a formation of a layer composed of both hyaline cartilage and fibrocartilage with the higher modulus of elasticity when compared to the control saline group. These results suggest that application of CS could be an effective treatment for tissue degenerative defects.

In a clinical trial for treatment of lower back pain, Klein et al. used a solution of glucosamine and CS combined with hypertonic dextrose and dimethylsulfoxide (DMSO) for an intradiscal injection treatment of 30 patients with chronic lower back pain [52]. Significant improvement in patients with moderate levels of back pain was observed after 1-year follow up based on post-treatment Roland-Morris disability score. However, little or no improvement was observed in patients with severe cases of disc degeneration. This may indicate that proposed approach could be more beneficial for people with mild cases of lower back pain.

Positive effects of these pilot studies, lack of complications and serious side effects warrant further evaluations of this approach including comprehensive biomechanical testing.

CS in Cellular Treatments of Degenerated Tissue

Much attention has been paid to cellular-based approaches to repair degenerated tissue. In general, these approaches involve isolation of particular cells of interest, expansion in culture and either injecting them back into a degenerated segment or seeding them into a biomaterial scaffold, which is further implanted/delivered into a tissue where cells produce new extracellular matrix thus helping to repair damaged site. For example, autologous disc "chondrocyte" transplantation was investigated in 2 years trial by Meisel et al. with the results showing a clinically significant reduction in lower back pain [53, 54]. Autologous chondrocyte implantation was also shown to be effective for cartilage repair [55, 56]. However cellular therapy can have complications arising from the highly aggressive degenerative microenvironment of the intervertebral disc (poor nutritional supply [57, 58], hypoxic [59-61], inflammatory [62, 63] and aggressive mechanical environment [64-66]), potential leakage of chondrocytes, periosteal complications in cartilage [67, 68]. Therefore, focus has shifted to a combination of cells and three-dimensional scaffolds.

Different natural and synthetic materials such as types I and II collagen based hydrogels, chitosan-alginate composite gels, poly(glycolic acid), poly(lactic-acid), to name a few, have been used in cellular delivery strategies both *in vitro* and *in vivo* [69-75]. In addition, GAGs were shown to play a crucial role in chondrogenesis promoting secretion of PGs as well as type II collagen associated with healthy hyaline cartilage [29-31, 76]. This makes CS a potential good cellular carrier which closely mimics natural extracellular matrix, can promote formation of hyaline cartilage *in vivo* (as opposed to undesirable fibrocartilaginous matrix), and newly secreted proteoglycans at the site of CS scaffold implantation can potentially help to compensate for GAG loss occurring in tissue with age and degeneration. This application would require fabrication of CS scaffolds that are further reviewed in the following section.

CS Scaffolds and Gels for Treatment of Tissue Degeneration

A significant body of research is focused on application of CS and CS-modified scaffolds (including mixtures with collagen, hyaluronic acid, gelatin, synthetic polymers) for restoration of degenerated tissue. Scaffolds have been widely used in tissue engineering to alter tissue mechanical properties and restore functionality: scaffolds can directly contribute to tissue compressive stiffness, serve as delivery vehicles for cells and growth factors, provide support for cell migration during tissue re-modeling and adhesion between an implant and native tissue.

Incorporation of a natural component of the extracellular matrix, chondroitin sulfate, into a scaffold can potentially provide an additional increase in local tissue hydration and affect bioactivity. In addition, having CS chemically bound in a form of a hydrogel/scaffold or an adhesive layer can prolong its lifetime at a delivery site, minimize migration out of the tissue and improve scaffold integration.

Cross-Linked and Functionalized CS

Individual CS molecules can be either cross-linked to form a hydrogel or functionalized to improve further integration of CS into an existing matrix. Presence of hydroxyl and carboxyl groups on CS opens a lot of potential pathways for chemical modification of CS including reaction between –COOH and primary amines mediated with 1-ethyl-3-(-3-dimethylaminopropyl) carbodiimide (EDC) and N-hydroxysuccinimide (NHS), reaction between -OH and epoxides, oxidation to form aldehydes which could be further reacted with amines [77].

Cross-linkable CS has been extensively investigated by the Elisseeff's group at the Johns Hopkins University [78-80]. One example of their work includes modification of CS with glycidyl methacrylate (GMa) via reaction between a hydroxyl group on CS and an epoxide on GMa. Resulting macronomer was UV cross-linked via pendant double bonds on CS to form CS-GMa hydrogel and was also co-polymerized with different fractions of poly(ethyleneoxide-diacrylate) (PEO-DA) to modify mechanical properties of the scaffold. Resulting hydrogels were shown to have no cytotoxic effects and their elastic properties and swelling degree were a function of PEO-DA polymer fraction. This potentially allows adjustment of hydrogel properties to meet clinical requirements based on a particular tissue being treated.

In another project, carboxyl groups on CS were modified with NHS to promote further reaction with primary amines. A six-arm poly(ethylene-glycol) with terminal primary amine groups was further used as a cross-linker to form a CS hydrogel which was studied in a sub-Q mouse model and was shown to have minimal inflammatory response [80].

Recent publication in Nature Materials by Elisseeff's group describes CS being modified with glycidyl methacrylate (as described above) and further oxidized to create aldehyde groups which could help to bind functionalized CS material to tissue via chemical reaction with primary amine in cartilage [81]. In this approach, CS in not directly cross-linked to form a hydrogel implant but rather serves as an intermediate adhesive layer between tissue and acrylate-base polymer graft with which it connects via polymerization of pendant acrylate groups on disaccharides. Cytocompatibility tests for the new adhesive confirmed cell viability in both polymer graft-hydrogel and a cartilage layer. *In vivo* implantation studies (mice model) also showed promising results of cell-loaded hydrogel being successfully bonded to cartilage via CS adhesive while encapsulated cells produced type II collagen and matrix proteoglycans facilitating neo-cartilage formation. Application of this newly developed CS adhesive can potentially help to overcome common issues with hydrogel implantation for tissue regeneration by improving integration between biomaterial scaffold and native cartilage. This will help to increase mechanical performance (due to improved scaffold stability within the tissue, i.e. material being hold in place), as well as neo-cartilage formation (due to a presence of an additional adhesive connective layer between biomaterial and tissue). This approach was further evaluated in human cadaveric joints and a pilot human clinical trial (knee microfracture) where the majority of patients reported significant decrease in severity of knee pain after implantation of a scaffold modified with CS adhesive [82].

CS-Based Scaffolds

In order to vary CS hydrogel mechanical properties and more closely mimic extracellular matrix (being inspired by the neat organization of natural tissue), researchers have worked on fabrication of various CS-based scaffolds, where CS molecules are integrated with other extracellular components, such as collagen and hyaluronic acid. Often, these scaffolds do not possess appropriate mechanical strength so different cross-linking methods are employed to alter matrix stiffness and pore size. Polymers, like poly(vinyl alcohol), poly(L-lactic acid), poly(glycolic acid) have been used to achieve systematic variation in scaffold mechanical properties. In combination with CS providing good cellular support, it allows fabrication of hydrophilic, bioactive materials with optimized mechanical characteristics.

While it is impossible to review all recent research activities in this field, several examples of CS-based scaffolds are summarized in Table 1.

CS Based Biomimetic Proteoglycans

In previously described efforts, CS chains remained disordered achieving only part of their mechanical potential via osmotic swelling properties and integration within an existing matrix [78, 80, 81, 91, 95, 96]. Bottle brush architecture is essential for electrostatic forces between CS bristles and resulting contribution to compressive resistance of the tissue. These electrostatic interactions gained by the ultra-structural organization of CS into the bottle brush architecture cannot be achieved using strategies mentioned above. Therefore, fabrication of proteoglycan mimic based on CS has begun to receive increased attention.

Table 1. Selective examples of CS-based scaffolds

Scaffold	Description	Study
Poly(L-lactide)-g-CS blend with Poly(L-lactide)	Poly(L-lactide) was grafted onto CS via chemical bonding and further mixed with unreacted poly(L-lactide). Increased expressions of type II collagen and aggrecan by encapsulated chondrocytes.	Lee et al. [83]
Poly(γ-glutamic acid)-g-CS-blend-poly(ε-caprolactone)	Inclusion of poly(γ-glutamic acid)-g-CS into PCL scaffold led to increased water binding capacity and reduced degradation of the scaffold.	Chang et al. [84]
CS-Poly(vinyl alcohol) hydrogels	Photo-polymerized CS-PVA hydrogels were shown to possess mechanical properties superior to homopolymer gels of CS and PVA.	Bryant et al. [85]
Poly(lactic-co-glycolic acid)-gelatin/chondroitin/hyaluronate	Improved proliferation of mesenchymal stem cells as compared to pure PLGA scaffolds (rabbit model, full-thickness cartilage defect) Positive results on cartilage regeneration when scaffold was implanted with TGF-β3 growth factor encapsulated (rabbit model).	Fan et al. [86] Fan et al. [87]
CS-dermatan sulfate (DS)-chitosan	Scaffolds were fabricated via EDC/NHS crosslinking. While addition of CS/DS generally enhanced GAG and collagen production by cells, the magnitude of that effect was dependent on CS/DS ratios used for scaffold fabrication.	
Type II collagen - CS	EDC/NHS cross-linking improved mechanical stability of a collagen-CS scaffold as well as proliferation of encapsulated cells.	Cao et al. [88]
Type II collagen-CS-hyaluronan	Scaffolds were cross-linked by genipin and showed increased expression of genes of type II collagen and aggrecan by encapsulated chondrocytes (as compared to collagen only scaffolds).	Ko et al. [89, 90]
Type I Collagen-CS-hyaluronan	CS and HA were first cross-linked with adipic acid dihydrazide followed up by the cross-linking reaction with collagen using genipin. New scaffolds had superior mechanical properties, reduced degradation as compared to collagen only scaffolds, while cell proliferation was not significantly different.	Zhang et al. [91]
Concentrated type I collagen-CS	Collagen-CS scaffolds with high concentration (4x) of collagen were obtained by centrifugation and exhibited 30x fold improvement in mechanical properties, as compared to conventional unconcentrated scaffolds.	Liang 2010 et al.[92]
Gelatin-CS-Hyaluronan	Gelatin, CS and HA were cross-linked with EDC in concentrations mimicking natural ECM composition in cartilage. *In vitro* secretion of ECM and type I collagen by encapsulated chondrocytes.	Chang et al. [93]
Gelatin-CS-Hyaluronan	Gelatin, CS and HA were used in concentrations mimicking composition of nucleus pulposus of the intervertebral disc and cross-linked with glutaraldehyde. *In vitro* studies confirmed preservation of viability and proliferation of encapsulated human NP cells.	Yang et al. [94]
Collagen-Aggrecan mimic (CS-Hyaluronic acid)	CS was first chemically bonded with HA via functionalization with HA-specific binding peptide and mixed with Type I collagen to fabricate ECM constructs. Chemical bonding of CS and HA significantly improved compressive stiffness of constructs and their resistance to degradation as compared to uncross-linked mixture of CS/HA/collagen. Incorporation of aggrecan mimic enhanced type II collagen expression (*in vitro*) that could be further improved by pre-alignment of collagen fibers in the construct.	Bernhard at el. [95] Sharma et al. [96]

While in the recent study by Bernhard et al. [95], described above, design of aggrecan mimic was attempted, bottle-brush architecture again was not achieved since CS was linked to HA via functional groups along the CS chain and not through a terminal end.

A potential pathway to mimic an actual architecture of natural aggrecan molecule, however, can be envisioned based on a recent study by Sarkar et al. [97, 98]. In this study, several commercially available CS sources were analyzed, and one source was identified as containing a terminal primary amine functional group. The reaction kinetics between this terminal group on CS and different amine-reactive vinyl monomers (acrylic acid and allyl glycidyl ether) was studied, and successful conjugation of CS via terminal end onto an epoxide functionalized surface was confirmed.

Conclusion

Chondroitin sulfate is an important natural biomacromolecule and a structural unit of the most abundant proteoglycan in tissue, aggrecan. CS is essential for proper tissue hydration and its elastic properties, interaction between different components of the extracellular matrix, and may also affect cellular activity. Unfortunately, as our tissues degenerate as result of either age or trauma, CS proteoglycans are being lost which could result in a host of mechanical, hydration and nutritional deficits to tissue function. In this regard, CS has been extensively studied as a therapeutic agent that can help to halt or even reverse tissue degeneration. While the oral administration of CS is the only treatment that is currently being used clinically, its efficacy has been under a debate. However, with research activities focused on development of new strategies (local delivery, cellular, scaffolds), we are poised to see some exciting scientific findings in the future that could translate into new clinical therapies.

References

[1]   Ng, L; et al., Individual cartilage aggrecan macromolecules and their constituent glycosaminoglycans visualized via atomic force microscopy. *Journal of Structural Biology*, 2003, 143(3), 242-257.

[2]   Nap, RJ; Szleifer, I. Structure and Interactions of Aggrecans: Statistical Thermodynamic Approach. *Biophysical Journal*, 2008, 95(10), 4570-4583.

[3]   Volpi, N. *Chondroitin sulfate: structure, role and pharmacological activity*. Vol. 53. 2006, Academic Press.

[4]   Yao Jiong, W; et al. The interaction of versican with its binding partners. Cell research, 2005, 15(7), 483-494.

[5]   Dours-Zimmermann, MT; Zimmermann, DR. A novel glycosaminoglycan attachment domain identified in two alternative splice variants of human versican. *Journal of Biological Chemistry*, 1994, 269(52), 32992-32998.

[6]   Roughley, PJ; Lee, ER. Cartilage proteoglycans: structure and potential functions. *Microscopy research and technique*, 1994, 28(5), 385-397.

[7]   Roughley, PJ; et al. The structure and degradation of aggrecan in human intervertebral disc. *European Spine Journal*, 2006. 15, 326-332.

[8]   Dudhia, J. Aggrecan, aging and assembly in articular cartilage. *Cellular and molecular life sciences*, 2005. 62(19), 2241-2256.

[9]   Kiani, C; et al. Structure and function of aggrecan. *Cell Research*, 2002, 12(1), 19-32.

[10] Buschmann, MD; Grodzinsky, AJ. A molecular model of proteoglycan-associated electrostatic forces in cartilage mechanics. *J Biomech Eng*, 1995, 117(2), 179-92.

[11] Vertel, BM; The ins and outs of aggrecan. *Trends in Cell Biology*, 1995, 5(12), 458-464.

[12] Roughley, P. Biology of intervertebral disc aging and degeneration: involvement of the extracellular matrix. *Spine*, 2004, 29(23), 2691.

[13] Johnstone, B; Bayliss, MT. The Large Proteoglycans of the Human Intervertebral Disc-Changes in their Biosynthesis and Structure with Age, Topography and Pathology. *Spine*, 1995, 20, 674-684.

[14] Mizuguchi, S; et al. Chondroitin proteoglycans are involved in cell division of Caenorhabditis elegans. *Nature*, 2003, 423(6938), 443-448.

[15] Gama, CI; et al. Sulfation patterns of glycosaminoglycans encode molecular recognition and activity. *Nature chemical biology*, 2006, 2(9), 467-473.

[16] Weiler, C; et al. 2002 SSE Award Competition in Basic Science: expression of major matrix metalloproteinases is associated with intervertebral disc degradation and resorption. *European Spine Journal*, 2002, 11(4), 308-320.

[17] Roberts, S; et al. Matrix metalloproteinases and aggrecanase: their role in disorders of the human intervertebral disc. *Spine*, 2000. 25(23), 3005.

[18] Goupille, P; et al. Matrix metalloproteinases: the clue to intervertebral disc degeneration? *Spine*, 1998. 23(14), 1612.

[19] Le Maitre, C; et al. Matrix synthesis and degradation in human intervertebral disc degeneration. *Biochemical Society Transactions*, 2007, 35, 652-655.

[20] Huang, K; Wu, L. Aggrecanase and aggrecan degradation in osteoarthritis: a review. *Journal of International Medical Research*, 2008, 36(6), 1149-1160.

[21] Atlas, SJ; Deyo, RA. Evaluating and managing acute low back pain in the primary care setting. *J Gen Intern Med*, 2001, 16(2), 120-31.

[22] Felson, DT; et al. Osteoarthritis: new insights. Part 1: the disease and its risk factors. *Annals of internal medicine*, 2000, 133(8), 635-646.

[23] Helmick, CG; et al. Estimates of the prevalence of arthritis and other rheumatic conditions in the United States: Part I. *Arthritis & Rheumatism*, 2008, 58(1), 15-25.

[24] Medtech-Insights, Report # A606 - U.S. Surgical Procedure Volumes: Windhover Information, 2007.

[25] Zhang, W; et al. OARSI recommendations for the management of hip and knee osteoarthritis, Part II: OARSI evidence-based, expert consensus guidelines. *Osteoarthritis and cartilage*, 2008, 16(2), 137-162.

[26] Jordan, K; et al. EULAR Recommendations 2003: an evidence based approach to the management of knee osteoarthritis: Report of a Task Force of the Standing Committee for International Clinical Studies Including Therapeutic Trials (ESCISIT). *Annals of the Rheumatic Diseases*, 2003, 62(12), 1145-1155.

[27] Zhang, W; et al. EULAR evidence based recommendations for the management of hip osteoarthritis: report of a task force of the EULAR Standing Committee for International Clinical Studies Including Therapeutics (ESCISIT). *Annals of the Rheumatic Diseases*, 2005, 64(5), 669-681.

[28] Monfort, J; et al. Biochemical basis of the effect of chondroitin sulphate on osteoarthritis articular tissues. *Annals of the rheumatic diseases*, 2008, 67(6), 735-740.

[29] Lippiello, L; et al. In vivo chondroprotection and metabolic synergy of glucosamine and chondroitin sulfate. *Clinical Orthopaedics and Related Research*, 2000, 381, 229-240.

[30] Schwartz, NB; Dorfman, A. Stimulation of chondroitin sulfate proteoglycan production by chondrocytes in monolayer. *Connective tissue research*, 1975, 3(2-3), 115-122.

[31] Wang, L; et al. Influence of polysulphated polysaccharides and hydrocortisone on the extracellular matrix metabolism of human articular chondrocytes in vitro. *Clinical and experimental rheumatology*, 2002, 20(5), 669.

[32] Monfort, J; et al. Chondroitin sulfate and hyaluronic acid (500-730 kda) inhibit stromelysin-1 synthesis in human osteoarthritic chondrocytes. *Drugs under experimental and clinical research*, 2005, 31(2), 71-76.

[33] Tahiri, K; et al. Natural chondroitin sulphates increase aggregation of proteoglycan complexes and decrease adamts-5 expression in interleukin 1β-treated chondrocytes. *Annals of the rheumatic diseases*, 2008, 67(5), 696-702.

[34] Chan, P; et al. Glucosamine and chondroitin sulfate regulate gene expression and synthesis of nitric oxide and prostaglandin E (2) in articular cartilage explants. Osteoarthritis and cartilage/OARS, *Osteoarthritis Research Society*, 2005. 13(5), 387.

[35] Chan, P-S; Caron, JP; Orth, MW. Short-term gene expression changes in cartilage explants stimulated with interleukin beta plus glucosamine and chondroitin sulfate. *The Journal of rheumatology*, 2006, 33(7), 1329-1340.

[36] Uebelhart, D; et al. Effects of oral chondroitin sulfate on the progression of knee osteoarthritis: a pilot study. *Osteoarthritis and cartilage*, 1998, 6, 39-46.

[37] Wildi, LM; et al. Chondroitin sulphate reduces both cartilage volume loss and bone marrow lesions in knee osteoarthritis patients starting as early as 6 months after initiation of therapy: a randomised, double-blind, placebo-controlled pilot study using MRI. *Annals of the rheumatic diseases*, 2011, 70(6), 982-989.

[38] Hochberg, M. Structure-modifying effects of chondroitin sulfate in knee osteoarthritis: an updated meta-analysis of randomized placebo-controlled trials of 2-year duration. *Osteoarthritis and cartilage*, 2010, 18, S28-S31.

[39] Leeb, BF; et al. A metaanalysis of chondroitin sulfate in the treatment of osteoarthritis. *The Journal of rheumatology*, 2000, 27(1), 205.

[40] Reichenbach, S; et al. Meta-analysis: chondroitin for osteoarthritis of the knee or hip. *Annals of internal medicine*, 2007, 146(8), 580-590.

[41] Trial, G. The NIH Glucosamine/Chondroitin Arthritis Intervention Trial (GAIT). *J Pain Palliat Care Pharmacother*, 2008, 22(1), 39-43.

[42] Sawitzke, AD; et al. Clinical efficacy and safety of glucosamine, chondroitin sulphate, their combination, celecoxib or placebo taken to treat osteoarthritis of the knee: 2-year results from GAIT. *Annals of the rheumatic diseases*, 2010, 69(8), 1459-1464.

[43] van Blitterswijk, WJ; van de Nes, JC; Wuisman, PI. Glucosamine and chondroitin sulfate supplementation to treat symptomatic disc degeneration: biochemical rationale and case report. *BMC Complementary and Alternative Medicine*, 2003, 3(1), 2.

[44] Leffler, CT; et al. Glucosamine, chondroitin, and manganese ascorbate for degenerative joint disease of the knee or low back: a randomized, double-blind, placebo-controlled pilot study. *Military Medicine*, 1999, 164(2), 85-91.

[45] Volpi, N. Oral bioavailability of chondroitin sulfate (Condrosulf) and its constituents in healthy male volunteers. Osteoarthritis and cartilage/OARS, *Osteoarthritis Research Society*, 2002, 10(10), 768.

[46] Ronca, F; et al. Anti-inflammatory activity of chondroitin sulfate. *Osteoarthritis and Cartilage*, 1998, 6(Supplement 1), 14-21.

[47] Henrotin, Y; et al. Chondroitin sulfate in the treatment of osteoarthritis: from in vitro studies to clinical recommendations. *Therapeutic Advances in Musculoskeletal Disease*, 2010, 2(6), 335-348.

[48] Gerwin, N; Hops, C; Lucke, A. Intraarticular drug delivery in osteoarthritis. *Advanced Drug Delivery Reviews*, 2006, 58(2), 226-242.

[49] Strauss, EJ; et al. Hyaluronic Acid Viscosupplementation and Osteoarthritis Current Uses and Future Directions. *The American Journal of Sports Medicine*, 2009, 37(8), 1636-1644.

[50] Uebelhart, D; et al. Protective effect of exogenous chondroitin 4, 6-sulfate in the acute degradation of articular cartilage in the rabbit. *Osteoarthritis and cartilage*, 1998, 6, 6-13.

[51] Hui, JH; et al. Intra-articular delivery of chondroitin sulfate for the treatment of joint defects in rabbit model. *Journal of molecular histology*, 2007, 38(5), 483-489.

[52] Klein, RG; et al. Biochemical injection treatment for discogenic low back pain: a pilot study. *The spine journal: official journal of the North American Spine Society*, 2003, 3(3), 220.

[53] Meisel, HJ; et al. Clinical experience in cell-based therapeutics: Disc chondrocyte transplantation: A treatment for degenerated or damaged intervertebral disc. *Biomolecular engineering*, 2007, 24(1), 5-21.

[54] Meisel, HJ; et al. Clinical experience in cell-based therapeutics: intervention and outcome. *European spine journal*, 2006, 15, 397-405.

[55] Peterson, L; et al. Autologous Chondrocyte Implantation A Long-term Follow-up. *The American Journal of Sports Medicine*, 2010, 38(6), 1117-1124.

[56] Peterson, L; et al. Autologous chondrocyte transplantation biomechanics and long-term durability. *The American Journal of Sports Medicine*, 2002, 30(1), 2-12.

[57] Urban, JPG; Smith, S; Fairbank, JCT. Nutrition of the intervertebral disc. *Spine*, 2004, 29(23), 2700-2709.

[58] Bibby, SRS; Urban, JPG. Effect of nutrient deprivation on the viability of intervertebral disc cells. *European spine journal*, 2004, 13(8), 695-701.

[59] Roughley, PJ. Biology of intervertebral disc aging and degeneration: involvement of the extracellular matrix. *Spine*, 2004, 29(23), 2691.

[60] Bartels, EM; et al. Oxygen and lactate concentrations measured in vivo in the intervertebral discs of patients with scoliosis and back pain. *Spine*, 1998, 23(1), 1-7.

[61] Ishihara, H; Urban, JPG. Effects of low oxygen concentrations and metabolic inhibitors on proteoglycan and protein synthesis rates in the intervertebral disc. *Journal of Orthopaedic Research*, 2005, 17(6), 829-835.

[62] Burke, J; et al. Intervertebral discs which cause low back pain secrete high levels of proinflammatory mediators. Journal of Bone & Joint Surgery, *British Volume*, 2002. 84(2), 196-201.

[63] Kang, JD; et al. Toward a biochemical understanding of human intervertebral disc degeneration and herniation: contributions of nitric oxide, interleukins, prostaglandin E2, and matrix metalloproteinases. *Spine*, 1997, 22(10), 1065-1073.

[64] Hutton, WC; et al. The effect of hydrostatic pressure on intervertebral disc metabolism. *Spine*, 1999, 24(15), 1507.

[65] Lotz, J; et al. Mechanobiology of the intervertebral disc. *Biochemical Society Transactions*, 2002. 30, 853-858.

[66] Lotz, JC; Chin, JR. Intervertebral disc cell death is dependent on the magnitude and duration of spinal loading. *Spine*, 2000, 25(12), 1477-1483.

[67] Brittberg, M. Autologous chondrocyte transplantation. Clinical Orthopaedics and Related Research, 1999, 367, S147-S155.

[68] Minas, T; Chiu, R. Autologous chondrocyte implantation. *The American journal of knee surgery*, 2000, 13(1), 41.

[69] Chevallay, B; Herbage, D. Collagen-based biomaterials as 3D scaffold for cell cultures: applications for tissue engineering and gene therapy. *Medical and Biological Engineering and Computing*, 2000, 38(2), 211-218.

[70] Calderon, L; et al. Type II collagen-hyaluronan hydrogel-a step towards a scaffold for intervertebral disc tissue engineering. 2010.

[71] Li, Z; Zhang, M. Chitosan–alginate as scaffolding material for cartilage tissue engineering. *Journal of Biomedical Materials Research Part A*, 2005, 75(2), 485-493.

[72] Ushida, T; et al. Three-dimensional seeding of chondrocytes encapsulated in collagen gel into PLLA scaffolds. *Cell transplantation*, 2002, 11(5), 489-494.

[73] Chen, G; et al. Tissue engineering of cartilage using a hybrid scaffold of synthetic polymer and collagen. *Tissue Engineering*, 2004, 10(3-4), 323-330.

[74] Moran, JM; Pazzano, D; Bonassar, LJ. Characterization of polylactic acid-polyglycolic acid composites for cartilage tissue engineering. *Tissue engineering*, 2003, 9(1), 63-70.

[75] Freed, L; et al. Neocartilage formation in vitro and in vivo using cells cultured on synthetic biodegradable polymers. *Journal of Biomedical Materials Research*, 1993, 27(1), 11-23.

[76] Nishimoto, S; et al. Effect of chondroitin sulfate and hyaluronic acid on gene expression in a three-dimensional culture of chondrocytes. *Journal of bioscience and bioengineering*, 2005, 100(1), 123-126.

[77] Hermanson, GT. *Bioconjugate techniques*. 1996, Academic press.

[78] Li, Q; et al. Photocrosslinkable polysaccharides based on chondroitin sulfate. *Journal of Biomedical Materials Research*, 2004, 68(1), 28-33.

[79] Li, Q; Wang, D-a; Elisseeff, JH. Heterogeneous-phase reaction of glycidyl methacrylate and chondroitin sulfate: Mechanism of ring-opening-transesterification competition. *Macromolecules*, 2003, 36, 2556-2562.

[80] Strehin, I; et al. A versatile pH sensitive chondroitin sulfate–PEG tissue adhesive and hydrogel. *Biomaterials*, 2010, 31(10), 2788-2797.

[81] Wang, DA; et al. Multifunctional chondroitin sulphate for cartilage tissue–biomaterial integration. *Nature materials*, 2007, 6(5), 385-392.

[82] Sharma, B; et al. Human Cartilage Repair with a Photoreactive Adhesive-Hydrogel Composite. *Science translational medicine*, 2013, 5(167), 167ra6-167ra6.

[83]   Lee, C-T; Huang, C-P; Lee, Y-D. Biomimetic porous scaffolds made from poly (L-lactide)-g-chondroitin sulfate blend with poly (L-lactide) for cartilage tissue engineering. *Biomacromolecules*, 2006, 7(7), 2200-2209.

[84]   Chang, K-Y; et al. Fabrication and characterization of poly (γ-glutamic acid)-graft-chondroitin sulfate/polycaprolactone porous scaffolds for cartilage tissue engineering. *Acta biomaterialia*, 2009, 5(6), 1937-1947.

[85]   Bryant, SJ; et al. Synthesis and characterization of photopolymerized multifunctional hydrogels: water-soluble poly (vinyl alcohol) and chondroitin sulfate macromers for chondrocyte encapsulation. *Macromolecules*, 2004, 37(18), 6726-6733.

[86]   Fan, H; et al. Cartilage regeneration using mesenchymal stem cells and a PLGA–gelatin/chondroitin/hyaluronate hybrid scaffold. *Biomaterials*, 2006, 27(26), 4573-4580.

[87]   Fan, H; et al. TGF-β3 immobilized PLGA-gelatin/chondroitin sulfate/hyaluronic acid hybrid scaffold for cartilage regeneration. *Journal of Biomedical Materials Research Part A*, 2010, 95(4), 982-992.

[88]   Cao, H; Xu, S-Y. EDC/NHS-crosslinked type II collagen-chondroitin sulfate scaffold: characterization and in vitro evaluation. *Journal of Materials Science: Materials in Medicine*, 2008, 19(2), 567-575.

[89]   Ko, C-S; et al. Type II collagen-chondroitin sulfate-hyaluronan scaffold cross-linked by genipin for cartilage tissue engineering. *Journal of bioscience and bioengineering*, 2009, 107(2), 177-182.

[90]   Ko, C; et al. Genipin cross-linking of type II collagen-chondroitin sulfate-hyaluronan scaffold for articular cartilage therapy. *Journal of Medical and Biological Engineering*, 2007, 27(1), 7.

[91]   Zhang, L; et al. Preparation of collagen–chondroitin sulfate–hyaluronic acid hybrid hydrogel scaffolds and cell compatibility in vitro. *Carbohydrate polymers*, 2011, 84(1), 118-125.

[92]   Liang, WH; et al. Concentrated collagen-chondroitin sulfate scaffolds for tissue engineering applications. *Journal of Biomedical Materials Research Part A*, 2010, 94(4), 1050-1060.

[93]   Chang, C-H; et al. Gelatin–chondroitin–hyaluronan tri-copolymer scaffold for cartilage tissue engineering. *Biomaterials*, 2003, 24(26), 4853-4858.

[94]   Yang, SH; et al. An In-vitro Study on Regeneration of Human Nucleus Pulposus by Using Gelatin/Chondroitin-6-Sulfate/Hyaluronan Tri-copolymer Scaffold. *Artificial organs*, 2005, 29(10), 806-814.

[95]   Bernhard, JC; Panitch, A. Synthesis and characterization of an aggrecan mimic. *Acta biomaterialia*, 2012, 8(4), 1543-1550.

[96]   Sharma, S; Panitch, A; Neu, CP. Incorporation of an Aggrecan Mimic Prevents Proteolytic Degradation of Anisotropic Cartilage Analogs. *Acta Biomaterialia*, 2012.

[97]   Sarkar, S. Synthesis and characterization of a chondroitin sulfate based hybrid bio/synthetic biomimetic aggrecan macromolecule., in Biomedical Engineering 2011, Drexel University: Philadelphia, PA.

[98]   Sarkar, S; et al. Terminal-end functionalization of chondroitin sulfate for the synthesis of biomimetic proteoglycans. *Carbohydrate Polymers*, 2012.

In: Chondroitin Sulfate
Editor: Vitor H. Pomin

ISBN: 978-1-62808-490-0
© 2013 Nova Science Publishers, Inc.

Chapter 10

Chondroitin Sulfate Proteoglycan Abnormalities in Schizophrenia

Harry Pantazopoulos[1,2] and Sabina Berretta[1,2,3]
[1]Department of Psychiatry, Harvard Medical School, Boston, MA, US
[2]Translational Neuroscience Laboratory, Mclean Hospital, Belmont, MA, US
[3]Program in Neuroscience, Harvard Medical School, Boston, MA, US

Abstract

Schizophrenia is a chronic psychiatric illness known to affect approximately 1% of the population. Genetic and early life environmental factors conjure to disrupt distinct neuronal and glial populations in several cortical and subcortical brain regions. The resulting clinical symptoms emerge in late adolescence to early adulthood, preceded by a prodromal syndrome. Recent evidence points to a role for chondroitin sulfate proteoglycans (CSPGs) in the pathophysiology of schizophrenia. Our group has shown large increases of CSPG expression in glial cells accompanied by reductions of perineuronal nets (PNNs) in the medial temporal lobe of subjects with schizophrenia. Similar findings in the prefrontal cortex and olfactory epithelium suggest that CSPG abnormalities may be widespread in this disease. Genetic studies reporting associations of polymorphisms for specific CSPG genes, including PTPRZ1, neuroglycan-C and neurocan with schizophrenia, and recent animal studies examining the effects of abnormal CSPG expression or sulfation on brain development and function, lend further support for CSPG abnormalities in this disorder. In this chapter we discuss these findings and their potential relevance to core aspects of the pathophysiology of schizophrenia, such as brain development, myelination and regulation of key neurotransmitter systems including the glutamatergic, GABAergic and dopaminergic systems. We put forth the hypothesis that altered CSPG expression may contribute to a number of critical components of the pathophysiology of schizophrenia, including altered neuronal migration and connectivity, neural circuit plasticity, synaptic regulation, and electrical oscillatory rhythms observed in this disorder.

Introduction

In recent years, significant advances have been made toward our understanding of the pathophysiology of schizophrenia. Although much remains to be done, as a field we have now identified key brain regions, neurotransmitters and cell systems affected in this disorder. Extracellular matrix molecules, and chondroitin sulfate proteoglycans (CSPGs) in particular, have been recently shown to represent novel, and very promising, players in the pathophysiology of schizophrenia. In light of their role in the developing and adult brain, CSPGs bear the potential to link many seemingly unrelated aspects of neuronal and glial disturbances. Here, we provide a brief overview of the clinical and pathophysiological characteristics of this disorder; in this context, we then discuss current evidence for CSPG abnormalities and their potential pathophysiological implications for schizophrenia.

Schizophrenia: an Overview

Schizophrenia is a severe and often disabling psychiatric syndrome, characterized by a complex symptomatology. Positive symptoms, such as hallucinations, delusions, disorganized speech, abnormal psychomotor behavior (agitation, catatonia), are typically accompanied to various degrees by negative symptoms, including restricted affect, avolition, anhedonia and asociality [1]. The clinical onset of schizophrenia typically occurs between 16 to 30 years of age, and is preceded by a prodromal state characterized by social withdrawal, anxiety, irritability, cognitive decline, attention difficulty and unusual thoughts [2-8]. Relapses, increased suicide risk, worsening of positive, cognitive and, particularly, negative symptoms and repeated hospitalizations are observed in the majority of patients over the course of several years. Sustained recovery occurs in approximately 20-35% of people, while the remaining patients show little or no improvement.

Growing evidence supports the view that schizophrenia is a neurodevelopmental disorder, arising from complex genetic vulnerabilities involving large numbers of genes, each with weak effects [9], in combination with environmental factors likely to occur during fetal and early postnatal life. Several candidate vulnerability genes for schizophrenia, including neuregulin [10-12], dysbindin-1, COMT [13-22], and DISC1 [23-30], are known to play a role in brain development, notably neuronal migration through the regulation of cell to cell and cell to matrix interactions [31]. Early exposure to environmental predisposing factors, such as maternal stress and birth complications, contribute to increased vulnerability for schizophrenia. The long-term effects of these factors may be mediated by epigenetic mechanisms, such as histone modification and DNA methylation, both found to be abnormal in schizophrenia [32-45]. Furthermore, the often protracted prodromal period occurs during late postnatal brain development, coinciding with late stage maturation of synaptic connections and axonal myelination. Together with early neurobiological deficits observed in subjects at risk for schizophrenia, this observation suggests a progressive disruption of brain development that may culminate with the clinical onset of the disease [2-8, 46-52].

Postmortem and brain imaging studies have implicated a number of interconnected brain regions in schizophrenia [53-68]. Abnormalities affecting glutamatergic, GABAergic and dopaminergic neurotransmission, as well as distinct neuronal and glial cell types have been detected in several brain regions, including the hippocampus, entorhinal cortex, amygdala, dorsolateral prefrontal cortex, anterior cingulate gyrus and thalamus. Not surprisingly, the functional roles of these brain regions are highly relevant to the symptomatology and functional impairment observed in schizophrenia. The hippocampus is involved in episodic memory storage and context related cognitive processing [69-73]; the entorhinal cortex gates cortical and subcortical inputs to the hippocampus and participates in sensory integration and memory processing [74-77]; the amygdala plays a key role in the attribution of salience/emotional valence, associative learning, anxiety and stress response [78-92]; the dorsolateral prefrontal cortex is involved in working memory and executive cognitive functions [93-98]; components of the thalamus, such as the mediodorsal nucleus, contribute to associative learning and working memory (Jones E.G. The thalamus 2nd edition New York, Cambridge University Press, 2007) [99-103]; the anterior cingulate cortex is involved in the regulation of attention, motivation, and response selection [104-106]. Several neuronal populations within each of these regions are affected in schizophrenia. Distinct populations of inhibitory GABAergic interneurons play a key role in intrinsic information processing and the generation of oscillatory rhythms, which in turn have been found to be altered in schizophrenia [57, 107-120]. Abnormalities affecting glutamate ionotropic and metabotropic receptors have been reported, although a predominant role of NMDA receptors has been long suspected and validated by growing evidence [121-125]. Dopaminergic neurotransmission abnormalities have been detected in the prefrontal cortex, striatum and amygdala [126-130] (Markota et al., manuscript in preparation). More recently, the involvement of glial cells, astrocytes, and oligodendrocytes in particular, in the pathophysiology of schizophrenia has also been reported [131-144]. Astrocytes take an active role in a broad variety of brain functions, including uptake and release of neurotransmitters, integration of synaptic activity and regulation of the blood-brain barrier [145-147]. Oligodendrocytes are the myelinating cells of the CNS. Axon myelination is a key aspect of brain development. It allows fast saltatory nerve conduction and affects axonal transport processes and neuronal functions [148].

In this context, abnormalities affecting extracellular matrix molecules chondroitin sulfate proteoglycans (CSPGs) in schizophrenia represent a novel and unexpected finding in this disorder [149-154]. CSPGs interact with each of the neurotransmitter systems implicated in this disease, and contribute to critical neurodevelopmental functions [155-159]. During early brain developmental stages, CSPGs play critical roles in neuronal migration and axonal guidance [155-159]. Their regulation of neural functions continues during postnatal development and adult life. During late postnatal development, CSPGs contribute to the maturation of perineuronal nets (PNNs), of which they are major components (**Figure 1**). PNNs are specialized extracellular matrix aggregates that envelop subpopulations of neurons and regulate neuronal plasticity, synaptic formation and electrophysiological maturation [160-162]. Interestingly, in a rodent model, PTPRZ1 overexpression resulted in deficits in the GABAergic, glutamatergic, and dopaminergic neurotransmitter systems, as well as delayed maturation of oligodendrocytes and behavioral deficits associated with schizophrenia [163]. We propose that a disruption of CSPG expression may represent a critical factor in the pathophysiology of this disorder, linking together a variety of key neural abnormalities. In this chapter, we discuss current evidence for the involvement of CSPGs in neurodevelopmental aspects of the pathophysiology of schizophrenia, and their potential impact on distinct neural cell populations and neurotransmitter systems.

1. Evidence for CSPG Abnormalities in Schizophrenia

Rapidly mounting evidence points to abnormal CSPG expression in schizophrenia. Recent findings from our group have shown marked increases of glial cells expressing CSPGs (419 to 1560 percent) in the amygdala and superficial layers of the entorhinal cortex of subjects with schizophrenia [153] (**Figure 2**). In healthy human subjects, the vast majority of these cells were found to express the astrocytic marker glial fibrillary acidic protein (GFAP), indicating that they correspond to a subpopulation of astrocytes [164]. Numbers of GFAP immunoreactive astrocytes were not increased in subjects with schizophrenia, a finding consistent with previous reports showing that astrocytosis is not present in this disorder [165-168]. Increases of CSPG-positive glial cells were accompanied by significant reductions of CSPG-positive PNNs in the lateral nucleus of the amygdala and in superficial layers of the lateral entorhinal cortex [153]. Therefore, increased CSPG expression in glial cells was accompanied by a more spatially segregated PNN reduction. CSPG-positive glial cell increases and PNN decreases did not correlate with duration of illness and they were not affected by other variables including age, gender, cause of death and treatment with antipsychotic drugs [153]. Therefore, these changes may be present early on in the disease and reflect some of the core aspects of its pathophysiology.

PNN decreases were also found in layers 3 through 5 of the prefrontal cortex [169] and increases of CSPG glia have been reported in layers 2 through 4 of this region in subjects with schizophrenia [152]. Thus, CSPG expression abnormalities in schizophrenia may be widespread, shared by several cortical and subcortical brain regions. Notably, PNNs in the prefrontal cortex of human subjects were shown to continue maturing until late adolescence [169], potentially coinciding with the age of onset of schizophrenia.

CSPG abnormalities were also recently detected in the olfactory epithelium (Pantazopoulos et al., submitted for publication). The olfactory epithelium, located in the nasal cavity, is unique in that neuronal differentiation, migration and axon outgrowth occur robustly throughout life, and are at least in part regulated by CSPGs [170]. Abnormal expression of these molecules observed in postmortem olfactory epithelium of subjects with schizophrenia are consistent with neuronal lineage abnormalities observed in the same subject cohort [171], and suggest that CSPGs may represent a contributing factor. Notably, schizophrenic subjects and first-degree relatives experience deficits in olfactory identification [172-177], possibly due to anomalous connections between olfactory sensory neurons in the olfactory epithelium to the olfactory bulb. Anomalous CSPG expression in the olfactory epithelium may contribute to altered maturation of olfactory sensory neurons and their odor-specific connectivity with the olfactory bulb, ultimately affecting olfactory identification.

Finally, genetic studies have reported associations of polymorphisms for specific CSPG genes including PTPRZ1 [151], neuroglycan-C [150] and neurocan [149] with schizophrenia, suggesting that abnormal CSPG expression may be due, at least in part, to genetic factors. It is worth noting that other extracellular matrix molecules, including semaphorin 3a, and reelin [178-182], have also been found to be affected in schizophrenia, suggesting a broader involvement of the extracellular matrix in this disorder.

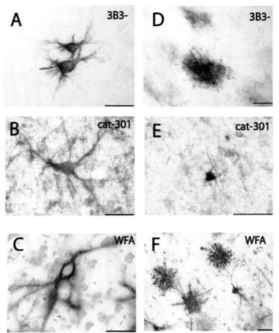

Photomicrographs of PNNs (A-C) and glial cells (D-F) in the normal human amygdala. PNNs and glia
cells in A and D, respectively, were detected using antibodies raised against CS isomers containing
penultimate 6-sulphated N-Acetyl-galactosamine (3B3; gift from Dr. B. Caterson, Cardiff
University, U.K.), while antibodies raised against the aggrecan core protein (cat-301) were using in
B and E. CSPGs can also be detected using the lectin *wisteria floribunda agglutinin* (WFA), as
shown by PNNs and glial cells depicted in C and F, respectively. Note the difference in size and
labeling distribution of CSPG-positive glial cells in D, E, and F, which may reflect different
intracellular distribution or expression in distinct cell types. Scale bars = 50 μm.

Figure 1. CSPG-positive PNNs and glial cells in the normal human amygdala.

2. Neurodevelopmental Abnormalities in Schizophrenia: Potential Role of CSPG Dysregulation

Pathological evidence for the neurodevelopmental nature of schizophrenia is based in
great part on cytoarchitectonic anomalies and heterotopic neuron displacement strongly
suggestive of disrupted neuronal migration, reported in several brain regions [183-186, 193-
199]. In the entorhinal cortex of subjects with schizophrenia, cytoarchitectonic abnormalities
of the superficial layers include invaginations of the surface, decreased neuron density and
poorly formed neuronal clusters in layer II with putative displacement of these neurons
deeper into layer III [184, 185]. Notably, increases of CSPG-positive glial cells were most
pronounced in layer II of the entorhinal cortex of schizophrenic subjects [153], largely
overlapping with layer II cell clusters. We put forth that enduring CSPG expression
abnormalities in the superficial layers of the entorhinal cortex may contribute to a disruption
of neuronal migration and incorrect cell cluster formation in schizophrenia (Figure 3).

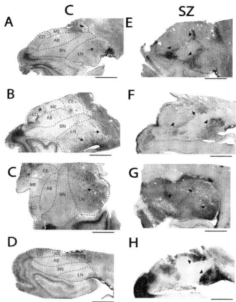

High resolution photocomposites depicting sections from the amygdala of four pairs of control (A-D) and schizophrenic subjects (E-H). Sections were stained with the lectin WFA to label CSPGs and counterstained with methyl green. Areas with prevalent CSPG-positive PNN densities are marked with arrows, while those with prevalent CSPG-positive glial cell densities are marked with arrow heads. In subjects with schizophrenia, CSPG-positive glial cells were markedly increased, while CSPG-positive glial cells were decreased. This is reflected by an overall increase of CSPG labeling in subjects with schizophrenia (E-H) with respect to controls, and a shift from PNN to glial CSPG labeling. *Abbreviations:* AB, accessory basal nucleus; BN, basal nucleus; C, control subjects; CE, central nucleus; CO, cortical nucleus; LN, lateral nucleus; ME, medial nucleus; SZ, subjects with schizophrenia. Scale bar = 4 mm.

Figure 2. CSPG expression abnormalities in the amygdala of subjects with schizophrenia.

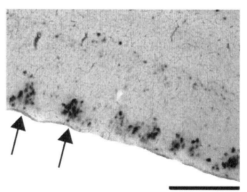

Photomicrograph showing the superficial layers of the entorhinal cortex in a section stained with WFA from a subject with schizophrenia. Marked increases in the number of CSPG expressing glial cells were observed in clusters within the superficial layer of the entorhinal cortex, corresponding to layer 2 cell islands, known to project to the hippocampus [159]. Cytoarchitectonic abnormalities in this layer have been consistently reported in subjects with schizophrenia [173], suggesting that a disruption of CSPG expression in glial cells in this layer may impact on cell migration in the entorhinal cortex of subjects with schizophrenia. Scale bar, 1 mm.

Figure 3. Increases of CSPG-positive glial cells in the superficial layers of the entorhinal cortex in subjects with schizophrenia.

Heterotopic neuron displacement, and more specifically increase of interstitial white matter neurons, was also detected in the frontal, parietal and temporal cortical lobes, and interpreted as a failure of these neurons to migrate into the cortical grey matter [187-192]. In support of this interpretation, an increase of interneurons expressing somatostatin in the superficial white matter was accompanied by reduced somatostatin mRNA in the gray matter [193]. Notably, in the superior temporal gyrus, an increase of interstitial white matter neurons was accompanied by a reduction of neurons expressing reelin mRNA in layer I and superficial white matter [194], adding further support for the hypothesis that abnormal expression of extracellular matrix molecules, possibly including CSPGs, may contribute to altered neuronal migration in schizophrenia. During early brain developmental stages, CSPGs containing oversulfated CS chains contribute to the guidance of neurons and axons to their proper locations [155, 156]. Chondroitin-4 sulfated (CS-4) CSPGs interact with the secreted membrane protein semaphorin 3a to guide the migration of cortical interneurons originating from the ganglionic eminence [195]. Semaphorin 3a has reported to be increased in schizophrenia [178]. This increase was correlated with decreases of reelin and synaptic markers, indicating that increased CSPGs and semaphorin 3a, may contribute to altered neuronal migration in schizophrenia.

Further evidence for the neurodevelopmental nature of this disorder originates from imaging and postmortem findings consistent with altered connectivity, or 'mis-wiring', in schizophrenia. Some of these studies are discussed below, in the context of dopaminergic innervation and myelination abnormalities. It is worth to mention here that findings indicating a disruption of axon fasciculation in the entorhinal cortex [196] strongly suggest a disruption of axonal guidance, another key CSPG function [156, 197-209], and overlap in distribution with CSPG-positive glia and PNN abnormalities in schizophrenia [153].

3. Neurotransmitter System Abnormalities in Schizophrenia: Potential Role of CSPG Dysregulation

3.1. GABAergic and Glutamatergic Neurotransmission

Findings showing the involvement of inhibitory, GABAergic, interneurons are among of the most solid in schizophrenia. Reduction of glutamic acid decarboxylase (GAD), the synthesizing enzyme of GABA, decreased numbers of GABAergic interneurons, and in particular interneurons expressing the calcium binding protein parvalbumin (PVB), and decreased PVB terminals have been reported in several brain regions [40, 57, 58, 66, 179, 210-215]. PVB-positive neurons are a subpopulation of GABAergic neurons with distinct fast-firing properties [216-220]. They form dense axo-somatic contacts onto projection neurons [221, 222], and thus have the ability to powerfully inhibit information outflow from the regions affected [223]. In addition, PVB-positive neurons have been shown to generate gamma-oscillatory rhythms, synchronized neural activity thought to provide the temporal structure for learning and information integration and to be disrupted in schizophrenia [107, 111, 113, 216, 224, 117-120]. Altered gamma oscillations in this disorder have been postulated to contribute to cognitive and memory deficits and, speculatively, to disturb developmental synaptic reorganization processes know to occur during late adolescence [120, 225]. PVB-positive neurons are predominantly associated with PNNs, which contribute to multiple aspects of neuronal activity. First, the formation of PNNs around PVB-positive neurons during late postnatal life represents a key aspect of the maturation of these neurons [162, 226-233]. Increased expression levels of CSPGs, such as aggrecan, coincide with the maturation of electrophysiological properties of neurons [160], while degradation of PNNs by ChABC results in reduced inhibition of excitatory pyramidal cells in the hippocampus [234]. PNN maturation around PVB-positive neurons closes developmental critical periods, establishing an adult, typically restricted, form of plasticity [161, 235, 236]. In particular, in the amygdala, where PNNs were found to be markedly decreased in schizophrenia, PNN maturation contributes to the transition between juvenile and adult forms of emotion-related plasticity, as exemplified by the effects of CSPG digestion on the resilience of fear memory in a rodent model. Notably, fear extinction and context-dependent recall were found to be disrupted in subjects with schizophrenia in conjunction with anomalous amygdala activation [237, 238]. Second, PNNs are postulated to help maintain the ionic homeostasis necessary to support PVB-positive neurons' distinct fast-firing properties [229, 234, 239-241], and to control the availability of glutamatergic ionic receptors to the postsynaptic membrane specialization and the composition of the NMDA receptor subunits, thus powerfully controlling the excitatory synapse maturation and target neuron responsivity to glutamate neurotransmission [242, 243]. In turn, PNN formation is an activity-dependent process [236, 244-246]. Decreased NMDA receptors may therefore contribute to decreases of PNNs in schizophrenia [211, 247-253]. Third, PNNs have been shown to regulate the sprouting and pruning of synapses, thus controlling powerful mechanisms mediating plasticity. Notably, reductions of synaptic spines and abnormal expression of presynaptic proteins represents one of the most solid findings in schizophrenia [254-264]. Together, these findings raise the possibility that loss of, or failure to develop, PNNs in subjects with schizophrenia may contribute to interneuron-related dysfunction, including anomalous electrophysiological and neurochemical maturation and responsivity to glutamatergic inputs. In turn, these changes are likely to contribute to abnormal oscillatory rhythms observed in this disorder [117-120].

3.2. Dopaminergic System

Dopamine was one of the first neurotransmitters to be implicated in the pathogenesis of schizophrenia. Initial findings on reserpine, and observations that dopamine D2 receptors are targeted by antipsychotics and symptoms of schizophrenia are improved by dopamine antagonists and exacerbated by dopamine releasing agents, led to the hypothesis that dopaminergic transmission may be altered in schizophrenia [265-272]. Recent views postulate that dopaminergic transmission may be reduced in the prefrontal cortex, while enhanced in the ventral striatum/nucleus accumbens [129, 126-128, 130]. A similar enhancement in the amygdala is supported by recent findings from our group (Markota et al., manuscript in preparation). Consistent with these findings, higher levels of dopamine have been reported in the amygdala, caudate nucleus, and nucleus accumbens in subjects with schizophrenia, [128-130, 273]. While a state of hypodopaminergia in the prefrontal cortex may contribute to impairment of working memory and cognitive functions observed in schizophrenia, enhanced dopaminergic transmission in the ventral striatum and amygdala has been postulated to disrupt salience attribution and error prediction mechanisms, speculatively contributing to psychotic symptoms [274-279].

CSPG abnormalities may contribute, and/or interact with, dopaminergic abnormalities in several ways. During development, CSPGs have been shown to promote neurite outgrowth of dopaminergic neurons [280] and to guide dopaminergic axons to their target regions [281-284]. Altered CSPG expression in developmental stages may result in abnormal development of dopaminergic innervation in the brain of subjects with schizophrenia. Furthermore, it is conceivable that altered CSPG expression in the extracellular matrix may impact on neurotransmitter diffusibility in the extracellular space [285]. In subjects with schizophrenia, volume diffusion of excess dopamine overflowing from the synaptic space in the striatum and amygdala, postulated on the basis of evidence for hyperdopaminergia in these regions [128-130, 273], may be impacted by extracellular matrix abnormalities which may affect the likelihood of reaching poorly regulated extrasynaptic dopamine D2 receptors [286]. It is also worth noting that PVB-positive neurons represent one of the main targets of dopaminergic innervation in the amygdala [287]. Loss of PNNs in schizophrenia is predicted to profoundly affect their synaptic inputs, presumably including dopaminergic contacts. Finally, it has been reported that degradation of PNNs in the rodent hippocampus results in increased activity of ventral tegmental area dopaminergic neurons [234]. Thus, CSPGs disruption may have an indirect effect on dopaminergic transmission in schizophrenia, affecting intrinsic hippocampal activity and ultimately its impact on dopaminergic neurons in the ventral tegmental area [234].

4. Glial Cell Dysfunction in Schizophrenia: Potential Contributions of CSPGs

4.1. Oligodendrocytes

Myelin abnormalities have been consistently reported in schizophrenia. Together, altered expression of key myelin components such as sphingomyelin, galactocerebrosides, myelin-associated glycoprotein, decreased numbers of oligodendrocytes, altered expression of oligodendrocyte-related genes, reduction of myelin compactness and increased density of concentric lamellar bodies, point to a significant disruption of myelination in this disorder [288-305]. Decreased expression of multiple genes associated with the integrity of the nodes of Ranvier has been reported in subjects with schizophrenia [306, 307]. Finally, typical and atypical antipsychotic drugs, including haloperidol, quetiapine, olanzapine and clozapine, have been shown to promote proliferation of oligodendrocyte progenitor cells and possibly contribute to re-myelination [308-313].

We postulate that a disruption of CSPG expression in schizophrenia may impact on several aspect of the myelination process. Brevican expression in immature oligodendrocytes postnatally coincides with the extension of membrane processes ensheathing axon fibers [314]. Together with tenascin-R and phosphacan, brevican is present at the nodes of Ranvier of large diameter myelinated axons in the adult CNS, where it is thought to control the ECM composition [315]. The CSPG NG2 is expressed in oligodendrocyte progenitor cells. Although these cells are not directly involved in myelination, their number increases during re-myelination, possibly in response to cytokines and growth factors [316-328]. A disruption of CSPG expression, perhaps including brevican and NG2, may contribute to myelin defects reported in schizophrenia.

4.2. Astrocytes

Astrocytes perform a wide range of functions in the developing and adult brain, including modulation of neuronal maturation and synaptogenesis, regulation of the blood-brain barrier, ion and neurotransmitter buffering, release of neurotransmitters and growth factors and response to brain injury [147, 329]. Importantly, interactions between astrocytes and the extracellular matrix are at the core of several of these functions. Expression of the CSPGs brevican, aggrecan and phosphacan has been shown to regulate glial cell differentiation [330-333]. Conversely, astrocytes are considered to be the organizers of the brain extracellular matrix, and PNNs in particular [334]. More specifically, converging lines of evidence show that astrocyte-derived tenascins and CSPGs play a key role in regulating PNN formation and maintenance as well as fundamental synaptic functions [334].

While it is widely accepted that reactive astrocytosis is not present in schizophrenia [153, 165-168, 335], growing evidence indicates that abnormal astrocyte functions may contribute to the pathophysiology of this disorder. Altered expression and N-glycosylation of the glutamate transporters EAAT1 and EAAT2, expressed by astrocytes, has been reported in schizophrenia [135-137, 139, 336]. Increased levels of the calcium binding protein S100beta have been detected in the blood serum and cerebral spinal fluid of subjects with this disorder [134, 337-342]. S100beta, expressed primarily by astrocytes and some NG2 cells [343, 344], is involved in the proliferation and differentiation, migration, and maturation of astrocytes [338, 345-347]. Marked increases of CSPG positive glial cells in the amygdala and entorhinal cortex of subjects with schizophrenia [153] are consistent with a prominent glial pathology in schizophrenia and point to abnormalities of astrocyte-derived CSPGs as a contributing factor to key aspects of the pathophysiology of this disease, as discussed above.

Conclusion

In summary, schizophrenia is a neurodevelopmental disorder with a complex neuropathology involving several main neurotransmitter systems, neural cell populations and brain regions. CSPGs interact with each of these components and play critical roles in early and late stages of brain development, including neuronal migration, axon guidance, synapse maturation, and myelination, as well as adult functions, such as regulation of neuronal firing properties, regulation of plasticity and NMDA receptor availability at the postsynaptic space. Together, marked abnormalities affecting both CSPG-positive PNNs and glial cells, their distribution patterns in the brain, indirect evidence that these abnormalities may be inherent to the disease, and the relevance that CSPG functions bear to the pathophysiology of this disorder, raise the possibility that their disregulation may impact on developmental and adult brain functions known to be disrupted in schizophrenia.

Acknowledgment

The authors would like to thank Dr. Bruce Caterson, Ph.D. from the University of Cardiff, U.K. for producing and providing the 3B3 antibody, and for technical advice.

References

[1]   Washington D.C. Diagnostic and Statistical Manual of Mental Disorders 2000.

[2]   Kane, JM; Krystal, J; Correll, CU. Treatment models and designs for intervention research during the psychotic prodrome. *Schizophr Bull.*, 2003; 29(4), 747-56. PubMed PMID: 14989412. Epub 2004/03/03. eng.

[3]   Schultze-Lutter, F; Ruhrmann, S; Hoyer, C; Klosterkotter, J; Leweke, FM. The initial prodrome of schizophrenia: different duration, different underlying deficits? *Comprehensive psychiatry.*, 2007 Sep-Oct; 48(5), 479-88. PubMed PMID: 17707258. Epub 2007/08/21. eng.

[4]   Olsen, KA; Rosenbaum, B. Prospective investigations of the prodromal state of schizophrenia: review of studies. *Acta psychiatrica Scandinavica.*, 2006 Apr; 113(4), 247-72. PubMed PMID: 16638070. Epub 2006/04/28. eng.

[5]   Ruhrmann, S; Schultze-Lutter, F; Klosterkotter, J. Early detection and intervention in the initial prodromal phase of schizophrenia. *Pharmacopsychiatry.*, 2003 Nov; 36 Suppl 3:S162-7. PubMed PMID: 14677074. Epub 2003/12/17. eng.

[6]   Bechdolf, A; Schultze-Lutter, F; Klosterkotter, J. Self-experienced vulnerability, prodromal symptoms and coping strategies preceding schizophrenic and depressive relapses. *Eur Psychiatry.*, 2002 Nov; 17(7), 384-93. PubMed PMID: 12547304. Epub 2003/01/28. eng.

[7]   Preda, A; Miller, TJ; Rosen, JL; Somjee, L; McGlashan, TH; Woods, SW. Treatment histories of patients with a syndrome putatively prodromal to schizophrenia. *Psychiatr Serv.*, 2002 Mar; 53(3), 342-4. PubMed PMID: 11875232. Epub 2002/03/05. eng.

[8]   Klosterkotter, J; Hellmich, M; Steinmeyer, EM; Schultze-Lutter, F. Diagnosing schizophrenia in the initial prodromal phase. *Arch Gen Psychiatry.*, 2001 Feb; 58(2), 158-64. PubMed PMID: 11177117. Epub 2001/02/15. eng.

[9]   Purcell, SM; Wray, NR; Stone, JL; Visscher, PM; O'Donovan, MC; Sullivan, PF; et al. Common polygenic variation contributes to risk of schizophrenia and bipolar disorder. *Nature.*, 2009 Aug 6; 460(7256), 748-52. PubMed PMID: 19571811. Epub 2009/07/03. eng.

[10]   Yang, JZ; Si, TM; Ruan, Y; Ling, YS; Han, YH; Wang, XL; et al. Association study of neuregulin 1 gene with schizophrenia. *Mol Psychiatry.*, 2003 Jul; 8(7), 706-9. PubMed PMID: 12874607. Epub 2003/07/23. eng.

[11]   Stefansson, H; Sarginson, J; Kong, A; Yates, P; Steinthorsdottir, V; Gudfinnsson, E; et al. Association of neuregulin 1 with schizophrenia confirmed in a Scottish population. *Am J Hum Genet.*, 2003 Jan; 72(1), 83-7. PubMed PMID: 12478479. Pubmed Central PMCID: 420015. Epub 2002/12/13. eng.

[12]   Stefansson, H; Sigurdsson, E; Steinthorsdottir, V; Bjornsdottir, S; Sigmundsson, T; Ghosh, S; et al. Neuregulin 1 and susceptibility to schizophrenia. *Am J Hum Genet.*

2002 Oct; 71(4), 877-92. PubMed PMID: 12145742. Pubmed Central PMCID: 378543. Epub 2002/07/30. eng.

[13] DeRosse, P; Funke, B; Burdick, KE; Lencz, T; Ekholm, JM; Kane, JM; et al. Dysbindin genotype and negative symptoms in schizophrenia. *Am J Psychiatry.*, 2006 Mar; 163(3), 532-4. PubMed PMID: 16513878. Epub 2006/03/04. eng.

[14] Schwab, SG; Knapp, M; Mondabon, S; Hallmayer, J; Borrmann-Hassenbach, M; Albus, M; et al. Support for association of schizophrenia with genetic variation in the 6p22.3 gene, dysbindin, in sib-pair families with linkage and in an additional sample of triad families. *Am J Hum Genet.* 2003 Jan; 72(1), 185-90. PubMed PMID: 12474144. Pubmed Central PMCID: 378624. Epub 2002/12/11. eng.

[15] Straub, RE; Jiang, Y; MacLean, CJ; Ma, Y; Webb, BT; Myakishev, MV; et al. Genetic variation in the 6p22.3 gene DTNBP1, the human ortholog of the mouse dysbindin gene, is associated with schizophrenia. *Am J Hum Genet.*, 2002 Aug; 71(2), 337-48. PubMed PMID: 12098102. Pubmed Central PMCID: 379166. Epub 2002/07/05. eng.

[16] Allen, NC; Bagade, S; McQueen, MB; Ioannidis, JP; Kavvoura, FK; Khoury, MJ; et al. Systematic meta-analyses and field synopsis of genetic association studies in schizophrenia: the SzGene database. *Nat Genet.* 2008 Jul; 40(7), 827-34. PubMed PMID: 18583979. Epub 2008/06/28. eng.

[17] Paterlini, M; Zakharenko, SS; Lai, WS; Qin, J; Zhang, H; Mukai, J; et al. Transcriptional and behavioral interaction between 22q11.2 orthologs modulates schizophrenia-related phenotypes in mice. *Nat Neurosci.* 2005 Nov; 8(11), 1586-94. PubMed PMID: 16234811. Epub 2005/10/20. eng.

[18] Glatt, SJ; Faraone, SV; Tsuang, MT. Association between a functional catechol O-methyltransferase gene polymorphism and schizophrenia: meta-analysis of case-control and family-based studies. *Am J Psychiatry.* 2003 Mar; 160(3), 469-76. PubMed PMID: 12611827. Epub 2003/03/04. eng.

[19] Fan, JB; Chen, WY; Tang, JX; Li, S; Gu, NF; Feng, GY; et al. Family-based association studies of COMT gene polymorphisms and schizophrenia in the Chinese population. *Mol Psychiatry.*, 2002; 7(5), 446-7. PubMed PMID: 12082558. Epub 2002/06/26. eng.

[20] Herken, H; Erdal, ME. Catechol-O-methyltransferase gene polymorphism in schizophrenia: evidence for association between symptomatology and prognosis. *Psychiatr Genet.*, 2001 Jun; 11(2), 105-9. PubMed PMID: 11525417. Epub 2001/08/30. eng.

[21] Kotler, M; Barak, P; Cohen, H; Averbuch, IE; Grinshpoon, A; Gritsenko, I; et al. Homicidal behavior in schizophrenia associated with a genetic polymorphism determining low catechol O-methyltransferase (COMT) activity. *American journal of medical genetics.*, 1999 Dec 15; 88(6), 628-33. PubMed PMID: 10581481. Epub 1999/12/03. eng.

[22] Lachman, HM; Morrow, B; Shprintzen, R; Veit, S; Parsia, SS; Faedda, G; et al. Association of codon 108/158 catechol-O-methyltransferase gene polymorphism with the psychiatric manifestations of velo-cardio-facial syndrome. *American journal of medical genetics.*, 1996 Sep 20; 67(5), 468-72. PubMed PMID: 8886163. Epub 1996/09/20. eng.

[23] Millar, JK; Wilson-Annan, JC; Anderson, S; Christie, S; Taylor, MS; Semple, CA; et al. Disruption of two novel genes by a translocation co-segregating with schizophrenia.

Hum Mol Genet., 2000 May 22; 9(9), 1415-23. PubMed PMID: 10814723. Epub 2000/05/18. eng.

[24] Miyoshi, K; Honda, A; Baba, K; Taniguchi, M; Oono, K; Fujita, T; et al. Disrupted-In-Schizophrenia 1, a candidate gene for schizophrenia, participates in neurite outgrowth. *Mol Psychiatry.*, 2003 Jul; 8(7), 685-94. PubMed PMID: 12874605. Epub 2003/07/23. eng.

[25] Callicott, JH; Straub, RE; Pezawas, L; Egan, MF; Mattay, VS; Hariri, AR; et al. Variation in DISC1 affects hippocampal structure and function and increases risk for schizophrenia. *Proc Natl Acad Sci U S A.*, 2005 Jun 14; 102(24), 8627-32. PubMed PMID: 15939883. Pubmed Central PMCID: 1143583. Epub 2005/06/09. eng.

[26] Millar, JK; James, R; Christie, S; Porteous, DJ. Disrupted in schizophrenia 1 (DISC1), subcellular targeting and induction of ring mitochondria. *Mol Cell Neurosci.* 2005 Dec; 30(4), 477-84. PubMed PMID: 16209927. Epub 2005/10/08. eng.

[27] Hamshere, ML; Bennett, P; Williams, N; Segurado, R; Cardno, A; Norton, N; et al. Genomewide linkage scan in schizoaffective disorder: significant evidence for linkage at 1q42 close to DISC1, and suggestive evidence at 22q11 and 19p13. *Arch Gen Psychiatry.*, 2005 Oct; 62(10), 1081-8. PubMed PMID: 16203953. Epub 2005/10/06. eng.

[28] Weinberger, DR. Genetic mechanisms of psychosis: in vivo and postmortem genomics. *Clinical therapeutics.*, 2005; 27 Suppl A:S8-15. PubMed PMID: 16198200. Epub 2005/10/04. eng.

[29] Hennah, W; Tuulio-Henriksson, A; Paunio, T; Ekelund, J; Varilo, T; Partonen, T; et al. A haplotype within the DISC1 gene is associated with visual memory functions in families with a high density of schizophrenia. *Mol Psychiatry.*, 2005 Dec; 10(12), 1097-103. PubMed PMID: 16103888. Epub 2005/08/17. eng.

[30] Niwa, M; Kamiya, A; Murai, R; Kubo, K; Gruber, AJ; Tomita, K; et al. Knockdown of DISC1 by in utero gene transfer disturbs postnatal dopaminergic maturation in the frontal cortex and leads to adult behavioral deficits. *Neuron.*, 2010 Feb 25; 65(4), 480-9. PubMed PMID: 20188653. Pubmed Central PMCID: 3084528. Epub 2010/03/02. eng.

[31] Hattori, T; Shimizu, S; Koyama, Y; Yamada, K; Kuwahara, R; Kumamoto, N; et al. DISC1 regulates cell-cell adhesion, cell-matrix adhesion and neurite outgrowth. *Mol Psychiatry.*, 2010 Aug; 15(8), 778, 98-809. PubMed PMID: 20479754. Epub 2010/05/19. eng.

[32] Gebicke-Haerter, PJ. Epigenetics of schizophrenia. *Pharmacopsychiatry.*, 2012 May; 45 Suppl 1, S42-8. PubMed PMID: 22565234. Epub 2012/05/18. eng.

[33] Chen, Y; Zhang, J; Zhang, L; Shen, Y; Xu, Q. Effects of MAOA promoter methylation on susceptibility to paranoid schizophrenia. *Human genetics.*, 2012 Jul; 131(7), 1081-7. PubMed PMID: 22198720. Epub 2011/12/27. eng.

[34] Tamura, Y; Kunugi, H; Ohashi, J; Hohjoh, H. Epigenetic aberration of the human REELIN gene in psychiatric disorders. *Mol Psychiatry.*, 2007 Jun; 12(6), 519, 93-600. PubMed PMID: 17310238. Epub 2007/02/21. eng.

[35] Guidotti, A; Ruzicka, W; Grayson, DR; Veldic, M; Pinna, G; Davis, JM; et al. S-adenosyl methionine and DNA methyltransferase-1 mRNA overexpression in psychosis. *Neuroreport.*, 2007 Jan 8; 18(1), 57-60. PubMed PMID: 17259861. Epub 2007/01/30. eng.

[36] Grayson, DR; Jia, X; Chen, Y; Sharma, RP; Mitchell, CP; Guidotti, A; et al. Reelin promoter hypermethylation in schizophrenia. *Proc Natl Acad Sci U S A.*, 2005 Jun 28; 102(26), 9341-6. PubMed PMID: 15961543. Pubmed Central PMCID: 1166626. Epub 2005/06/18. eng.

[37] Veldic, M; Caruncho, HJ; Liu, WS; Davis, J; Satta, R; Grayson, DR; et al. DNA-methyltransferase 1 mRNA is selectively overexpressed in telencephalic GABAergic interneurons of schizophrenia brains. *Proc Natl Acad Sci U S A.*, 2004 Jan 6; 101(1), 348-53. PubMed PMID: 14684836. Pubmed Central PMCID: 314188. Epub 2003/12/20. eng.

[38] Houston, I; Peter, CJ; Mitchell, A; Straubhaar, J; Rogaev, E; Akbarian, S. Epigenetics in the human brain. *Neuropsychopharmacology.*, 2013 Jan; 38(1), 183-97. PubMed PMID: 22643929. Pubmed Central PMCID: 3521991. Epub 2012/05/31. eng.

[39] Connor, CM; Akbarian, S. DNA methylation changes in schizophrenia and bipolar disorder. *Epigenetics.*, 2008 Mar-Apr; 3(2), 55-8. PubMed PMID: 18398310. Epub 2008/04/10. eng.

[40] Huang, HS; Akbarian, S. GAD1 mRNA expression and DNA methylation in prefrontal cortex of subjects with schizophrenia. *PLoS One.*, 2007; 2(8), e809. PubMed PMID: 17726539. Pubmed Central PMCID: 1950080. Epub 2007/08/30. eng.

[41] Akbarian, S; Ruehl, MG; Bliven, E; Luiz, LA; Peranelli, AC; Baker, SP; et al. Chromatin alterations associated with down-regulated metabolic gene expression in the prefrontal cortex of subjects with schizophrenia. *Arch Gen Psychiatry.*, 2005 Aug; 62(8), 829-40. PubMed PMID: 16061760.

[42] Stadler, F; Kolb, G; Rubusch, L; Baker, SP; Jones, EG; Akbarian, S. Histone methylation at gene promoters is associated with developmental regulation and region-specific expression of ionotropic and metabotropic glutamate receptors in human brain. *J Neurochem.*, 2005 Jul; 94(2), 324-36. PubMed PMID: 15998284.

[43] Kurita, M; Holloway, T; Garcia-Bea, A; Kozlenkov, A; Friedman, AK; Moreno, JL; et al. HDAC2 regulates atypical antipsychotic responses through the modulation of mGlu2 promoter activity. *Nat Neurosci.*, 2012 Sep; 15(9), 1245-54. PubMed PMID: 22864611. Pubmed Central PMCID: 3431440. Epub 2012/08/07. eng.

[44] Tang, B; Dean, B; Thomas, EA. Disease- and age-related changes in histone acetylation at gene promoters in psychiatric disorders. *Transl Psychiatry.*, 2011; 1:e64. PubMed PMID: 22832356. Pubmed Central PMCID: 3305989. Epub 2011/01/01. eng.

[45] Kundakovic, M; Chen, Y; Guidotti, A; Grayson, DR. The reelin and GAD67 promoters are activated by epigenetic drugs that facilitate the disruption of local repressor complexes. *Mol Pharmacol.*, 2009 Feb; 75(2), 342-54. PubMed PMID: 19029285. Pubmed Central PMCID: 2684898. Epub 2008/11/26. eng.

[46] Jessen, F; Scherk, H; Traber, F; Theyson, S; Berning, J; Tepest, R; et al. Proton magnetic resonance spectroscopy in subjects at risk for schizophrenia. *Schizophr Res.*, 2006 Oct; 87(1-3), 81-8. PubMed PMID: 16842971. Epub 2006/07/18. eng.

[47] Cannon, TD. Clinical and genetic high-risk strategies in understanding vulnerability to psychosis. *Schizophr Res.*, 2005 Nov 1; 79(1), 35-44. PubMed PMID: 16054805. Epub 2005/08/02. eng.

[48] Huang, JT; Leweke, FM; Tsang, TM; Koethe, D; Kranaster, L; Gerth, CW; et al. CSF metabolic and proteomic profiles in patients prodromal for psychosis. *PLoS One.*, 2007;

2(8), e756. PubMed PMID: 17712404. Pubmed Central PMCID: 1942084. Epub 2007/08/23. eng.

[49] Gudlowski, Y; Ozgurdal, S; Witthaus, H; Gallinat, J; Hauser, M; Winter, C; et al. Serotonergic dysfunction in the prodromal, first-episode and chronic course of schizophrenia as assessed by the loudness dependence of auditory evoked activity. *Schizophr Res.*, 2009 Apr; 109(1-3), 141-7. PubMed PMID: 19268544. Epub 2009/03/10. eng.

[50] Stone, JM; Day, F; Tsagaraki, H; Valli, I; McLean, MA; Lythgoe, DJ; et al. Glutamate dysfunction in people with prodromal symptoms of psychosis: relationship to gray matter volume. *Biol Psychiatry.*, 2009 Sep 15; 66(6), 533-9. PubMed PMID: 19559402. Epub 2009/06/30. eng.

[51] Fusar-Poli, P; Howes, OD; Allen, P; Broome, M; Valli, I; Asselin, MC; et al. Abnormal frontostriatal interactions in people with prodromal signs of psychosis: a multimodal imaging study. *Arch Gen Psychiatry.*, 2010 Jul; 67(7), 683-91. PubMed PMID: 20603449. Epub 2010/07/07. eng.

[52] Witthaus, H; Mendes, U; Brune, M; Ozgurdal, S; Bohner, G; Gudlowski, Y; et al. Hippocampal subdivision and amygdalar volumes in patients in an at-risk mental state for schizophrenia. *J Psychiatry Neurosci.*, 2010 Jan; 35(1), 33-40. PubMed PMID: 20040244. Pubmed Central PMCID: 2799502. Epub 2009/12/31. eng.

[53] Velakoulis, D; Wood, SJ; Wong, MT; McGorry, PD; Yung, A; Phillips, L; et al. Hippocampal and amygdala volumes according to psychosis stage and diagnosis: a magnetic resonance imaging study of chronic schizophrenia, first-episode psychosis, and ultra-high-risk individuals. *Arch Gen Psychiatry.*, 2006 Feb; 63(2), 139-49. PubMed PMID: 16461856. Epub 2006/02/08. eng.

[54] Taylor, SF; Kang, J; Brege, IS; Tso, IF; Hosanagar, A; Johnson, TD. Meta-analysis of functional neuroimaging studies of emotion perception and experience in schizophrenia. *Biol Psychiatry.*, 2012 Jan 15; 71(2), 136-45. PubMed PMID: 21993193. Pubmed Central PMCID: 3237865. Epub 2011/10/14. eng.

[55] Szeszko, PR; Goldberg, E; Gunduz-Bruce, H; Ashtari, M; Robinson, D; Malhotra, AK; et al. Smaller anterior hippocampal formation volume in antipsychotic-naive patients with first-episode schizophrenia. *Am J Psychiatry.*, 2003 Dec; 160(12), 2190-7. PubMed PMID: 14638589. Epub 2003/11/26. eng.

[56] Simpson, MD; Slater, P; Deakin, JF; Royston, MC; Skan, WJ. Reduced GABA uptake sites in the temporal lobe in schizophrenia. *Neurosci Lett.*, 1989 Dec 15; 107(1-3), 211-5. PubMed PMID: 2616032. Epub 1989/12/15. eng.

[57] Konradi, C; Yang, CK; Zimmerman, EI; Lohmann, KM; Gresch, P; Pantazopoulos, H; et al. Hippocampal interneurons are abnormal in schizophrenia. *Schizophr Res.*, 2011 Sep; 131(1-3), 165-73. PubMed PMID: 21745723. Pubmed Central PMCID: 3159834. Epub 2011/07/13. eng.

[58] Heckers, S; Stone, D; Walsh, J; Shick, J; Koul, P; Benes, FM. Differential hippocampal expression of glutamic acid decarboxylase 65 and 67 messenger RNA in bipolar disorder and schizophrenia. *Arch Gen Psychiatry.*, 2002 Jun; 59(6), 521-9. PubMed PMID: 12044194.

[59] Heckers, S; Rauch, SL; Goff, D; Savage, CR; Schacter, DL; Fischman, AJ; et al. Impaired recruitment of the hippocampus during conscious recollection in

schizophrenia. *Nat Neurosci.*, 1998 Aug; 1(4), 318-23. PubMed PMID: 10195166. Epub 1999/04/09. eng.

[60] Benes, FM; Kwok, EW; Vincent, SL; Todtenkopf, MS. A reduction of nonpyramidal cells in sector CA2 of schizophrenics and manic depressives. *Biol Psychiatry.*, 1998 Jul 15; 44(2), 88-97. PubMed PMID: 9646890.

[61] Benes, FM; Khan, Y; Vincent, SL; Wickramasinghe, R. Differences in the subregional and cellular distribution of GABAA receptor binding in the hippocampal formation of schizophrenic brain. *Synapse.*, 1996 Apr; 22(4), 338-49. PubMed PMID: 8867028. Epub 1996/04/01. eng.

[62] Meador-Woodruff, JH; Clinton, SM; Beneyto, M; McCullumsmith, RE. Molecular abnormalities of the glutamate synapse in the thalamus in schizophrenia. *Ann N Y Acad Sci.*, 2003 Nov; 1003:75-93. PubMed PMID: 14684436. Epub 2003/12/20. eng.

[63] Guller, Y; Ferrarelli, F; Shackman, AJ; Sarasso, S; Peterson, MJ; Langheim, FJ; et al. Probing thalamic integrity in schizophrenia using concurrent transcranial magnetic stimulation and functional magnetic resonance imaging. *Arch Gen Psychiatry.*, 2012 Jul; 69(7), 662-71. PubMed PMID: 22393203. Pubmed Central PMCID: 3411883. Epub 2012/03/07. eng.

[64] Sodhi, MS; Simmons, M; McCullumsmith, R; Haroutunian, V; Meador-Woodruff, JH. Glutamatergic gene expression is specifically reduced in thalamocortical projecting relay neurons in schizophrenia. *Biol Psychiatry.* 2011 Oct 1; 70(7), 646-54. PubMed PMID: 21549355. Pubmed Central PMCID: 3176961. Epub 2011/05/10. eng.

[65] Ananth, H; Popescu, I; Critchley, HD; Good, CD; Frackowiak, RS; Dolan, RJ. Cortical and subcortical gray matter abnormalities in schizophrenia determined through structural magnetic resonance imaging with optimized volumetric voxel-based morphometry. *Am J Psychiatry.* 2002 Sep; 159(9), 1497-505. PubMed PMID: 12202269. Epub 2002/08/31. eng.

[66] Lewis, DA; Cruz, DA; Melchitzky, DS; Pierri, JN. Lamina-specific deficits in parvalbumin-immunoreactive varicosities in the prefrontal cortex of subjects with schizophrenia: evidence for fewer projections from the thalamus. *Am J Psychiatry.* 2001; 158(9), 1411-22.

[67] Benes, FM; Todtenkopf, MS; Logiotatos, P; Williams, M. Glutamate decarboxylase(65)-immunoreactive terminals in cingulate and prefrontal cortices of schizophrenic and bipolar brain. *Journal of chemical neuroanatomy.*, 2000 Dec; 20(3-4), 259-69. PubMed PMID: 11207424.

[68] Benes, FM; McSparren, J; Bird, ED; SanGiovanni, JP; Vincent, SL. Deficits in small interneurons in prefrontal and cingulate cortices of schizophrenic and schizoaffective patients. *Arch Gen Psychiatry.*, 1991; 48(11), 996-1001.

[69] Burgess, N; Maguire, EA; O'Keefe, J. The human hippocampus and spatial and episodic memory. *Neuron.* 2002 Aug 15; 35(4), 625-41. PubMed PMID: 12194864. Epub 2002/08/27. eng.

[70] Brown, TI; Ross, RS; Keller, JB; Hasselmo, ME; Stern, CE. Which way was I going? Contextual retrieval supports the disambiguation of well learned overlapping navigational routes. *J Neurosci.*, 2010 May 26; 30(21), 7414-22. PubMed PMID: 20505108. Pubmed Central PMCID: 2905880. Epub 2010/05/28. eng.

[71] Leutgeb, S; Leutgeb, JK; Barnes, CA; Moser, EI; McNaughton, BL; Moser, MB. Independent codes for spatial and episodic memory in hippocampal neuronal

ensembles. *Science.*, 2005 Jul 22; 309(5734), 619-23. PubMed PMID: 16040709. Epub 2005/07/26. eng.

[72] Wood, ER; Dudchenko, PA; Eichenbaum, H. The global record of memory in hippocampal neuronal activity. *Nature.*, 1999; 397(6720), 613-6.

[73] O'Keefe, J; Burgess, N. Geometric determinants of the place fields of hippocampal neurons. *Nature.*, 1996 May 30; 381(6581), 425-8. PubMed PMID: 8632799. Epub 1996/05/30. eng.

[74] Suh, J; Rivest, AJ; Nakashiba, T; Tominaga, T; Tonegawa, S. Entorhinal cortex layer III input to the hippocampus is crucial for temporal association memory. *Science.* 2011 Dec 9; 334(6061), 1415-20. PubMed PMID: 22052975. Epub 2011/11/05. eng.

[75] Boutros, NN; Mears, R; Pflieger, ME; Moxon, KA; Ludowig, E; Rosburg, T. Sensory gating in the human hippocampal and rhinal regions: regional differences. *Hippocampus.*, 2008; 18(3), 310-6. PubMed PMID: 18064708. Epub 2007/12/08. eng.

[76] Remondes, M; Schuman, EM. Direct cortical input modulates plasticity and spiking in CA1 pyramidal neurons. *Nature.* 2002 Apr 18; 416(6882), 736-40. PubMed PMID: 11961555. Epub 2002/04/19. eng.

[77] Flach, KA; Adler, LE; Gerhardt, GA; Miller, C; Bickford, P; MacGregor, RJ. Sensory gating in a computer model of the CA3 neural network of the hippocampus. *Biol Psychiatry.* 1996 Dec 15; 40(12), 1230-45. PubMed PMID: 8959288. Epub 1996/12/15. eng.

[78] Debiec, J; Diaz-Mataix, L; Bush, DE; Doyere, V; Ledoux, JE. The amygdala encodes specific sensory features of an aversive reinforcer. *Nat Neurosci.*, 2010 May; 13(5), 536-7. PubMed PMID: 20348916. Pubmed Central PMCID: 2860669. Epub 2010/03/30. eng.

[79] LeDoux, J. The amygdala. *Curr Biol.*, 2007 Oct 23; 17(20), R868-74. PubMed PMID: 17956742. Epub 2007/10/25. eng.

[80] Phelps, EA; LeDoux, JE. Contributions of the amygdala to emotion processing: from animal models to human behavior. *Neuron.*, 2005 Oct 20; 48(2), 175-87. PubMed PMID: 16242399. Epub 2005/10/26. eng.

[81] LeDoux, J. The emotional brain, fear, and the amygdala. *Cell Mol Neurobiol.*, 2003 Oct; 23(4-5), 727-38. PubMed PMID: 14514027.

[82] Blanchard, C; Blanchard, R; Fellous, JM; Guimaraes, FS; Irwin, W; Ledoux, JE; et al. The brain decade in debate: III. Neurobiology of emotion. *Brazilian journal of medical and biological research = Revista brasileira de pesquisas medicas e biologicas / Sociedade Brasileira de Biofisica* [et al]. 2001 Mar; 34(3), 283-93. PubMed PMID: 11262578. Epub 2001/03/23. eng.

[83] Tye, KM; Prakash, R; Kim, SY; Fenno, LE; Grosenick, L; Zarabi, H; et al. Amygdala circuitry mediating reversible and bidirectional control of anxiety. *Nature.* 2011 Mar 17; 471(7338), 358-62. PubMed PMID: 21389985. Pubmed Central PMCID: 3154022. Epub 2011/03/11. eng.

[84] Meyer-Lindenberg, A. Behavioural neuroscience: Genes and the anxious brain. *Nature.* 2010 Aug 12; 466(7308), 827-8. PubMed PMID: 20703297. Epub 2010/08/13. eng.

[85] Zhou, Z; Zhu, G; Hariri, AR; Enoch, MA; Scott, D; Sinha, R; et al. Genetic variation in human NPY expression affects stress response and emotion. *Nature.*, 2008 Apr 24; 452(7190), 997-1001. PubMed PMID: 18385673. Pubmed Central PMCID: 2715959. Epub 2008/04/04. eng.

[86] Gur, RE; McGrath, C; Chan, RM; Schroeder, L; Turner, T; Turetsky, BI; et al. An fMRI study of facial emotion processing in patients with schizophrenia. *Am J Psychiatry.*, 2002 Dec; 159(12), 1992-9. PubMed PMID: 12450947. Epub 2002/11/27. eng.

[87] Rotshtein, P; Malach, R; Hadar, U; Graif, M; Hendler, T. Feeling or features: different sensitivity to emotion in high-order visual cortex and amygdala. *Neuron.*, 2001 Nov 20; 32(4), 747-57. PubMed PMID: 11719213. Epub 2001/11/24. eng.

[88] Garavan, H; Pendergrass, JC; Ross, TJ; Stein, EA; Risinger, RC. Amygdala response to both positively and negatively valenced stimuli. *Neuroreport.*, 2001 Aug 28; 12(12), 2779-83. PubMed PMID: 11522965. Epub 2001/08/28. eng.

[89] Paradiso, S; Johnson, DL; Andreasen, NC; O'Leary, DS; Watkins, GL; Ponto, LL; et al. Cerebral blood flow changes associated with attribution of emotional valence to pleasant, unpleasant, and neutral visual stimuli in a PET study of normal subjects. *Am J Psychiatry.*, 1999 Oct; 156(10), 1618-29. PubMed PMID: 10518175. Epub 1999/10/13. eng.

[90] Sergerie, K; Chochol, C; Armony, JL. The role of the amygdala in emotional processing: a quantitative meta-analysis of functional neuroimaging studies. *Neurosci Biobehav Rev.*, 2008; 32(4), 811-30. PubMed PMID: 18316124. Epub 2008/03/05. eng.

[91] Gosselin, N; Peretz, I; Johnsen, E; Adolphs, R. Amygdala damage impairs emotion recognition from music. *Neuropsychologia.*, 2007 Jan 28; 45(2), 236-44. PubMed PMID: 16970965. Epub 2006/09/15. eng.

[92] Lanteaume, L; Khalfa, S; Regis, J; Marquis, P; Chauvel, P; Bartolomei, F. Emotion induction after direct intracerebral stimulations of human amygdala. *Cereb Cortex.*, 2007 Jun; 17(6), 1307-13. PubMed PMID: 16880223. Epub 2006/08/02. eng.

[93] Petrides, M. The role of the mid-dorsolateral prefrontal cortex in working memory. *Experimental brain research Experimentelle Hirnforschung Experimentation cerebrale.*, 2000 Jul; 133(1), 44-54. PubMed PMID: 10933209. Epub 2000/08/10. eng.

[94] Kane, MJ; Engle, RW. The role of prefrontal cortex in working-memory capacity, executive attention, and general fluid intelligence: an individual-differences perspective. *Psychonomic bulletin & review.*, 2002 Dec; 9(4), 637-71. PubMed PMID: 12613671. Epub 2003/03/05. eng.

[95] Miller, EK; Erickson, CA; Desimone, R. Neural mechanisms of visual working memory in prefrontal cortex of the macaque. *J Neurosci.*, 1996 Aug 15; 16(16), 5154-67. PubMed PMID: 8756444. Epub 1996/08/15. eng.

[96] Miller, EK; Cohen, JD. An integrative theory of prefrontal cortex function. *Annual review of neuroscience.* 2001; 24:167-202. PubMed PMID: 11283309. Epub 2001/04/03. eng.

[97] Fuster, JM. Executive frontal functions. *Experimental brain research Experimentelle Hirnforschung Experimentation cerebrale.* 2000 Jul; 133(1), 66-70. PubMed PMID: 10933211. Epub 2000/08/10. eng.

[98] Arnsten, AF; Li, BM. Neurobiology of executive functions: catecholamine influences on prefrontal cortical functions. *Biol Psychiatry.*, 2005 Jun 1; 57(11), 1377-84. PubMed PMID: 15950011. Epub 2005/06/14. eng.

[99] Sherman, SM. The thalamus is more than just a relay. *Curr Opin Neurobiol.*, 2007 Aug; 17(4), 417-22. PubMed PMID: 17707635. Pubmed Central PMCID: 2753250. Epub 2007/08/21. eng.

[100] Sherman, SM. Thalamic relays and cortical functioning. *Prog Brain Res.*, 2005; 149:107-26. PubMed PMID: 16226580. Epub 2005/10/18. eng.

[101] Ervin, FR; Mark, VH. Stereotactic thalamotomy in the human. Part II. Physiologic observations on the human thalamus. *Arch Neurol.*, 1960 Oct; 3:368-80. PubMed PMID: 13697294. Epub 1960/10/01. eng.

[102] Pinault, D. The thalamic reticular nucleus: structure, function and concept. *Brain Res Brain Res Rev.*, 2004 Aug; 46(1), 1-31. PubMed PMID: 15297152. Epub 2004/08/07. eng.

[103] Pinault, D; Pumain, R. Ectopic action potential generation: its occurrence in a chronic epileptogenic focus. *Experimental brain research Experimentelle Hirnforschung Experimentation cerebrale.*, 1985; 60(3), 599-602. PubMed PMID: 3935471. Epub 1985/01/01. eng.

[104] Devinsky, O; Morrell, MJ; Vogt, BA. Contributions of anterior cingulate cortex to behaviour. *Brain.*, 1995 Feb; 118 (Pt 1), 279-306. PubMed PMID: 7895011. Epub 1995/02/01. eng.

[105] Bush, G; Vogt, BA; Holmes, J; Dale, AM; Greve, D; Jenike, MA; et al. Dorsal anterior cingulate cortex: a role in reward-based decision making. *Proc Natl Acad Sci U S A.*, 2002 Jan 8; 99(1), 523-8. PubMed PMID: 11756669. Pubmed Central PMCID: 117593. Epub 2002/01/05. eng.

[106] Bush, G; Luu, P; Posner, MI. Cognitive and emotional influences in anterior cingulate cortex. *Trends Cogn Sci.*, 2000 Jun; 4(6), 215-22. PubMed PMID: 10827444. Epub 2000/05/29. Eng.

[107] Volman, V; Behrens, MM; Sejnowski, TJ. Downregulation of parvalbumin at cortical GABA synapses reduces network gamma oscillatory activity. *J Neurosci.*, 2011 Dec 7; 31(49), 18137-48. PubMed PMID: 22159125. Pubmed Central PMCID: 3257321. Epub 2011/12/14. eng.

[108] Lewis, DA; Curley, AA; Glausier, JR; Volk, DW. Cortical parvalbumin interneurons and cognitive dysfunction in schizophrenia. *Trends Neurosci.*, 2012 Jan; 35(1), 57-67. PubMed PMID: 22154068. Pubmed Central PMCID: 3253230. Epub 2011/12/14. eng.

[109] Gonzalez-Burgos, G; Fish, KN; Lewis, DA. GABA neuron alterations, cortical circuit dysfunction and cognitive deficits in schizophrenia. *Neural plasticity.*, 2011; 2011:723184. PubMed PMID: 21904685. Pubmed Central PMCID: 3167184. Epub 2011/09/10. eng.

[110] Brockmann, MD; Poschel, B; Cichon, N; Hanganu-Opatz, IL. Coupled oscillations mediate directed interactions between prefrontal cortex and hippocampus of the neonatal rat. *Neuron.*, 2011 Jul 28; 71(2), 332-47. PubMed PMID: 21791291. Epub 2011/07/28. eng.

[111] Sohal, VS. Insights into cortical oscillations arising from optogenetic studies. *Biol Psychiatry.*, 2012 Jun 15; 71(12), 1039-45. PubMed PMID: 22381731. Pubmed Central PMCID: 3361599. Epub 2012/03/03. eng.

[112] Carlen, M; Meletis, K; Siegle, JH; Cardin, JA; Futai, K; Vierling-Claassen, D; et al. A critical role for NMDA receptors in parvalbumin interneurons for gamma rhythm induction and behavior. *Mol Psychiatry.*, 2012 May; 17(5), 537-48. PubMed PMID: 21468034. Pubmed Central PMCID: 3335079. Epub 2011/04/07. eng.

[113] Sohal, VS; Zhang, F; Yizhar, O; Deisseroth, K. Parvalbumin neurons and gamma rhythms enhance cortical circuit performance. *Nature.*, 2009 Jun 4; 459(7247), 698-702. PubMed PMID: 19396159. Epub 2009/04/28. eng.

[114] Benes, FM; Berretta, S. GABAergic interneurons: implications for understanding schizophrenia and bipolar disorder. *Neuropsychopharmacology.*, 2001 Jul; 25(1), 1-27. PubMed PMID: 11377916. Epub 2001/05/30. eng.

[115] Benes, FM. Altered glutamatergic and GABAergic mechanisms in the cingulate cortex of the schizophrenic brain. *Arch Gen Psychiatry.*, 1995 Dec; 52(12), 1015-8; discussion 9-24. PubMed PMID: 7492253. Epub 1995/12/01. eng.

[116] Beasley, CL; Reynolds, GP. Parvalbumin-immunoreactive neurons are reduced in the prefrontal cortex of schizophrenics. *Schizophr Res.*, 1997 Apr 11; 24(3), 349-55. PubMed PMID: 9134596. Epub 1997/04/11. eng.

[117] Uhlhaas, PJ; Singer, W. Abnormal neural oscillations and synchrony in schizophrenia. *Nature reviews Neuroscience.*, 2010 Feb; 11(2), 100-13. PubMed PMID: 20087360. Epub 2010/01/21. eng.

[118] Spencer, KM; Niznikiewicz, MA; Shenton, ME; McCarley, RW. Sensory-evoked gamma oscillations n chronic schizophrenia. *Biological psychiatry.*, 2008 Apr 15; 63(8), 744-7. PubMed PMID: 18083143. Pubmed Central PMCID: 2330275. Epub 2007/12/18. eng.

[119] Lewis, DA; Cho, RY; Carter, CS; Eklund, K; Forster, S; Kelly, MA; et al. Subunit-selective modulation of GABA type A receptor neurotransmission and cognition in schizophrenia. *The American journal of psychiatry.*, 2008 Dec; 165(12), 1585-93. PubMed PMID: 18923067. Pubmed Central PMCID: 2876339. Epub 2008/10/17. eng.

[120] Woo, TU; Spencer, K; McCarley, RW. Gamma oscillation deficits and the onset and early progression of schizophrenia. *Harvard review of psychiatry.*, 2010 Jun; 18(3), 173-89. PubMed PMID: 20415633. Pubmed Central PMCID: 2860612. Epub 2010/04/27. eng.

[121] Meador-Woodruff, JH; Healy, DJ. Glutamate receptor expression in schizophrenic brain. *Brain Res Brain Res Rev.*, 2000 Mar; 31(2-3), 288-94. PubMed PMID: 10719155. Epub 2000/03/17. eng.

[122] Ghose, S; Gleason, KA; Potts, BW; Lewis-Amezcua, K; Tamminga, CA. Differential expression of metabotropic glutamate receptors 2 and 3 in schizophrenia: a mechanism for antipsychotic drug action? *Am J Psychiatry.*, 2009 Jul; 166(7), 812-20. PubMed PMID: 19487395. Pubmed Central PMCID: 2860261. Epub 2009/06/03. eng.

[123] Harrison, PJ; Lyon, L; Sartorius, LJ; Burnet, PW; Lane, TA. The group II metabotropic glutamate receptor 3 (mGluR3, mGlu3, GRM3), expression, function and involvement in schizophrenia. *J Psychopharmacol.*, 2008 May; 22(3), 308-22. PubMed PMID: 18541626. Epub 2008/06/11. eng.

[124] Javitt, DC. Glutamatergic theories of schizophrenia. *Isr J Psychiatry Relat Sci.*, 2010; 47(1), 4-16. PubMed PMID: 20686195. Epub 2010/08/06. eng.

[125] Coyle, JT; Balu, D; Benneyworth, M; Basu, A; Roseman, A. Beyond the dopamine receptor: novel therapeutic targets for treating schizophrenia. *Dialogues Clin Neurosci.*, 2010; 12(3), 359-82. PubMed PMID: 20954431. Pubmed Central PMCID: 3181979. Epub 2010/10/20. eng.

[126] Howes, OD; Kapur, S. The dopamine hypothesis of schizophrenia: version III--the final common pathway. *Schizophr Bull.*, 2009 May; 35(3), 549-62. PubMed PMID: 19325164. Pubmed Central PMCID: 2669582. Epub 2009/03/28. eng.

[127] Toda, M; Abi-Dargham, A. Dopamine hypothesis of schizophrenia: making sense of it all. *Curr Psychiatry Rep.*, 2007 Aug; 9(4), 329-36. PubMed PMID: 17880866. Epub 2007/09/21. eng.

[128] Reynolds, GP. Increased concentrations and lateral asymmetry of amygdala dopamine in schizophrenia. *Nature.*, 1983 Oct 6-12; 305(5934), 527-9. PubMed PMID: 6621699. Epub 1983/10/06. eng.

[129] Owen, F; Cross, AJ; Crow, TJ; Longden, A; Poulter, M; Riley, GJ. Increased dopamine-receptor sensitivity in schizophrenia. *Lancet.*, 1978 Jul 29; 2(8083), 223-6. PubMed PMID: 79025. Epub 1978/07/29. eng.

[130] Mackay, AV; Iversen, LL; Rossor, M; Spokes, E; Bird, E; Arregui, A; et al. Increased brain dopamine and dopamine receptors in schizophrenia. *Arch Gen Psychiatry.*, 1982 Sep; 39(9), 991-7. PubMed PMID: 7115016. Epub 1982/09/01. eng.

[131] Steiner, J; Schroeter, ML; Schiltz, K; Bernstein, HG; Muller, UJ; Richter-Landsberg, C; et al. Haloperidol and clozapine decrease S100B release from glial cells. *Neuroscience.*, 2010 Jun 2; 167(4), 1025-31. PubMed PMID: 20226844. Epub 2010/03/17. eng.

[132] Steiner, J; Bernstein, HG; Bielau, H; Farkas, N; Winter, J; Dobrowolny, H; et al. S100B-immunopositive glia is elevated in paranoid as compared to residual schizophrenia: a morphometric study. *J Psychiatr Res.*, 2008 Aug; 42(10), 868-76. PubMed PMID: 18001771. Epub 2007/11/16. eng.

[133] Matute, C; Melone, M; Vallejo-Illarramendi, A; Conti, F. Increased expression of the astrocytic glutamate transporter GLT-1 in the prefrontal cortex of schizophrenics. *Glia.*, 2005 Feb; 49(3), 451-5. PubMed PMID: 15494981. Epub 2004/10/21. eng.

[134] Rothermundt, M; Falkai, P; Ponath, G; Abel, S; Burkle, H; Diedrich, M; et al. Glial cell dysfunction in schizophrenia indicated by increased S100B in the CSF. *Mol Psychiatry.*, 2004 Oct; 9(10), 897-9. PubMed PMID: 15241436. Epub 2004/07/09. eng.

[135] Spangaro, M; Bosia, M; Zanoletti, A; Bechi, M; Cocchi, F; Pirovano, A; et al. Cognitive dysfunction and glutamate reuptake: effect of EAAT2 polymorphism in schizophrenia. *Neurosci Lett.*, 2012 Aug 1; 522(2), 151-5. PubMed PMID: 22728822. Epub 2012/06/26. eng.

[136] Bauer, D; Haroutunian, V; Meador-Woodruff, JH; McCullumsmith, RE. Abnormal glycosylation of EAAT1 and EAAT2 in prefrontal cortex of elderly patients with schizophrenia. *Schizophr Res.*, 2010 Mar; 117(1), 92-8. PubMed PMID: 19716271. Pubmed Central PMCID: 2822023. Epub 2009/09/01. eng.

[137] Bauer, D; Gupta, D; Harotunian, V; Meador-Woodruff, JH; McCullumsmith, RE. Abnormal expression of glutamate transporter and transporter interacting molecules in prefrontal cortex in elderly patients with schizophrenia. *Schizophr Res.*, 2008 Sep; 104(1-3), 108-20. PubMed PMID: 18678470. Pubmed Central PMCID: 2656372. Epub 2008/08/06. eng.

[138] Huerta, I; McCullumsmith, RE; Haroutunian, V; Gimenez-Amaya, JM; Meador-Woodruff, JH. Expression of excitatory amino acid transporter interacting protein transcripts in the thalamus in schizophrenia. *Synapse.*, 2006 Jun 1; 59(7), 394-402. PubMed PMID: 16485262.

[139] Smith, RE; Haroutunian, V; Davis, KL; Meador-Woodruff, JH. Expression of excitatory amino acid ransporter transcripts in the thalamus of subjects with schizophrenia. *Am J Psychiatry.*, 2001 Sep; 158(9), 1393-9. PubMed PMID: 11532723. Epub 2001/09/05. eng.

[140] Martins-de-Souza, D. Proteome and transcriptome analysis suggests oligodendrocyte dysfunction in schizophrenia. *J Psychiatr Res.*, 2010 Feb; 44(3), 149-56. PubMed PMID: 19699489. Epub 2009/08/25. eng.

[141] Hoistad, M; Segal, D; Takahashi, N; Sakurai, T; Buxbaum, JD; Hof, PR. Linking white and grey matter in schizophrenia: oligodendrocyte and neuron pathology in the prefrontal cortex. *Front Neuroanat.*, 2009; 3:9. PubMed PMID: 19636386. Pubmed Central PMCID: 2713751. Epub 2009/07/29. eng.

[142] Bernstein, HG; Steiner, J; Bogerts, B. Glial cells in schizophrenia: pathophysiological significance and possible consequences for therapy. *Expert Rev Neurother.*, 2009 Jul; 9(7), 1059-71. PubMed PMID: 19589054. Epub 2009/07/11. eng.

[143] Segal, D; Koschnick, JR; Slegers, LH; Hof, PR. Oligodendrocyte pathophysiology: a new view of schizophrenia. *Int J Neuropsychopharmacol.*, 2007 Aug; 10(4), 503-11. PubMed PMID: 17291369. Epub 2007/02/13. eng.

[144] Davis, KL; Stewart, DG; Friedman, JI; Buchsbaum, M; Harvey, PD; Hof, PR; et al. White matter changes in schizophrenia: evidence for myelin-related dysfunction. *Arch Gen Psychiatry.*, 2003 May; 60(5), 443-56. PubMed PMID: 12742865. Epub 2003/05/14. eng.

[145] Wiese, S; Karus, M; Faissner, A. Astrocytes as a source for extracellular matrix molecules and cytokines. *Frontiers in pharmacology.*, 2012; 3:120. PubMed PMID: 22740833. Pubmed Central PMCID: 3382726. Epub 2012/06/29. eng.

[146] Sofroniew, MV; Vinters, HV. Astrocytes: biology and pathology. *Acta Neuropathol.*, 2010 Jan; 119(1), 7-35. PubMed PMID: 20012068. Pubmed Central PMCID: 2799634. Epub 2009/12/17. eng.

[147] Halassa, MM; Fellin, T; Haydon, PG. The tripartite synapse: roles for gliotransmission in health and disease. *Trends Mol Med.*, 2007 Feb; 13(2), 54-63. PubMed PMID: 17207662.

[148] Bradl, M; Lassmann, H. Oligodendrocytes: biology and pathology. *Acta Neuropathol.* 2010 Jan; 119(1), 37-53. PubMed PMID: 19847447. Pubmed Central PMCID: 2799635. Epub 2009/10/23. eng.

[149] Muhleisen, TW; Mattheisen, M; Strohmaier, J; Degenhardt, F; Priebe, L; Schultz, CC; et al. Association between schizophrenia and common variation in neurocan (NCAN), a genetic risk factor for bipolar disorder. *Schizophr Res.*, 2012 Jun; 138(1), 69-73. PubMed PMID: 22497794. Epub 2012/04/14. eng.

[150] So, HC; Fong, PY; Chen, RY; Hui, TC; Ng, MY; Cherny, SS; et al. Identification of neuroglycan C and interacting partners as potential susceptibility genes for schizophrenia in a Southern Chinese population. *Am J Med Genet B Neuropsychiatr Genet.*, Jan 5; 153B(1), 103-13. PubMed PMID: 19367581. Epub 2009/04/16. eng.

[151] Buxbaum, JD; Georgieva, L; Young, JJ; Plescia, C; Kajiwara, Y; Jiang, Y; et al. Molecular dissection of NRG1-ERBB4 signaling implicates PTPRZ1 as a potential schizophrenia susceptibility gene. *Molecular psychiatry.* 2008 Feb; 13(2), 162-72. PubMed PMID: 17579610. Epub 2007/06/21. eng.

[152] Mauney, S; Kim, SS; Pantazopoulos, H; Berretta, S; Woo, TU. Perineuronal net abnormalities in the prefrontal cortex in schizophrenia. *Society for Neuroscience.*, 2011; Washingon, D.C.

[153] Pantazopoulos, H; Woo, TU; Lim, MP; Lange, N; Berretta, S. Extracellular matrix-glial abnormalities in the amygdala and entorhinal cortex of subjects diagnosed with schizophrenia. *Arch Gen Psychiatry.*, 2010 Feb; 67(2), 155-66. PubMed PMID: 20124115. Epub 2010/02/04. eng.

[154] Pantazopoulos, H; Boyer-Boiteau, A; Holbrook, EH; Jang, W; Arnold, SE; Berretta, S. Proteoglycan Abnormalities In Olfactory Epithelium Tissue From Schizophrenic Subjects. *Brain and behavior.*, 2013; In Press.

[155] Maeda, N; Ishii, M; Nishimura, K; Kamimura, K. Functions of chondroitin sulfate and heparan sulfate in the developing brain. *Neurochemical research.*, 2011 Jul; 36(7), 1228-40. PubMed PMID: 21110089. Epub 2010/11/27. eng.

[156] Maeda, N; Fukazawa, N; Ishii, M. Chondroitin sulfate proteoglycans in neural development and plasticity. *Front Biosci.*, 2010; 15:626-44. PubMed PMID: 20036837. Epub 2009/12/29. eng.

[157] Garwood, J; Heck, N; Reichardt, F; Faissner, A. Phosphacan short isoform, a novel non-proteoglycan variant of phosphacan/receptor protein tyrosine phosphatase-beta, interacts with neuronal receptors and promotes neurite outgrowth. *J Biol Chem.*, 2003 Jun 27; 278(26), 24164-73. PubMed PMID: 12700241. Epub 2003/04/18. eng.

[158] Dobbertin, A; Rhodes, KE; Garwood, J; Properzi, F; Heck, N; Rogers, JH; et al. Regulation of RPTPbeta/phosphacan expression and glycosaminoglycan epitopes in injured brain and cytokine-reated glia. *Mol Cell Neurosci.*, 2003 Dec; 24(4), 951-71. PubMed PMID: 14697661. Epub 2003/12/31. eng.

[159] Wu, Y; Sheng, W; Chen, L; Dong, H; Lee, V; Lu, F; et al. Versican V1 isoform induces neuronal differentiation and promotes neurite outgrowth. *Mol Biol Cell.*, 2004 May; 15(5), 2093-104. PubMed PMID: 14978219. Pubmed Central PMCID: 404007. Epub 2004/02/24. eng.

[160] Kalb, RG; Hockfield, S. Molecular evidence for early activity-dependent development of hamster motor neurons. *J Neurosci.*, 1988 Jul; 8(7), 2350-60. PubMed PMID: 3249230. Epub 1988/07/01. eng.

[161] Gogolla, N; Caroni, P; Luthi, A; Herry, C. Perineuronal nets protect fear memories from erasure. *Science.*, 2009 Sep 4; 325(5945), 1258-61. PubMed PMID: 19729657. Epub 2009/09/05. eng.

[162] Sugiyama, S; Di Nardo, AA; Aizawa, S; Matsuo, I; Volovitch, M; Prochiantz, A; et al. Experience-dependent transfer of Otx2 homeoprotein into the visual cortex activates postnatal plasticity. *Cell.*, 2008 Aug 8; 134(3), 508-20. PubMed PMID: 18692473. Epub 2008/08/12. eng.

[163] Takahashi, N; Sakurai, T; Bozdagi-Gunal, O; Dorr, NP; Moy, J; Krug, L; et al. Increased expression of receptor phosphotyrosine phosphatase-beta/zeta is associated with molecular, cellular, behavioral and cognitive schizophrenia phenotypes. *Transl Psychiatry.*, 2011; 1:e8. PubMed PMID: 22832403. Pubmed Central PMCID: 3309478. Epub 2011/01/01. eng.

[164] Pantazopoulos, H; Murray, EA; Berretta, S. Total number, distribution, and phenotype of cells expressing chondroitin sulfate proteoglycans in the normal human amygdala. *Brain Res.*, 2008 May 1; 1207:84-95. PubMed PMID: 18374308.

[165] Harrison, PJ. The neuropathology of schizophrenia. A critical review of the data and their nterpretation. *Brain.*, 1999 Apr; 122 (Pt 4), 593-624. PubMed PMID: 10219775. Epub 1999/04/29. eng.

[166] Bogerts, B. The neuropathology of schizophrenic diseases: historical aspects and present knowledge. *Eur Arch Psychiatry Clin Neurosci.*, 1999; 249 Suppl 4:2-13. PubMed PMID: 10654104. Epub 2000/02/02. eng.

[167] Falkai, P; Honer, WG; David, S; Bogerts, B; Majtenyi, C; Bayer, TA. No evidence for astrogliosis in brains of schizophrenic patients. A post-mortem study. *Neuropathol Appl Neurobiol.*, 1999 Feb; 25(1), 48-53. PubMed PMID: 10194775. Epub 1999/04/09. eng.

[168] Arnold, SE. Neurodevelopmental abnormalities in schizophrenia: insights from neuropathology. *Dev Psychopathol.*, 1999 Summer; 11(3), 439-56. PubMed PMID: 10532618. Epub 1999/10/26. eng.

[169] Mauney, SA.; Athanas, KM, Pantazopoulos H., Shaskan, Passeri E., Berretta S., Woo, TU. Developmental Patterns of Perineuronal Nets in the Human Prefrontal Cortex and their Deficit in Schizophrenia. *Biological Psychiatry*, 2013; *in press.*

[170] Sirko, S; von Holst, A; Weber, A; Wizenmann, A; Theocharidis, U; Gotz, M; et al. Chondroitin sulfates are required for fibroblast growth factor-2-dependent proliferation and maintenance in neural stem cells and for epidermal growth factor-dependent migration of their progeny. *Stem Cells.*, 2010 Apr; 28(4), 775-87. PubMed PMID: 20087964. Epub 2010/01/21. eng.

[171] Arnold, SE; Han, LY; Moberg, PJ; Turetsky, BI; Gur, RE; Trojanowski, JQ; et al. Dysregulation of olfactory receptor neuron lineage in schizophrenia. *Archives of general psychiatry.*, 2001 Sep; 58(9), 829-35. PubMed PMID: 11545665. Epub 2001/09/26. eng.

[172] Ugur, T; Weisbrod, M; Franzek, E; Pfuller, U; Sauer, H. Olfactory impairment in monozygotic twins discordant for schizophrenia. *Eur Arch Psychiatry Clin Neurosci.*, 2005 Apr; 255(2), 94-8. PubMed PMID: 15812602. Epub 2005/04/07. eng.

[173] Brewer, WJ; Wood, SJ; McGorry, PD; Francey, SM; Phillips, LJ; Yung, AR; et al. Impairment of olfactory identification ability in individuals at ultra-high risk for psychosis who later develop schizophrenia. *Am J Psychiatry.*, 2003 Oct; 160(10), 1790-4. PubMed PMID: 14514492. Epub 2003/09/30. eng.

[174] Brewer, WJ; Pantelis, C; Anderson, V; Velakoulis, D; Singh, B; Copolov, DL; et al. Stability of olfactory identification deficits in neuroleptic-naive patients with first-episode psychosis. *Am J Psychiatry.*, 2001 Jan; 158(1), 107-15. PubMed PMID: 11136641. Epub 2001/01/04. eng.

[175] Good, KP; Martzke, JS; Frankland, BW; Kopala, LC. Deterioration of olfactory identification abilities in patients with schizophrenia. *Am J Psychiatry.*, 1998 Oct; 155(10), 1463-4. PubMed PMID: 9766790. Epub 1998/10/10. eng.

[176] Purdon, SE. Olfactory identification and Stroop interference converge in schizophrenia. *J Psychiatry Neurosci.*, 1998 May; 23(3), 163-71. PubMed PMID: 9595890. Pubmed Central PMCID: 1188923. Epub 1998/05/22. eng.

[177] Kopala, LC; Clark, C; Hurwitz, T. Olfactory deficits in neuroleptic naive patients with schizophrenia. *Schizophr Res.*, 1993 Jan; 8(3), 245-50. PubMed PMID: 8094630. Epub 1993/01/01. eng.

[178] Eastwood, SL; Law, AJ; Everall, IP; Harrison, PJ. The axonal chemorepellant semaphorin 3A is ncreased in the cerebellum in schizophrenia and may contribute to its

synaptic pathology. *Mol Psychiatry.*, 2003 Feb; 8(2), 148-55. PubMed PMID: 12610647. Epub 2003/03/01. eng.

[179] Guidotti, A; Auta, J; Davis, JM; Di-Giorgi-Gerevini, V; Dwivedi, Y; Grayson, DR; et al. Decrease in reelin and glutamic acid decarboxylase67 (GAD67) expression in schizophrenia and bipolar disorder: a postmortem brain study. *Arch Gen Psychiatry.*, 2000 Nov; 57(11), 1061-9. PubMed PMID: 11074872.

[180] Habl, G; Schmitt, A; Zink, M; von Wilmsdorff, M; Yeganeh-Doost, P; Jatzko, A; et al. Decreased reelin expression in the left prefrontal cortex (BA9) in chronic schizophrenia patients. *Neuropsychobiology.*, 2012; 66(1), 57-62. PubMed PMID: 22797278. Epub 2012/07/17. eng.

[181] Harvey, L; Boksa, P. A stereological comparison of GAD67 and reelin expression in the hippocampal stratum oriens of offspring from two mouse models of maternal inflammation during pregnancy. *Neuropharmacology.*, 2012 Mar; 62(4), 1767-76. PubMed PMID: 22178614. Epub 2011/12/20. eng.

[182] Impagnatiello, F; Guidotti, AR; Pesold, C; Dwivedi, Y; Caruncho, H; Pisu, MG; et al. A decrease of reelin expression as a putative vulnerability factor in schizophrenia. *Proc Natl Acad Sci U S A.*, 1998; 95(26), 15718-23.

[183] Falkai, P; Schneider-Axmann, T; Honer, WG. Entorhinal cortex pre-alpha cell clusters in schizophrenia: quantitative evidence of a developmental abnormality. *Biol Psychiatry.*, 2000 Jun 1; 47(11), 937-43. PubMed PMID: 10838061. Epub 2000/06/06. eng.

[184] Arnold, SE; Ruscheinsky, DD; Han, LY. Further evidence of abnormal cytoarchitecture of the entorhinal cortex in schizophrenia using spatial point pattern analyses. *Biol Psychiatry.*, 1997 Oct 15; 42(8), 639-47. PubMed PMID: 9325556. Epub 1997/11/05. eng.

[185] Arnold, SE; Hyman, BT; Van Hoesen, GW; Damasio, AR. Some cytoarchitectural abnormalities of the entorhinal cortex in schizophrenia. *Arch Gen Psychiatry.*, 1991 Jul; 48(7), 625-32. PubMed PMID: 2069493. Epub 1991/07/01. eng.

[186] Eastwood, SL. The synaptic pathology of schizophrenia: is aberrant neurodevelopment and plasticity to blame? *Int Rev Neurobiol.*, 2004; 59:47-72. PubMed PMID: 15006484. Epub 2004/03/10. eng.

[187] Akbarian, S; Bunney, WE Jr.; Potkin, SG; Wigal, SB; Hagman, JO; Sandman, CA; et al. Altered distribution of nicotinamide-adenine dinucleotide phosphate-diaphorase cells in frontal lobe of schizophrenics implies disturbances of cortical development. *Arch Gen Psychiatry.*, 1993; 50(3), 169-77.

[188] Akbarian, S; Kim, JJ; Potkin, SG; Hetrick, WP; Bunney, WE Jr.; Jones, EG. Maldistribution of interstitial neurons in prefrontal white matter of the brains of schizophrenic patients. *Arch Gen Psychiatry.*, 1996; 53(5), 425-36.

[189] Anderson, SA; Volk, DW; Lewis, DA. Increased density of microtubule associated protein 2-immunoreactive neurons in the prefrontal white matter of schizophrenic subjects. *Schizophr Res.*, 1996 May; 19(2-3), 111-9. PubMed PMID: 8789909. Epub 1996/05/01. eng.

[190] Akbarian, S; ViÒuela, A; Kim, JJ; Potkin, SG; Bunney, WE Jr.; Jones, EG. Distorted distribution of nicotinamide-adenine dinucleotide phosphate-diaphorase neurons in temporal lobe of schizophrenics implies anomalous cortical development. *Arch Gen Psychiatry.*, 1993; 50(3), 178-87.

[191] Kirkpatrick, B; Conley, RC; Kakoyannis, A; Reep, RL; Roberts, RC. Interstitial cells of the white matter in the inferior parietal cortex in schizophrenia: An unbiased cell-counting study. *Synapse.*, 1999 Nov; 34(2), 95-102. PubMed PMID: 10502308. Epub 1999/09/29. eng.

[192] Eastwood, SL; Harrison, PJ. Interstitial white matter neurons express less reelin and are abnormally distributed in schizophrenia: towards an integration of molecular and morphologic aspects of the neurodevelopmental hypothesis. *Mol Psychiatry.*, 2003 Sep; 8(9), 821-31. PubMed PMID: 12931209.

[193] Yang, Y; Fung, SJ; Rothwell, A; Tianmei, S; Weickert, CS. Increased interstitial white matter neuron density in the dorsolateral prefrontal cortex of people with schizophrenia. *Biol Psychiatry.*, 2011 Jan 1; 69(1), 63-70. PubMed PMID: 20974464. Pubmed Central PMCID: 3005941. Epub 2010/10/27. eng.

[194] Eastwood, SL; Harrison, PJ. Interstitial white matter neurons express less reelin and are abnormally distributed in schizophrenia: towards an integration of molecular and morphologic aspects of the neurodevelopmental hypothesis. *Mol Psychiatry.*, 2003 Sep; 8(9), 769, 821-31. PubMed PMID: 12931209. Epub 2003/08/22. eng.

[195] Zimmer, G; Schanuel, SM; Burger, S; Weth, F; Steinecke, A; Bolz, J; et al. Chondroitin sulfate acts in concert with semaphorin 3A to guide tangential migration of cortical interneurons in the ventral elencephalon. *Cereb Cortex.*, 2010 Oct; 20(10), 2411-22. PubMed PMID: 20071458. Epub 2010/01/15. eng.

[196] Longson, D; Deakin, JF; Benes, FM. Increased density of entorhinal glutamate-immunoreactive vertical fibers in schizophrenia. *J Neural Transm.*, 1996; 103(4), 503-7. PubMed PMID: 9617791. Epub 1996/01/01. eng.

[197] Wang, H; Katagiri, Y; McCann, TE; Unsworth, E; Goldsmith, P; Yu, ZX; et al. Chondroitin-4-sulfation negatively regulates axonal guidance and growth. *J Cell Sci.*, 2008 Sep 15; 121(Pt 18), 3083-91. PubMed PMID: 18768934. Pubmed Central PMCID: 2562295. Epub 2008/09/05. eng.

[198] de Wit, J; Verhaagen, J. Proteoglycans as modulators of axon guidance cue function. *Adv Exp Med Biol.*, 2007; 600:73-89. PubMed PMID: 17607948. Epub 2007/07/05. eng.

[199] Kantor, DB; Chivatakarn, O; Peer, KL; Oster, SF; Inatani, M; Hansen, MJ; et al. Semaphorin 5A is a bifunctional axon guidance cue regulated by heparan and chondroitin sulfate proteoglycans. *Neuron.*, 2004 Dec 16; 44(6), 961-75. PubMed PMID: 15603739. Epub 2004/12/18. eng.

[200] Ichijo, H. Proteoglycans as cues for axonal guidance in formation of retinotectal or retinocollicular projections. *Mol Neurobiol.*, 2004 Aug; 30(1), 23-33. PubMed PMID: 15247486. Epub 2004/07/13. eng.

[201] Chau, CH; Shum, DK; Li, H; Pei, J; Lui, YY; Wirthlin, L; et al. Chondroitinase ABC enhances axonal regrowth through Schwann cell-seeded guidance channels after spinal cord injury. *Faseb J.*, 2004 Jan; 18(1), 194-6. PubMed PMID: 14630702. Epub 2003/11/25. eng.

[202] Walz, A; Anderson, RB; Irie, A; Chien, CB; Holt, CE. Chondroitin sulfate disrupts axon pathfinding in the optic tract and alters growth cone dynamics. *J Neurobiol.*, 2002 Nov 15; 53(3), 330-42. PubMed PMID: 12382261. Epub 2002/10/17. eng.

[203] Becker, CG; Becker, T. Repellent guidance of regenerating optic axons by chondroitin sulfate glycosaminoglycans in zebrafish. *J Neurosci.*, 2002 Feb 1; 22(3), 842-53. PubMed PMID: 11826114. Epub 2002/02/05. eng.

[204] Anderson, RB; Walz, A; Holt, CE; Key, B. Chondroitin sulfates modulate axon guidance in embryonic Xenopus brain. *Dev Biol.*, 1998 Oct 15; 202(2), 235-43. PubMed PMID: 9769175. Epub 1998/10/14. eng.

[205] Tuttle, R; Braisted, JE; Richards, LJ; O'Leary, DD. Retinal axon guidance by region-specific cues in diencephalon. *Development.*, 1998 Mar; 125(5), 791-801. PubMed PMID: 9449662. Epub 1998/05/09. eng.

[206] Powell, EM; Fawcett, JW; Geller, HM. Proteoglycans provide neurite guidance at an astrocyte boundary. *Mol Cell Neurosci.*, 1997; 10(1-2), 27-42. PubMed PMID: 9361286. Epub 1997/01/01. eng.

[207] Treloar, HB; Nurcombe, V; Key, B. Expression of extracellular matrix molecules in the embryonic rat olfactory pathway. *J Neurobiol.*, 1996 Sep; 31(1), 41-55. PubMed PMID: 9120435. Epub 1996/09/01. eng.

[208] Landolt, RM; Vaughan, L; Winterhalter, KH; Zimmermann, DR. Versican is selectively expressed in embryonic tissues that act as barriers to neural crest cell migration and axon outgrowth. *Development.*, 1995 Aug; 121(8), 2303-12. PubMed PMID: 7671797. Epub 1995/08/01. eng.

[209] Dou, CL; Levine, JM. Inhibition of neurite growth by the NG2 chondroitin sulfate proteoglycan. *J Neurosci.*, 1994 Dec; 14(12), 7616-28. PubMed PMID: 7996200. Epub 1994/12/01. eng.

[210] Benes, FM. Relationship of GAD(67) regulation to cell cycle and DNA repair in GABA neurons in the adult hippocampus: bipolar disorder versus schizophrenia. *Cell Cycle.*, 2010 Feb 15; 9(4), 625-7. PubMed PMID: 20107308. Epub 2010/01/29. eng.

[211] Woo, TU; Walsh, JP; Benes, FM. Density of glutamic acid decarboxylase 67 messenger RNA-containing neurons that express the N-methyl-D-aspartate receptor subunit NR2A in the anterior cingulate cortex in schizophrenia and bipolar disorder. *Arch Gen Psychiatry.*, 2004 Jul; 61(7), 649-57. PubMed PMID: 15237077. Epub 2004/07/09. eng.

[212] Addington, AM; Gornick, M; Duckworth, J; Sporn, A; Gogtay, N; Bobb, A; et al. GAD1 (2q31.1), which encodes glutamic acid decarboxylase (GAD67), is associated with childhood-onset schizophrenia and cortical gray matter volume loss. *Mol Psychiatry.*, 2005 Jun; 10(6), 581-8. PubMed PMID: 15505639.

[213] Hashimoto, T; Volk, DW; Eggan, SM; Mirnics, K; Pierri, JN; Sun, Z; et al. Gene expression deficits in a subclass of GABA neurons in the prefrontal cortex of subjects with schizophrenia. *J Neurosci.*, 2003 Jul 16; 23(15), 6315-26. PubMed PMID: 12867516. Epub 2003/07/18. eng.

[214] Volk, DW; Austin, MC; Pierri, JN; Sampson, AR; Lewis, DA. Decreased glutamic acid decarboxylase67 messenger RNA expression in a subset of prefrontal cortical gamma-aminobutyric acid neurons in subjects with schizophrenia. *Arch Gen Psychiatry.*, 2000; 57(3), 237-45.

[215] Zhang, ZJ; Reynolds, GP. A selective decrease in the relative density of parvalbumin-immunoreactive neurons in the hippocampus in schizophrenia. *Schizophrenia research.*, 2002 May 1; 55(1-2), 1-10. PubMed PMID: 11955958. Epub 2002/04/17. eng.

[216] Gulyas, AI; Szabo, GG; Ulbert, I; Holderith, N; Monyer, H; Erdelyi, F; et al. Parvalbumin-containing fast-spiking basket cells generate the field potential oscillations

induced by cholinergic receptor activation in the hippocampus. *J Neurosci.*, 2010 Nov 10; 30(45), 15134-45. PubMed PMID: 21068319. Pubmed Central PMCID: 3044880. Epub 2010/11/12. eng.

[217] Kawaguchi, Y; Kondo, S. Parvalbumin, somatostatin and cholecystokinin as chemical markers for specific GABAergic interneuron types in the rat frontal cortex. *J Neurocytol.*, 2002 Mar-Jun; 31(3-5), 277-87. PubMed PMID: 12815247. Epub 2003/06/20. eng.

[218] Kawaguchi, Y. Distinct firing patterns of neuronal subtypes in cortical synchronized activities. *J Neurosci.*, 2001 Sep 15; 21(18), 7261-72. PubMed PMID: 11549736. Epub 2001/09/11. eng.

[219] Chow, A; Erisir, A; Farb, C; Nadal, MS; Ozaita, A; Lau, D; et al. K(+) channel expression distinguishes subpopulations of parvalbumin- and somatostatin-containing neocortical interneurons. *J Neurosci.*, 1999 Nov 1; 19(21), 9332-45. PubMed PMID: 10531438. Epub 1999/10/26. eng.

[220] Kawaguchi, Y; Kubota, Y. Correlation of physiological subgroupings of nonpyramidal cells with parvalbumin- and calbindinD28k-immunoreactive neurons in layer V of rat frontal cortex. *J Neurophysiol.*, 1993 Jul; 70(1), 387-96. PubMed PMID: 8395585. Epub 1993/07/01. eng.

[221] Pitkanen, A; Kemppainen, S. Comparison of the distribution of calcium-binding proteins and intrinsic connectivity in the lateral nucleus of the rat, monkey, and human amygdala. *Pharmacol Biochem Behav.*, 2002 Mar; 71(3), 369-77. PubMed PMID: 11830171. Epub 2002/02/07. eng.

[222] Sorvari, H; Miettinen, R; Soininen, H; Pitkanen, A. Parvalbumin-immunoreactive neurons make inhibitory synapses on pyramidal cells in the human amygdala: a light and electron microscopic study. *Neurosci Lett.*, 1996 Oct 18; 217(2-3), 93-6. PubMed PMID: 8916080. Epub 1996/10/18. eng.

[223] Rainnie, DG; Asprodini, EK; Shinnick-Gallagher, P. Inhibitory transmission in the basolateral amygdala. *J Neurophysiol.*, 1991 Sep; 66(3), 999-1009. PubMed PMID: 1684384. Epub 1991/09/01. eng.

[224] Cardin, JA; Carlen, M; Meletis, K; Knoblich, U; Zhang, F; Deisseroth, K; et al. Driving fast-spiking cells induces gamma rhythm and controls sensory responses. *Nature.*, 2009 Jun 4; 459(7247), 663-7. PubMed PMID: 19396156. Epub 2009/04/28. eng.

[225] Seidenbecher, T; Laxmi, TR; Stork, O; Pape, HC. Amygdalar and hippocampal theta rhythm synchronization during fear memory retrieval. *Science.*, 2003 Aug 8; 301(5634), 846-50. PubMed PMID: 12907806. Epub 2003/08/09. eng.

[226] Nowicka, D; Soulsby, S; Skangiel-Kramska, J; Glazewski, S. Parvalbumin-containing neurons, perineuronal nets and experience-dependent plasticity in murine barrel cortex. *Eur J Neurosci.*, 2009 Dec 3; 30(11), 2053-63. PubMed PMID: 20128844. Epub 2010/02/05. eng.

[227] Vidal, E; Bolea, R; Tortosa, R; Costa, C; Domenech, A; Monleon, E; et al. Assessment of calcium-binding proteins (Parvalbumin and Calbindin D-28K) and perineuronal nets in normal and scrapie-affected adult sheep brains. *Journal of virological methods.*, 2006 Sep; 136(1-2), 137-46. PubMed PMID: 16828173. Epub 2006/07/11. eng.

[228] Adams, I; Brauer, K; Arelin, C; Hartig, W; Fine, A; Mader, M; et al. Perineuronal nets in the rhesus monkey and human basal forebrain including basal ganglia. *Neuroscience.*, 2001; 108(2), 285-98. PubMed PMID: 11734361.

[229] Hartig, W; Singer, A; Grosche, J; Brauer, K; Ottersen, OP; Bruckner, G. Perineuronal nets in the rat medial nucleus of the trapezoid body surround neurons immunoreactive for various amino acids, calcium-binding proteins and the potassium channel subunit Kv3.1b. *Brain Res.*, 2001 Apr 27; 899(1-2), 123-33. PubMed PMID: 11311873.

[230] Haunso, A; Celio, MR; Margolis, RK; Menoud, PA. Phosphacan immunoreactivity is associated with perineuronal nets around parvalbumin-expressing neurones. *Brain Res.*, 1999 Jul 10; 834(1-2), 219-22. PubMed PMID: 10407120. Epub 1999/07/17. eng.

[231] Hartig, W; Brauer, K; Bigl, V; Bruckner, G. Chondroitin sulfate proteoglycan-immunoreactivity of lectin-labeled perineuronal nets around parvalbumin-containing neurons. *Brain Res.*, 1994 Jan 28; 635(1-2), 307-11. PubMed PMID: 8173967. Epub 1994/01/28. eng.

[232] Hartig, W; Brauer, K; Bruckner, G. Wisteria floribunda agglutinin-labelled nets surround parvalbumin-containing neurons. *Neuroreport.*, 1992 Oct; 3(10), 869-72. PubMed PMID: 1421090.

[233] Pantazopoulos, H; Lange, N; Hassinger, L; Berretta, S. Subpopulations of neurons expressing parvalbumin in the human amygdala. *J Comp Neurol.*, 2006 Jun 10; 496(5), 706-22. PubMed PMID: 16615121.

[234] Shah, A; Lodge, DJ. A loss of hippocampal perineuronal nets produces deficits in dopamine system function: relevance to the positive symptoms of schizophrenia. *Transl Psychiatry.*, 2013; 3:e215. PubMed PMID: 23321812. Pubmed Central PMCID: PMC3566725. Epub 2013/01/17. eng.

[235] Pizzorusso, T; Medini, P; Landi, S; Baldini, S; Berardi, N; Maffei, L. Structural and functional recovery from early monocular deprivation in adult rats. *Proc Natl Acad Sci U S A.*, 2006 May 30; 103(22), 8517-22. PubMed PMID: 16709670.

[236] Beurdeley, M; Spatazza, J; Lee, HH; Sugiyama, S; Bernard, C; Di Nardo, AA; et al. Otx2 binding to perineuronal nets persistently regulates plasticity in the mature visual cortex. *J Neurosci.*, 2012 Jul 4; 32(27), 9429-37. PubMed PMID: 22764251. Pubmed Central PMCID: 3419577. Epub 2012/07/06. eng.

[237] Holt, DJ; Coombs, G; Zeidan, MA; Goff, DC; Milad, MR. Failure of neural responses to safety cues in schizophrenia. *Arch Gen Psychiatry.*, 2012 Sep; 69(9), 893-903. PubMed PMID: 22945619. Epub 2012/09/05. eng.

[238] Holt, DJ; Lebron-Milad, K; Milad, MR; Rauch, SL; Pitman, RK; Orr, SP; et al. Extinction memory is impaired in schizophrenia. *Biol Psychiatry.*, 2009 Mar 15; 65(6), 455-63. PubMed PMID: 18986648. Epub 2008/11/07. eng.

[239] Morris, NP; Henderson, Z. Perineuronal nets ensheath fast spiking, parvalbumin-immunoreactive neurons in the medial septum/diagonal band complex. *Eur J Neurosci.*, 2000 Mar; 12(3), 828-38. PubMed PMID: 10762312.

[240] Hartig, W; Derouiche, A; Welt, K; Brauer, K; Grosche, J; Mader, M; et al. Cortical neurons immunoreactive for the potassium channel Kv3.1b subunit are predominantly surrounded by perineuronal nets presumed as a buffering system for cations. *Brain Res.*, 1999 Sep 18; 842(1), 15-29. PubMed PMID: 10526091.

[241] Celio, MR. Perineuronal nets of extracellular matrix around parvalbumin-containing neurons of the hippocampus. *Hippocampus.*, 1993; 3 Spec No:55-60. PubMed PMID: 8287112.

[242] Sinagra, M; Verrier, D; Frankova, D; Korwek, KM; Blahos, J; Weeber, EJ; et al. Reelin, very-low-density lipoprotein receptor, and apolipoprotein E receptor 2 control

somatic NMDA receptor composition during hippocampal maturation in vitro. *J Neurosci.*, 2005 Jun 29; 25(26), 6127-36. PubMed PMID: 15987942. Epub 2005/07/01. eng.

[243] Frischknecht, R; Heine, M; Perrais, D; Seidenbecher, CI; Choquet, D; Gundelfinger, ED. Brain extracellular matrix affects AMPA receptor lateral mobility and short-term synaptic plasticity. *Nat Neurosci.*, 2009 May 31. PubMed PMID: 19483686. Epub 2009/06/02. Eng.

[244] Sur, M; Frost, DO; Hockfield, S. Expression of a surface-associated antigen on Y-cells in the cat lateral geniculate nucleus is regulated by visual experience. *J Neurosci.*, 1988 Mar; 8(3), 874-82. PubMed PMID: 3346725. Epub 1988/03/01. eng.

[245] Kalb, RG; Hockfield, S. Large diameter primary afferent input is required for expression of the Cat-301 proteoglycan on the surface of motor neurons. *Neuroscience.*, 1990; 34(2), 391-401. PubMed PMID: 2333149. Epub 1990/01/01. eng.

[246] McRae, PA; Rocco, MM; Kelly, G; Brumberg, JC; Matthews, RT. Sensory deprivation alters aggrecan and perineuronal net expression in the mouse barrel cortex. *J Neurosci.*, 2007 May 16; 27(20), 5405-13. PubMed PMID: 17507562. Epub 2007/05/18. eng.

[247] Humphries, C; Mortimer, A; Hirsch, S; de Belleroche, J. NMDA receptor mRNA correlation with antemortem cognitive impairment in schizophrenia. *Neuroreport.*, 1996 Aug 12; 7(12), 2051-5. PubMed PMID: 8905723. Epub 1996/08/12. eng.

[248] Gao, XM; Sakai, K; Roberts, RC; Conley, RR; Dean, B; Tamminga, CA. Ionotropic glutamate receptors and expression of N-methyl-D-aspartate receptor subunits in subregions of human hippocampus: effects of schizophrenia. *Am J Psychiatry.*, 2000 Jul; 157(7), 1141-9. PubMed PMID: 10873924. Epub 2000/06/30. eng.

[249] Ibrahim, HM; Hogg, AJ Jr.; Healy, DJ; Haroutunian, V; Davis, KL; Meador-Woodruff, JH. Ionotropic glutamate receptor binding and subunit mRNA expression in thalamic nuclei in schizophrenia. *Am J Psychiatry.*, 2000 Nov; 157(11), 1811-23. PubMed PMID: 11058479. Epub 2000/11/04. eng.

[250] Zavitsanou, K; Ward, PB; Huang, XF. Selective alterations in ionotropic glutamate receptors in the anterior cingulate cortex in schizophrenia. *Neuropsychopharmacology.*, 2002 Nov; 27(5), 826-33. PubMed PMID: 12431856. Epub 2002/11/15. eng.

[251] Harrison, PJ; Law, AJ; Eastwood, SL. Glutamate receptors and transporters in the hippocampus in schizophrenia. *Ann N Y Acad Sci.*, 2003 Nov; 1003:94-101. PubMed PMID: 14684437. Epub 2003/12/20. eng.

[252] Woo, TU; Kim, AM; Viscidi, E. Disease-specific alterations in glutamatergic neurotransmission on inhibitory interneurons in the prefrontal cortex in schizophrenia. *Brain Res.*, 2008 Jul 7; 1218:267-77. PubMed PMID: 18534564. Pubmed Central PMCID: 2665281. Epub 2008/06/07. eng.

[253] Bitanihirwe, BK; Lim, MP; Kelley, JF; Kaneko, T; Woo, TU. Glutamatergic deficits and parvalbumin-containing inhibitory neurons in the prefrontal cortex in schizophrenia. *BMC Psychiatry.*, 2009; 9:71. PubMed PMID: 19917116. Pubmed Central PMCID: 2784456. Epub 2009/11/18. eng.

[254] Blennow, K; Davidsson, P; Gottfries, CG; Ekman, R; Heilig, M. Synaptic degeneration in thalamus in chizophrenia. *Lancet.*, 1996 Sep 7; 348(9028), 692-3. PubMed PMID: 8782788.

[255] Eastwood, SL; Harrison, PJ. Synaptic pathology in the anterior cingulate cortex in schizophrenia and mood disorders. A review and a Western blot study of

synaptophysin, GAP-43 and the complexins. *Brain Res Bull.*, 2001 Jul 15; 55(5), 569-78. PubMed PMID: 11576753. Epub 2001/09/29. eng.

[256] Hayashi-Takagi, A; Sawa, A. Disturbed synaptic connectivity in schizophrenia: convergence of genetic risk factors during neurodevelopment. *Brain Res Bull.*, 2010 Sep 30; 83(3-4), 140-6. PubMed PMID: 20433911. Epub 2010/05/04. eng.

[257] ohnson, RD; Oliver, PL; Davies, KE. SNARE proteins and schizophrenia: linking synaptic and neurodevelopmental hypotheses. *Acta Biochim Pol.*, 2008; 55(4), 619-28. PubMed PMID: 18985177. Epub 2008/11/06. eng.

[258] Landen, M; Davidsson, P; Gottfries, CG; Grenfeldt, B; Stridsberg, M; Blennow, K. Reduction of the small synaptic vesicle protein synaptophysin but not the large dense core chromogranins in the left thalamus of subjects with schizophrenia. *Biol Psychiatry.* 1999; 46(12), 1698-702.

[259] McGlashan, TH; Hoffman, RE. Schizophrenia as a disorder of developmentally reduced synaptic connectivity. *Arch Gen Psychiatry.*, 2000 Jul; 57(7), 637-48. PubMed PMID: 10891034. Epub 2000/07/13. eng.

[260] Broadbelt, K; Byne, W; Jones, LB. Evidence for a decrease in basilar dendrites of pyramidal cells in schizophrenic medial prefrontal cortex. *Schizophr Res.*, 2002 Nov 1; 58(1), 75-81. PubMed PMID: 12363393.

[261] Costa, E; Davis, J; Grayson, DR; Guidotti, A; Pappas, GD; Pesold, C. Dendritic spine hypoplasticity and downregulation of reelin and gabaergic tone in schizophrenia vulnerability. *Neurobiol Dis.*, 2001; 8(5), 723-42.

[262] Garey, LJ; Ong, WY; Patel, TS; Kanani, M; Davis, A; Mortimer, AM; et al. - Reduced dendritic spine density on cerebral cortical pyramidal neurons in schizophrenia [see comments]. *J Neurol Neurosurg Psychiatry.*, 1998; 65(4), 446-53.

[263] Glantz, LA; Lewis, DA. Decreased dendritic spine density on prefrontal cortical pyramidal neurons in schizophrenia [see comments]. *Arch Gen Psychiatry.*, 2000; 57(1), 65-73.

[264] Law, AJ; Weickert, CS; Hyde, TM; Kleinman, JE; Harrison, PJ. Reduced spinophilin but not microtubule-associated protein 2 expression in the hippocampal formation in schizophrenia and mood disorders: molecular evidence for a pathology of dendritic spines. *Am J Psychiatry.*, 2004 Oct; 161(10), 1848-55. PubMed PMID: 15465982.

[265] Creese, I; Burt, DR; Snyder, SH. Dopamine receptor binding predicts clinical and pharmacological potencies of antischizophrenic drugs. *Science.*, 1976; 192:596-8.

[266] Seeman, P; Schwarz, J; Chen, JF; Szechtman, H; Perreault, M; McKnight, GS; et al. Psychosis pathways converge via D2high dopamine receptors. *Synapse.*, 2006 Sep 15; 60(4), 319-46. PubMed PMID: 16786561.

[267] Seeman, P; Lee, T; Chau-Wong, M; Wong, K. Antipsychotic drug doses and neuroleptic/dopamine receptors. *Nature.*, 1976 Jun 24; 261(5562), 717-9. PubMed PMID: 945467.

[268] Seeman, P; Chau-Wong, M; Tedesco, J; Wong, K. Brain receptors for antipsychotic drugs and dopamine: direct binding assays. *Proc Natl Acad Sci U S A.*, 1975 Nov; 72(11), 4376-80. PubMed PMID: 1060115.

[269] Carlsson, A; Lindqvist, M. Effect of Chlorpromazine or Haloperidol on Formation of 3methoxytyramine and Normetanephrine in Mouse Brain. *Acta Pharmacol Toxicol* (Copenh). 1963; 20:140-4. PubMed PMID: 14060771.

[270] Sedvall, G. Monoamines and schizophrenia. *Acta Psychiatr Scand Suppl.*, 1990; 358:7-13. PubMed PMID: 1978495.

[271] Ellison, GD; Eison, MS. Continuous amphetamine intoxication: an animal model of the acute psychotic episode. *Psychol Med.*, 1983 Nov; 13(4), 751-61. PubMed PMID: 6320247.

[272] Lieberman, JA; Kinon, BJ; Loebel, AD. Dopaminergic mechanisms in idiopathic and drug-induced psychoses. *Schizophr Bull.*, 1990; 16(1), 97-110. PubMed PMID: 2185538.

[273] Reynolds, GP. Beyond the dopamine hypothesis. The neurochemical pathology of schizophrenia. *Br J Psychiatry.*, 1989 Sep; 155:305-16. PubMed PMID: 2692761. Epub 1989/09/01. eng.

[274] Kegeles, LS; Abi-Dargham, A; Frankle, WG; Gil, R; Cooper, TB; Slifstein, M; et al. Increased synaptic dopamine function in associative regions of the striatum in schizophrenia. *Arch Gen Psychiatry.*, 2010 Mar; 67(3), 231-9. PubMed PMID: 20194823. Epub 2010/03/03. eng.

[275] Heinz, A; Schlagenhauf, F. Dopaminergic dysfunction in schizophrenia: salience attribution revisited. *Schizophr Bull.*, 2010 May; 36(3), 472-85. PubMed PMID: 20453041. Pubmed Central PMCID: 2879696. Epub 2010/05/11. eng.

[276] Abi-Dargham, A; Xu, X; Thompson, JL; Gil, R; Kegeles, LS; Urban, N; et al. Increased prefrontal cortical D(1) receptors in drug naive patients with schizophrenia: a PET study with [(1)(1)C]NNC112. *J Psychopharmacol.*, 2012 Jun; 26(6), 794-805. PubMed PMID: 21768159. Epub 2011/07/20. eng.

[277] Aleman, A; Kahn, RS. Strange feelings: do amygdala abnormalities dysregulate the emotional brain in schizophrenia? *Prog Neurobiol.*, 2005 Dec; 77(5), 283-98. PubMed PMID: 16352388.

[278] Xing, G; Zhang, L; Russell, S; Post, R. Reduction of dopamine-related transcription factors Nurr1 and NGFI-B in the prefrontal cortex in schizophrenia and bipolar disorders. *Schizophr Res.*, 2006 May; 84(1), 36-56. PubMed PMID: 16631355.

[279] Pankow, A; Knobel, A; Voss, M; Heinz, A. Neurobiological correlates of delusion: beyond the salience attribution hypothesis. *Neuropsychobiology.*, 2012; 66(1), 33-43. PubMed PMID: 22797275. Epub 2012/07/17. eng.

[280] Sotogaku, N; Tully, SE; Gama, CI; Higashi, H; Tanaka, M; Hsieh-Wilson, LC; et al. Activation of phospholipase C pathways by a synthetic chondroitin sulfate-E tetrasaccharide promotes neurite outgrowth of dopaminergic neurons. *J Neurochem.*, 2007 Oct; 103(2), 749-60. PubMed PMID: 17680989. Epub 2007/08/08. eng.

[281] Gates, MA; Fillmore, H; Steindler, DA. Chondroitin sulfate proteoglycan and tenascin in the wounded adult mouse neostriatum in vitro: dopamine neuron attachment and process outgrowth. *J Neurosci.*, 1996 Dec 15; 16(24), 8005-18. PubMed PMID: 8987827.

[282] Charvet, I; Hemming, FJ; Feuerstein, C; Saxod, R. Transient compartmental expression of neurocan n the developing striatum of the rat. *J Neurosci Res.*, 1998 Mar 1; 51(5), 612-8. PubMed PMID: 9512005. Epub 1998/03/25. eng.

[283] Moon, LD; Asher, RA; Rhodes, KE; Fawcett, JW. Relationship between sprouting axons, proteoglycans and glial cells following unilateral nigrostriatal axotomy in the adult rat. *Neuroscience.*, 2002; 109(1), 101-17. PubMed PMID: 11784703. Epub 2002/01/11. eng.

[284] Li, HP; Homma, A; Sango, K; Kawamura, K; Raisman, G; Kawano, H. Regeneration of nigrostriatal dopaminergic axons by degradation of chondroitin sulfate is accompanied by elimination of the fibrotic scar and glia limitans in the lesion site. *J Neurosci Res.*, 2007 Feb 15; 85(3), 536-47. PubMed PMID: 17154415. Epub 2006/12/13. eng.

[285] Agnati, LF; Leo, G; Zanardi, A; Genedani, S; Rivera, A; Fuxe, K; et al. Volume transmission and wiring transmission from cellular to molecular networks: history and perspectives. *Acta Physiol* (Oxf)., 2006 May-Jun; 187(1-2), 329-44. PubMed PMID: 16734770.

[286] Carlsson, A; Carlsson, ML. A dopaminergic deficit hypothesis of schizophrenia: the path to discovery. *Dialogues Clin Neurosci.*, 2006; 8(1), 137-42. PubMed PMID: 16640125.

[287] Brinley-Reed, M; McDonald, AJ. Evidence that dopaminergic axons provide a dense innervation of specific neuronal subpopulations in the rat basolateral amygdala. *Brain Res.*, 1999; 850(1-2), 127-35.

[288] Hyde, TM; Ziegler, JC; Weinberger, DR. Psychiatric disturbances in metachromatic leukodystrophy. Insights into the neurobiology of psychosis. *Arch Neurol.*, 1992 Apr; 49(4), 401-6. PubMed PMID: 1532712. Epub 1992/04/01. eng.

[289] Schmitt, A; Wilczek, K; Blennow, K; Maras, A; Jatzko, A; Petroianu, G; et al. Altered thalamic membrane phospholipids in schizophrenia: a postmortem study. *Biol Psychiatry.*, 2004 Jul 1; 56(1), 41-5. PubMed PMID: 15219471. Epub 2004/06/29. eng.

[290] Uranova, N; Orlovskaya, D; Vikhreva, O; Zimina, I; Kolomeets, N; Vostrikov, V; et al. Electron microscopy of oligodendroglia in severe mental illness. *Brain Res Bull.*, 2001; 55(5), 597-610.

[291] Uranova, NA; Vostrikov, VM; Orlovskaya, DD; Rachmanova, VI. Oligodendroglial density in the prefrontal cortex in schizophrenia and mood disorders: a study from the Stanley Neuropathology Consortium. *Schizophr Res.*, 2004 Apr 1; 67(2-3), 269-75. PubMed PMID: 14984887.

[292] Hof, PR; Haroutunian, V; Friedrich, VL Jr.; Byne, W; Buitron, C; Perl, DP; et al. Loss and altered spatial distribution of oligodendrocytes in the superior frontal gyrus in schizophrenia. *Biol Psychiatry.*, 2003 Jun 15; 53(12), 1075-85. PubMed PMID: 12814859.

[293] Hof, PR; Haroutunian, V; Copland, C; Davis, KL; Buxbaum, JD. Molecular and cellular evidence for an oligodendrocyte abnormality in schizophrenia. *Neurochem Res.*, 2002 Oct; 27(10), 1193-200. PubMed PMID: 12462417.

[294] Flynn, SW; Lang, DJ; Mackay, AL; Goghari, V; Vavasour, IM; Whittall, KP; et al. Abnormalities of myelination in schizophrenia detected in vivo with MRI, and post-mortem with analysis of oligodendrocyte proteins. *Mol Psychiatry.*, 2003 Sep; 8(9), 811-20. PubMed PMID: 12931208.

[295] Hakak, Y; Walker, JR; Li, C; Wong, WH; Davis, KL; Buxbaum, JD; et al. Genome-wide expression analysis reveals dysregulation of myelination-related genes in chronic schizophrenia. *Proc Natl Acad Sci U S A.*, 2001 Apr 10; 98(8), 4746-51. PubMed PMID: 11296301. Pubmed Central PMCID: 31905. Epub 2001/04/11. eng.

[296] Tkachev, D; Mimmack, ML; Ryan, MM; Wayland, M; Freeman, T; Jones, PB; et al. Oligodendrocyte dysfunction in schizophrenia and bipolar disorder. *Lancet.*, 2003 Sep 6; 362(9386), 798-805. PubMed PMID: 13678875.

[297] Dwork, AJ; Mancevski, B; Rosoklija, G. White matter and cognitive function in schizophrenia. *Int J Neuropsychopharmacol.*, 2007 Aug; 10(4), 513-36. PubMed PMID: 17313699. Epub 2007/02/23. eng.

[298] Konrad, A; Winterer, G. Disturbed structural connectivity in schizophrenia primary factor in pathology or epiphenomenon? *Schizophr Bull.*, 2008 Jan; 34(1), 72-92. PubMed PMID: 17485733. Pubmed Central PMCID: 2632386. Epub 2007/05/09. eng.

[299] Sokolov, BP. Oligodendroglial abnormalities in schizophrenia, mood disorders and substance abuse. Comorbidity, shared traits, or molecular phenocopies? *Int J Neuropsychopharmacol.*, 2007 Aug; 10(4), 547-55. PubMed PMID: 17291372. Epub 2007/02/13. eng.

[300] Chan, MK; Tsang, TM; Harris, LW; Guest, PC; Holmes, E; Bahn, S. Evidence for disease and antipsychotic medication effects in post-mortem brain from schizophrenia patients. *Mol Psychiatry.*, 2010 Oct 5. PubMed PMID: 20921955. Epub 2010/10/06. Eng.

[301] Dean, B; Boer, S; Gibbons, A; Money, T; Scarr, E. Recent advances in postmortem pathology and neurochemistry in schizophrenia. *Curr Opin Psychiatry.*, 2009 Mar; 22(2), 154-60. PubMed PMID: 19553869. Epub 2009/06/26. eng.

[302] English, JA; Dicker, P; Focking, M; Dunn, MJ; Cotter, DR. 2-D DIGE analysis implicates cytoskeletal abnormalities in psychiatric disease. *Proteomics.*, 2009 Jun; 9(12), 3368-82. PubMed PMID: 19562803. Epub 2009/06/30. eng.

[303] Le-Niculescu, H; Balaraman, Y; Patel, S; Tan, J; Sidhu, K; Jerome, RE; et al. Towards understanding the schizophrenia code: an expanded convergent functional genomics approach. *Am J Med Genet B Neuropsychiatr Genet.* 2007 Mar 5; 144B(2), 129-58. PubMed PMID: 17266109. Epub 2007/02/03. eng.

[304] Martins-de-Souza, D. Proteome and transcriptome analysis suggests oligodendrocyte dysfunction in schizophrenia. *J Psychiatr Res.*, 2010 Feb; 44(3), 149-56. PubMed PMID: 19699489. Epub 2009/08/25. eng.

[305] Martins-de-Souza, D; Gattaz, WF; Schmitt, A; Maccarrone, G; Hunyadi-Gulyas, E; Eberlin, MN; et al. Proteomic analysis of dorsolateral prefrontal cortex indicates the involvement of cytoskeleton, oligodendrocyte, energy metabolism and new potential markers in schizophrenia. *J Psychiatr Res.*, 2009 Jul; 43(11), 978-86. PubMed PMID: 19110265. Epub 2008/12/27. eng.

[306] Roussos, P; Katsel, P; Davis, KL; Bitsios, P; Giakoumaki, SG; Jogia, J; et al. Molecular and genetic evidence for abnormalities in the nodes of Ranvier in schizophrenia. *Arch Gen Psychiatry.*, 2012 Jan; 69(1), 7-15. PubMed PMID: 21893642. Epub 2011/09/07. eng.

[307] Haroutunian, V; Roussos, P; Katsel, P; Siever, L; Davis, K; editors. The Node of Ranvier in Schizophrenia Postmortem Brain Tissue. *American College of Neuropsychopharmacology*; 2010; Miami Beach, Florida.

[308] Niu, J; Mei, F; Li, N; Wang, H; Li, X; Kong, J; et al. Haloperidol promotes proliferation but inhibits differentiation in rat oligodendrocyte progenitor cell cultures. *Biochemistry and cell biology = Biochimie et biologie cellulaire.*, 2010 Aug; 88(4), 611-20. PubMed PMID: 20651832. Epub 2010/07/24. eng.

[309] Wang, H; Xu, H; Niu, J; Mei, F; Li, X; Kong, J; et al. Haloperidol activates quiescent oligodendroglia precursor cells in the adult mouse brain. *Schizophr Res.*, 2010 Jun; 119(1-3), 164-74. PubMed PMID: 20346631. Epub 2010/03/30. eng.

[310] Bi, X; Zhang, Y; Yan, B; Fang, S; He, J; Zhang, D; et al. Quetiapine prevents oligodendrocyte and myelin loss and promotes maturation of oligodendrocyte progenitors in the hippocampus of global cerebral ischemia mice. *J Neurochem.*, 2012 Oct; 123(1), 14-20. PubMed PMID: 22817262. Epub 2012/07/24. eng.

[311] Zhang, Y; Zhang, H; Wang, L; Jiang, W; Xu, H; Xiao, L; et al. Quetiapine enhances oligodendrocyte regeneration and myelin repair after cuprizone-induced demyelination. *Schizophr Res.*, 2012 Jun; 138(1), 8-17. PubMed PMID: 22555017. Epub 2012/05/05. eng.

[312] Steiner, J; Sarnyai, Z; Westphal, S; Gos, T; Bernstein, HG; Bogerts, B; et al. Protective effects of haloperidol and clozapine on energy-deprived OLN-93 oligodendrocytes. *Eur Arch Psychiatry Clin Neurosci.*, 2011 Oct; 261(7), 477-82. PubMed PMID: 21328015. Epub 2011/02/18. eng.

[313] Yamauchi, T; Tatsumi, K; Makinodan, M; Kimoto, S; Toritsuka, M; Okuda, H; et al. Olanzapine increases cell mitotic activity and oligodendrocyte-lineage cells in the hypothalamus. *Neurochem Int.*, 2010 Nov; 57(5), 565-71. PubMed PMID: 20643174. Epub 2010/07/21. eng.

[314] Ogawa, T; Hagihara, K; Suzuki, M; Yamaguchi, Y. Brevican in the developing hippocampal fimbria: differential expression in myelinating oligodendrocytes and adult astrocytes suggests a dual role for brevican in central nervous system fiber tract development. *J Comp Neurol.*, 2001 Apr 9; 432(3), 285-95. PubMed PMID: 11246208.

[315] Bekku, Y; Rauch, U; Ninomiya, Y; Oohashi, T. Brevican distinctively assembles extracellular components at the large diameter nodes of Ranvier in the CNS. *J Neurochem.*, 2009 Mar; 108(5), 1266-76. PubMed PMID: 19141078. Epub 2009/01/15. eng.

[316] Keirstead, HS; Levine, JM; Blakemore, WF. Response of the oligodendrocyte progenitor cell population (defined by NG2 labelling) to demyelination of the adult spinal cord. *Glia.*, 1998 Feb; 22(2), 161-70. PubMed PMID: 9537836. Epub 1998/04/16. eng.

[317] Arnett, HA; Mason, J; Marino, M; Suzuki, K; Matsushima, GK; Ting, JP. TNF alpha promotes proliferation of oligodendrocyte progenitors and remyelination. *Nat Neurosci.*, 2001 Nov; 4(11), 1116-22. PubMed PMID: 11600888. Epub 2001/10/16. eng.

[318] McTigue, DM; Wei, P; Stokes, BT. Proliferation of NG2-positive cells and altered oligodendrocyte numbers in the contused rat spinal cord. *J Neurosci.*, 2001 May 15; 21(10), 3392-400. PubMed PMID: 11331369. Epub 2001/05/23. eng.

[319] Chang, A; Nishiyama, A; Peterson, J; Prineas, J; Trapp, BD. NG2-positive oligodendrocyte progenitor cells in adult human brain and multiple sclerosis lesions. *J Neurosci.*, 2000 Sep 1; 20(17), 6404-12. PubMed PMID: 10964946. Epub 2000/08/31. eng.

[320] Redwine, JM; Blinder, KL; Armstrong, RC. In situ expression of fibroblast growth factor receptors by oligodendrocyte progenitors and oligodendrocytes in adult mouse central nervous system. *J Neurosci Res.*, 1997 Oct 15; 50(2), 229-37. PubMed PMID: 9373032. Epub 1998/02/12. eng.

[321] VonDran, MW; Singh, H; Honeywell, JZ; Dreyfus, CF. Levels of BDNF impact oligodendrocyte lineage cells following a cuprizone lesion. *J Neurosci.*, 2011 Oct 5;

31(40), 14182-90. PubMed PMID: 21976503. Pubmed Central PMCID: 3203635. Epub 2011/10/07. eng.

[322] Aguirre, A; Dupree, JL; Mangin, JM; Gallo, V. A functional role for EGFR signaling in myelination and remyelination. *Nat Neurosci.*, 2007 Aug; 10(8), 990-1002. PubMed PMID: 17618276. Epub 2007/07/10. eng.

[323] Kumar, S; Biancotti, JC; Yamaguchi, M; de Vellis, J. Combination of growth factors enhances remyelination in a cuprizone-induced demyelination mouse model. *Neurochem Res.*, 2007 Apr-May; 32(4-5), 783-97. PubMed PMID: 17186374. Epub 2006/12/23. eng.

[324] Wilson, HC; Scolding, NJ; Raine, CS. Co-expression of PDGF alpha receptor and NG2 by oligodendrocyte precursors in human CNS and multiple sclerosis lesions. *Journal of neuroimmunology.*, 2006 Jul; 176(1-2), 162-73. PubMed PMID: 16753227. Epub 2006/06/07. eng.

[325] Polito, A; Reynolds, R. NG2-expressing cells as oligodendrocyte progenitors in the normal and demyelinated adult central nervous system. *J Anat.*, 2005 Dec; 207(6), 707-16. PubMed PMID: 16367798. Pubmed Central PMCID: 1571577. Epub 2005/12/22. eng.

[326] Reynolds, R; Dawson, M; Papadopoulos, D; Polito, A; Di Bello, IC; Pham-Dinh, D; et al. The response of NG2-expressing oligodendrocyte progenitors to demyelination in MOG-EAE and MS. *J Neurocytol.*, 2002 Jul-Aug; 31(6-7), 523-36. PubMed PMID: 14501221. Epub 2003/09/23. eng.

[327] Watanabe, M; Toyama, Y; Nishiyama, A. Differentiation of proliferated NG2-positive glial progenitor cells in a remyelinating lesion. *J Neurosci Res.*, 2002 Sep 15; 69(6), 826-36. PubMed PMID: 12205676. Epub 2002/09/03. eng.

[328] Moransard, M; Dann, A; Staszewski, O; Fontana, A; Prinz, M; Suter, T. NG2 expressed by macrophages and oligodendrocyte precursor cells is dispensable in experimental autoimmune encephalomyelitis. *Brain.*, 2011 May; 134(Pt 5), 1315-30. PubMed PMID: 21596769. Epub 2011/05/21. eng.

[329] Wang, DD; Bordey, A. The Astrocyte Odyssey. *Prog Neurobiol.*, 2008 Dec; 86(4), 342-67. PubMed PMID: 18948166. eng.

[330] Domowicz, MS; Sanders, TA; Ragsdale, CW; Schwartz, NB. Aggrecan is expressed by embryonic brain glia and regulates astrocyte development. *Developmental biology.* 2008 Mar 1; 315(1), 114-24. PubMed PMID: 18207138. Pubmed Central PMCID: 2408532. Epub 2008/01/22. eng.

[331] Seidenbecher, CI; Gundelfinger, ED; Bockers, TM; Trotter, J; Kreutz, MR. Transcripts for secreted and GPI-anchored brevican are differentially distributed in rat brain. *Eur J Neurosci.*, 1998 May; 10(5), 1621-30. PubMed PMID: 9751135. Epub 1998/09/29. eng.

[332] Ranjan, M; Hudson, LD. Regulation of tyrosine phosphorylation and protein tyrosine phosphatases during oligodendrocyte differentiation. *Mol Cell Neurosci.*, 1996 May; 7(5), 404-18. PubMed PMID: 8812065. Epub 1996/05/01. eng.

[333] Kabos, P; Matundan, H; Zandian, M; Bertolotto, C; Robinson, ML; Davy, BE; et al. Neural precursors express multiple chondroitin sulfate proteoglycans, including the lectican family. *Biochem Biophys Res Commun.*, 2004 Jun 11; 318(4), 955-63. PubMed PMID: 15147965. Epub 2004/05/19. eng.

[334] Faissner, A; Pyka, M; Geissler, M; Sobik, T; Frischknecht, R; Gundelfinger, ED; et al. Contributions of astrocytes to synapse formation and maturation - Potential functions of

the perisynaptic extracellular matrix. *Brain Res Rev.*, 2010 May; 63(1-2), 26-38. PubMed PMID: 20096729. Epub 2010/01/26. eng.

[335] Damadzic, R; Bigelow, LB; Krimer, LS; Goldenson, DA; Saunders, RC; Kleinman, JE; et al. A quantitative immunohistochemical study of astrocytes in the entorhinal cortex in schizophrenia, bipolar disorder and major depression: absence of significant astrocytosis. *Brain Res Bull.*, 2001 Jul 15; 55(5), 611-8. PubMed PMID: 11576757. Epub 2001/09/29. eng.

[336] Ohnuma, T; Augood, SJ; Arai, H; McKenna, PJ; Emson, PC. Expression of the human excitatory amino acid transporter 2 and metabotropic glutamate receptors 3 and 5 in the prefrontal cortex from normal individuals and patients with schizophrenia. *Brain Res Mol Brain Res.*, 1998 May; 56(1-2), 207-17. PubMed PMID: 9602129. Epub 1998/05/29. eng.

[337] Yelmo-Cruz, S; Morera-Fumero, AL; Abreu-Gonzalez, P. S100B and schizophrenia. *Psychiatry Clin Neurosci.*, 2013 Feb; 67(2), 67-75. PubMed PMID: 23438158. Epub 2013/02/27. eng.

[338] Rothermundt, M; Ponath, G; Arolt, V. S100B in schizophrenic psychosis. *Int Rev Neurobiol.*, 2004; 59:445-70. PubMed PMID: 15006498. Epub 2004/03/10. eng.

[339] Rothermundt, M; Ponath, G; Glaser, T; Hetzel, G; Arolt, V. S100B serum levels and long-term mprovement of negative symptoms in patients with schizophrenia. *Neuropsychopharmacology.*, 2004 May; 29(5), 1004-11. PubMed PMID: 14997170.

[340] Schroeter, ML; Abdul-Khaliq, H; Fruhauf, S; Hohne, R; Schick, G; Diefenbacher, A; et al. Serum S100B is increased during early treatment with antipsychotics and in deficit schizophrenia. *Schizophr Res.*, 2003 Aug 1; 62(3), 231-6. PubMed PMID: 12837519. Epub 2003/07/03. eng.

[341] Rothermundt, M; Missler, U; Arolt, V; Peters, M; Leadbeater, J; Wiesmann, M; et al. Increased S100B blood levels in unmedicated and treated schizophrenic patients are correlated with negative symptomatology. *Mol Psychiatry.*, 2001 Jul; 6(4), 445-9. PubMed PMID: 11443531. Epub 2001/07/10. eng.

[342] Lara, DR; Gama, CS; Belmonte-de-Abreu, P; Portela, LV; Goncalves, CA; Fonseca, M; et al. Increased serum S100B protein in schizophrenia: a study in medication-free patients. *J Psychiatr Res.*, 2001 Jan-Feb; 35(1), 11-4. PubMed PMID: 11287051. Epub 2001/04/05. eng.

[343] Sypecka, J; Sarnowska, A; Domanska-Janik, K. Crucial role of the local microenvironment in fate decision of neonatal rat NG2 progenitors. *Cell proliferation.*, 2009 Oct; 42(5), 661-71. PubMed PMID: 19614677. Epub 2009/07/21. eng.

[344] Hachem, S; Aguirre, A; Vives, V; Marks, A; Gallo, V; Legraverend, C. Spatial and temporal expression of S100B in cells of oligodendrocyte lineage. *Glia.*, 2005 Aug 1; 51(2), 81-97. PubMed PMID: 15782413. Epub 2005/03/23. eng.

[345] Brozzi, F; Arcuri, C; Giambanco, I; Donato, R. S100B Protein Regulates Astrocyte Shape and Migration via Interaction with Src Kinase: Implications for Astrocyte Development, Activation, and Tumor Growth. *J Biol Chem.*, 2009 Mar 27; 284(13), 8797-811. PubMed PMID: 19147496. Pubmed Central PMCID: 2659238. Epub 2009/01/17. eng.

[346] Raponi, E; Agenes, F; Delphin, C; Assard, N; Baudier, J; Legraverend, C; et al. S100B expression defines a state in which GFAP-expressing cells lose their neural stem cell potential and acquire a more mature developmental stage. *Glia.*, 2007 Jan 15; 55(2),

165-77. PubMed PMID: 17078026. Pubmed Central PMCID: 2739421. Epub 2006/11/02. eng.

[347] Donato, R. S100: a multigenic family of calcium-modulated proteins of the EF-hand type with intracellular and extracellular functional roles. *The international journal of biochemistry & cell biology.*, 2001 Jul; 33(7), 637-68. PubMed PMID: 11390274. Epub 2001/06/08. eng

In: Chondroitin Sulfate   ISBN: 978-1-62808-490-0
Editor: Vitor H. Pomin   © 2013 Nova Science Publishers, Inc.

Chapter 11

Structural Analysis of Chondroitin Sulfates and their Derivatives by ^{15}N-NMR Spectroscopy

Vitor H. Pomin[*]

Program of Glycobiology, Institute of Medical Biochemistry, and
University Hospital Clementino Fraga Filho, Federal University of Rio de Janeiro,
Rio de Janeiro, Brazil

Abstract

The structural studies of chondroitin sulfates (CSs) have mostly been based on the use of NMR spectroscopy particularly from the information of the [1]H- and ^{13}C-atoms. Nevertheless, a new scope has recently emerged. This concerns the extraction of data from the much less used isotope nitrogen-15. Despite its low abundance and very weak magnetic sensitivity, NMR technology has progressed, and nowadays research more based on the ^{15}N-nuclear properties has demonstrated to be relatively easy accomplishable for the retrieval of structural, conformational and dynamic information of CSs. The use of ^{15}N-related chemical shifts has proved to be quite diagnostic to the proper recognition of the CS types. Development of isotopic labeling methods for CS molecules has been implemented. Structural sequencing of sulfation patterns (4- and/or 6-substitutions), and anomeric ratio determination in CS-derived oligosaccharides were proved to be possible when analyses are focused on specific ^{15}N-chemical shifts. Moreover, this type of information can be achieved in a much simpler and straightforward way as compared to the more common NMR methods involving the [1]H- and/or ^{13}C-nuclei. The 3D-structural prediction of unsulfated CS determined by high-field ^{15}N-NMR points towards the conception of little effect of 4-sulfation on the backbone conformation. This chapter aims at describing the recent achievements made in structural analysis of CSs by the novel ^{15}N-NMR approach.

---

[*] Corresponding author: pominvh@bioqmed.ufrj.br.

Introduction

The application of nuclear magnetic resonance (NMR) spectroscopy in structural analysis of glycosaminoglycans (GAGs) has been primarily based on hydrogen-1 and/or carbon-13 atoms [1-5]. The complexity in interpret uni- and multi-dimensional NMR spectra of GAGs, involving either one of these isotopes, is very likely due to the low dispersion of the resultant signals aggravated with the structural heterogeneity of these molecules [1]. For example, in ^{1}H-NMR of the major naturally occurring GAGs, with exception of the most up-field methyl [1]H-signal from the acetyl groups around 2.0 ppm, the majority signals including the anomerics and those from the sugar rings are often squeezed between 6.0-3.0 ppm in the proton-chemical shift scale [1]. Even through 2D NMR spectra (used to spread the resonance overlap through the addition of another dimension) like the mostly exploited [1]H-^{13}C heteronuclear single quantum coherence (HSQC) experiments in which some structural components (methyl groups, anomerics, sulfation and glycosylation sites) become more identifiable because of their specific regions of cross-peaks, most of the [1]H-^{13}C resonances are yet condensed in a limited spectral window [6]. In reality, frequently just few of these components can be straightforwardly recognized even for the most homogeneous GAG types, and in cases that a more complete assignment is desired, other types of 2D NMR spectra are needed to allow reasonable interpretation. However, analysis of GAGs based on the magnetically less sensitive nuclei nitrogen-15 has become progressively more frequent within the last few years [1, 11-24]. And this new approach has been demonstrated that great efficiency for structural analysis besides reducing the NMR tendency of chemical shift degeneration commonly observed within the exploration of the commoner nuclei.

Chondroitin sulfates (CSs) are the most abundant GAG in the human body and together with heparan sulfate (HS), dermatan sulfate (DS), which is in turn a CS sub-type, and hyaluronic acid (HA), they contribute to build up the overall constitution of the extracellular matrices (ECM), either as composing side chains in cellular surface proteoglycans (CS, DS and HS), or as released free components of the ECM (mainly HA) [2]. Moreover, the GAGs heparin (Hp), HA and CS are also largely exploited as commercial bioproducts, as either an orally or intravenously administered drug in the case of Hp, as an ophthalmic solution in the case of HA and CS, or as an oral nutraceutical in the case of CS. These commercial applications are due to their respective biological properties, as anticoagulant/antithrombotic agents in the case of Hp [7], or as major forming structural components of the ECM in the globe of the eye and cornea in the case of HA and CS, and in cartilage tissues in the case of CS [10].

Given that all CS types have *N*-acetylgalactosamine (GalNAc) residues as a constituting member of their repeating disaccharide units (Figure 1) [1, 2], and that these amino sugar is directly or indirectly related to the overall and/or specific structural properties of such molecules as well as to the classification of their sub-families [CS-A is mostly 4-sulfated at the GalNAc unit; CS-B, also known as DS, has 4-sulfated GalNAc and iduronic acid (IdoA), sometimes 2-sulfated, as opposed to constituting glucuronic acid (GlcA) as normally found in the other CSs; CS-C is predominantly 6-sulfated; both CS-E and OSCS have 4,6-di-sulfated GalNAc units], it should be not surprising if a particular chemical group in one specific residue type, such as amide groups of GalNAc units, could serve as a useful molecular probe for the recognition of short- or long-range substitutions in different CS disaccharide units. In fact, previous works have been demonstrating that amide ^{15}N-related resonances, in 1D or 2D NMR spectra of CS disaccharides, oligosaccharides and even of the high molecular-weight native molecules, are very sensitive to structural features like anomeric configurations, glycosylation sites, hexosamine types, sulfation types and positions, neighboring uronate types, and conformational shapes [1, 11].

The main reason that has limited or impaired the use of ^{15}N-isotope in biomolecular NMR of GAGs in the past time is its low magnetic susceptibility (negative gyromagnetic ratio ten times lower than that of proton, and relativity receptivity, around 3.85×10^{-6} compared to 1.0 for proton) associated with its low natural abundance (~ 0.37%). Nowadays, however, technology has developed and NMR studies based on this nucleus have not only proved possible but also turned into a practice of more routine throughout the glycobiologists and NMR spectroscopists. This fact is mainly due to the progress and spread of modern NMR instruments with (ultra) high-magnetic fields, cryoprobe technology, the recent development of isotopic GAG-labeling strategies, together with the development of novel combinations of 2D pulse sequences for detection of specific ^{15}N-related magnetization transfer and coherences.

Through this chapter, we will summarize as a single document all the recent contributions made so far by ^{15}N-NMR spectroscopy on the structural studies of CS. We will also make a comparison in terms of advantageous versus disadvantageous characteristics of the NMR analysis using the much less used ^{15}N-isotope in relation to the commonest ^{1}H and ^{13}C-atoms.

^{15}N-NMR-Based Analysis of Unlabeled Naturally Occurring CS Polysaccharides

One of the major issues in the use of the commonest ^{1}H and ^{13}C-resonances in NMR analysis of CS is the chemical shift degeneracy originated by the low signal dispersion. This makes difficult both structural and spin assignments as well as proper identification of mixed samples or single samples containing the most heterogeneous structures. On the other hand, ^{15}N-NMR analysis of CS, especially those based on ^{15}N-HSQC spectrum can reduce drastically this tendency of resonance overlap since the resonances must come necessarily from the ^{1}H/^{15}N pairs of the acetyl amide groups from the GalNAc units rather than the anomeric and ring [1]H- and ^{13}C-atoms. This simpler resonance profile can be seen by the ^{15}N-HSQC spectra of the major CS types shown in figure 2. Moreover, structural determination can be straightforwardly accomplished when compared to the traditional nuclei.

For example, note at the panels A-D of figure 2 that 4-sulfated GalNAc units show amide resonances at the up-field ^{15}N-chemical shifts (somewhere between 120.5 and 121.0 ppm) as opposed to the down-field ^{15}N-chemical shifts of the 6-sulfated sites (somewhere between 121.5 and 122 ppm). The 4,6-di-sulfated GalNAc units, presented in oversulfated chondroitin sulfate (OSCS) for example, has showed a single amide resonance with a curious ^{15}N-chemical shift in the midway of the two mono-sulfated sites (~ 121.2 ppm) (Figure 2C). These resonances with different chemical shifts allow assignment and recognition of the sulfation types in a very quick and straightforward way. This differentiation allows rapid - assignment and distinction of the hexosamine types, which consequently enables the direct recognition of the GAG family in the analyzed sample. Observe that these resultant peaks are very unlikely to superimpose even in case of mixture samples, and therefore, the possible presence of minor species becomes feasible for diagnosis in procedures of quality control. The resonances from GalNAc units of CS and DS are also very distinguishable from each other. DS has down-field ^{1}H-resonance (~ 8.09 ppm) (Figure 2D) since their most GalNAc units are linked to IdoA units rather than linked to GlcA units as commonly found in CS-A and CS-C (Figures 2A and 2B) that in turn show up-field ^{1}H-chemical shift resonances at ~ 7.9 ppm. This is another clear differentiation based on ^{1}H-^{15}N pairs, and this allows easy identification of the sub-families of galactosaminoglycans (GalGs) which are composed of the GalNAc units as the hexosamine type. Nonetheless the IdoA-linked 4-sulfated GalNAc of DS has the equivalent upfield ^{15}N-chemical shift of those 4-sulfation-contained CS polymers like CS-A and CS-C (Figures 2A and 2B).

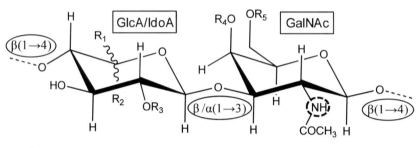

CS $\{R_1 = COO^-$ and $R_2 = H$ (β-D-GlcA); R_3, R_4 and $R_5 = H$ or SO_3^- (depending on the CS type)

DS $\{R_1 = COO^-$, $R_2 = H$ (β-D-GlcA) << $R_1 = H$, $R_2 = COO^-$ (α-L-IdoA); R_3, and $R_4 = H$ or SO_3^-, $R_4 = SO_3^-$ (mostly); $R_5 = H$

Figure 1. Representative structure of the CS disaccharide, and the possible variations that might occur accordingly to the CS sub-types.

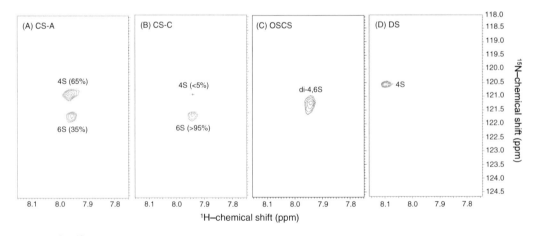

Figure 2. ^{1}H-^{15}N HSQC spectra at 25°C and pH 4.5 (800 MHz) of the GalGs chondroitin sulfates t the upper row: (A) CS-A, (B) CS-C, (C) oversulfated chondroitin sulfate (OSCS), and (D) DS, also known as CS-B, data modified from [1].

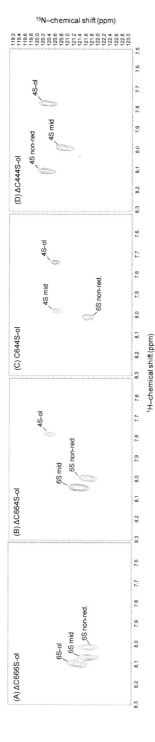

Figure 3. ^{15}N-HSQC spectra (800 MHz) of reduced CS hexasaccharides with different sulfation patterns obtained by either chondroitinases (A, B and D) or hyaluronidase (C) digestions. Data modified from [1]. The structures are the following: (A) ΔC666S-ol as ΔUA-(β1→3)-GalNAc-6S-(β1→4)-GlcA-(β1→3)-GalNAc-6S-(β1→4)-GlcA-(β1→3)-GalNAc-6S-ol; (B) ΔC6;6;4S-ol as ΔUA-(β1→3)-GalNAc-6S-(β1→4)-GlcA-(β1→3)-GalNAc-6S-(β1→4)-GlcA-(β1→3)-GalNAc-4S-ol; (C) C644S-ol as GlcA-(β1→3)-GalNAc-6S-(β1→4)-GlcA-(β1→3)-GalNAc-4S-(β1→4)-GlcA-(β1→3)-GalNAc-4S-ol; and (D) ΔC4;4;4S-ol as ΔUA-(β1→3)-GalNAc-4S-(β1→4)-GlcA-(β1→3)-GalNAc-4S-(β1→4)-GlcA-(β1→3)-GalNAc-4S-ol, where ΔUA = Δ^{4,5} unsaturated uronic acid; GalNAc = N-acetyl galactosamine; GlcA = glucuronic acid; S = sulfation group, in which the numbers before "S" represent the ring position; -ol stands for reduced sugars (open rings at the reducing-end termini) [6]. In the panels, 6S non-red., 6S mid, 6S-ol, 4S non-red., 4S mid, and 4S-ol belong respectively to the assignments of the amide ^{1}H-^{15}N pairs of 6-sulfated and 4-sulfated GalNAc from the non-reducing, middle, and reduced disaccharide units within the CS hexasaccharide chains.

^{15}N-NMR-Based Analysis of Chemically Well-Defined Unlabeled CS Oligosaccharides

Like native GAG polymers, structural characteristics of GAG oligosaccharides of well-defined sizes can also be easily revealed by ^{15}N-NMR experiments. For example, note the possibility of rapid characterization of the sulfation patterns in CS hexasaccharides through ^{15}N-HSQC spectra (Figure 3). These oligosaccharides were obtained from two different enzymatic digestions followed by reduction reaction with the strong reducing agent sodium borohydride in order to avoid possible ambiguities and complexities coming from the mutarotation of α/β-anomeric configurations in aqueous solution. From this novel ^{15}N-NMR approach, 6-sulfation can be simply distinguished away from 4-sulfated sites in all composing disaccharide units within the hexasaccharide chain (Figure 3). The former sulfation type in GalNAc units produce amide ^{1}H-^{15}N pairs at a more down-field ^{15}N-chemical shift than those 4-sulfated hexosamines (Figure 3). This rule based on different ^{15}N-chemical shifts of amides from 6- or 4-sulfated GalNAc units was also observed for CS disaccharide units (Figure 4). The cross-peak notation in the CS hexasaccharides enables additional recognition of the position of the disaccharides within the polymeric chain (see the assignments labeled as non-red, mid, and -ol, in Figure 3). In disaccharides, the diferential chemical shift position also allow notation of the anomeric signals, and the consequent volume peaks of these resonances can be useful to assess the anomeric ratio.

^{15}N-NMR-Based Analysis of ^{15}N-Enriched Cellular CS Polysaccharides

All the above-mentioned data (Figures 2-4) have been collected from compounds at natural abundance of magnetically sensitive isotopes. This is not an issue when we deal of material coming from commercially available sources. Concentrations of 15mg/mL can be reached and ^{15}N-HSQC spectra take no more than 3 hours at high-field NMR instruments, such as 800 or 900 MHz. Conversely, this concentration would be practically impossible to achieve when materials coming from cell extracts are the aim of analysis. Therefore, isotopic labeling strategies are demanded. Pomin, et al. (2010) [1], and the group of Professor Almond [11] have developed protocols for such regard. Figure 5 shows ^{15}N-HSQC spectra of extracts from two cell types. This methodology of ^{15}N-NMR combined with isotopically labeled materials has been proved quite useful for the retrieval of data concerning the screening of the GAG types and sub-types from cells in culture in a very straightforward way. For example, endothelial cells of mouse lung express both CS types (CS-A and CS-C) whereas Chinese hamster ovarian cells express only the CS-A. Nonetheless, this ^{15}N-NMR method has been proved very useful for rapid assessment of the GAG profile of cells as well as for diagnosis of the GAG features in differential cellular metabolic stages.

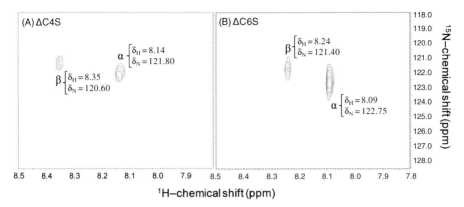

Figure 4. ^{1}H-^{15}N HSQC spectra of unreduced unsaturated 4-sulfated (A), and 6-sulfated (B) CS disaccharides, obtained at pH 4.5, and 25°C. They were obtained from an ABC-lyase digestion of the CS-A polysaccharide as documented in reference [6]. The α/β-signals arise from the mutarotation of anomerics in aqueous solution, in which the equilibrium is 6.5/3.5 ratio. Note the slight down-field ^{15}N-chemical shift of the amide resonances from the 6-sulfated disaccharides. Data modified from [1].

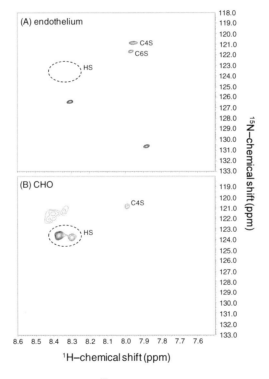

Figure 5. ^{15}N-gHSQC spectra of isotopically ^{15}N-labeled GAGs extracted isolated from (A) mouse lung endothelial cells, and of (B) chinese hamster ovarian (CHO) cells. HS, C4S, and C6S denote heparan sulfate, CS-A and CS-C, respectively.

^{15}N-NMR-Based Conformational Analysis of ^{15}N-Enriched CS Oligosaccharides

Based on ^{15}N-labeling protocol of CS extracted from cells in isotopically enriched media, a set of unsulfated CS molecules have been prepared. After enzymatic digestion, the released ^{15}N-enriched oligosaccharides were fractionated based on strong-anion exchange chromatography. Unsulfated CS 4-mers to 10-mers were produced [11]. The 1D ^{1}H-NMR spectrum of the tetrasaccharide is shown at figure 6. The large $^{1}J_{H-N}$ and small $^{3}J_{NH-H2}$ coupling constants were obtained for both GalNAc units and anormeric configurations. They are 92.74 Hz for $^{1}J_{H,N}$, and 9.39 Hz for $^{3}J_{NH-H2}$ of the GalNAc-1α; 91.57 Hz for $^{1}J_{H,N}$ and 9.69 Hz for $^{3}J_{NH-H2}$ of the GalNAc-1β; and 91.85 Hz for $^{1}J_{H,N}$, and 9.75 Hz for $^{3}J_{NH-H2}$ of the GalNAc-3. All these data suggest the same conformation of the amide groups regardless the position or anomeric configuration of the residues [11].

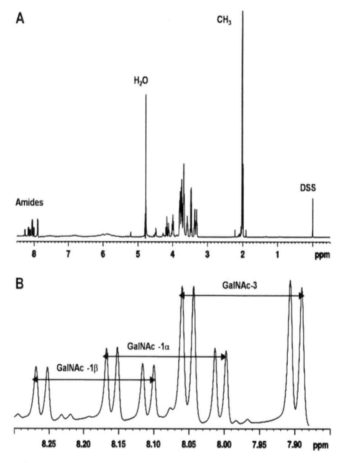

Figure 6. (A) The 1D ^{1}H-NMR spectrum of a ^{15}N-enriched unsulfated chondroitin tetrasaccharide. (B) The amide region is magnified. Resonances attributed to residues GalNAc-1α, GalNAc-1β and GalNAc-3, are labelled. The large (≈90 Hz) $^{1}J_{H,N}$ and small (≈10 Hz) $^{3}J_{HN,H2}$ couplings were obtained and they are described in the text. Data were acquired at 600 MHz, pH 6.0, 25 °C in 5–10% (v/v) D$_2$O and referenced relative to δ_{DSS} (^{1}H). Standard error: ^{1}H ±0.001 ppm. DSS stands for the standard 4,4-dimethyl-4-silapentane-1-sulfonic acid. Data from [11].

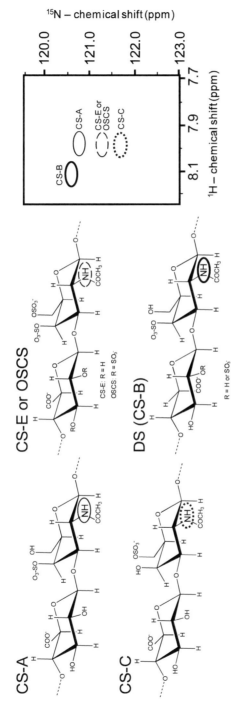

Figure 7. Structural representation of the most common chondroitin sulfate types and the typical position of their respective $^1H/^{15}N$-resonances in the ^{15}N-HSQC NMR spectrum. Note that these resonances are unlikely to overlap and they are very useful for diagnosis of the CS type, and their respective structural peculiarities.

Comparing the glycosidic torsion angles measured by both NMR spectroscopy and computational simulations of the ^{15}N-enriched unsulfated CS hexasaccharide [11] with a 4-sulfated CS pentasaccharide [12], the following values were obtained for the φ/Ψ dihedral angles: -73/-117, and -67/-124 for the β(1-4) glycosidic linkages of the ^{15}N-enriched unsulfated CS hexasaccharide, and 4-sulfated CS pentasaccharide, respectively; and -72/108, and -61/109 for the β(1-3) glycosidic linkages of the ^{15}N-enriched unsulfated CS hexasaccharide, and 4-sulfated CS pentasaccharide, respectively. This data has clearly proved that the 4-sulfation presence does not make a conformational change of the CS oligosaccharides in solution [11].

Conclusion

- The distinct ^{1}H-^{15}N resonances of CSs and DS allow quick characterization and respective identification of these CS sub-types when analyzed by ^{15}N-HSQC experiments [1] (see Figures 2 and 7);
- Structural sequencing of sulfation patterns (4- and/or 6-substituted) of CS-derived oligosaccharides of chemically well-defined structures is possible and can be achieved in a simpler and straightforward way, as compared to the more common NMR methods [1] (see Figure 3);
- Precise sulfation patterns, anomeric type and ratio can be determined in CS disaccharides, and these features can be achieved in a simpler and straightforward way, as compared to the more common NMR methods [1] (see Figure 4);
- Development of isotopic labeling methods for CS and DS [1], mainly by *in vivo* methods based on cell cultures grown in ^{15}N-precursors enriched media were implemented to allow observation of lower amounts of materials, especially those originated from cells (see Figure 5) [1, 11];
- The 3D-structural prediction of unsulfated CS determined by high-field ^{15}N-NMR points towards the conception of little effect of 4-sulfation on the backbone conformation (see Figure 6) [11].

References

[1]   Pomin, V. H., Sharp, J. S., Li, X., Wang, L. & Prestegard, J. H. (2010). *Anal Chem*, *82*, 4078-4088.
[2]   Pomin, V. H. & Park, Y. (2012). Chapter 1. In: Taylor JC (editor). *Advances in chemistry research*. Vol. *12*, 1st edition. Nova Publishers, New York, 1-64.
[3]   Guerrini, M., Naggi, A., Guglieri, S., Santarsiero, R. & Torri, G. (2005). *Anal Biochem*, *337*, 35-47.
[4]   Welti, D., Rees, D. A. & Welsh, E. J. (1979). *Eur J Biochem*, *94*, 505-514.
[5]   Hochuli, M., Wüthrich, K. & Steinmann, B. (2003). *NMR Biomed*, *16*, 224-236.
[6]   Pomin, V. H., Park, Y., Huang, R., Heiss, C., Sharp, J. S., Azadi, P. & Prestegard, J. H. (2012). *Glycobiology*, *22*, 826-836.
[7]   Guerrini, M., Beccati, D., Shriver, Z., et al. (2008). *Nat Biotechnol*, *26*, 669-675

[8] Kishimoto, T. K., Viswanathan, K., Ganguly, T. et al. (2008). *N Engl J Med, 358,* 2457-2467.

[9] Blossom, D. B., Kallen, A. J., Patel, P.R. et al. (2008). *N Engl J Med, 359,* 2674-2684

[10] Pomin, V. H., Piquet, A. A., Pereira, M. S. & Mourão, P. A. (2012). *Carbohydr Polym, 90,* 839-846.

[11] Sattelle, B. M., Shakeri, J., Roberts, I. S. & Almond, A. (2010). *Carbohydr Res, 345,* 291-302.

[12] Yu, F., Wolff, J. J., Amster, I. J. & Prestegard, J. H. (2007). *J Am Chem Soc, 129,* 13288-13297.

Index

B

C

G

H

J

K

L

M

N

O

P

T

Y

yield, 10, 11, 33, 46, 48, 60, 64, 82, 156

Z

zinc, 21